Current Advances in Spinal Diseases of Elderly Patients

Current Advances in Spinal Diseases of Elderly Patients

Editors

Takashi Hirai
Hiroaki Nakashima
Masayuki Miyagi
Shinji Takahashi
Masashi Uehara

MDPI • Basel • Beijing • Wuhan • Barcelona • Belgrade • Manchester • Tokyo • Cluj • Tianjin

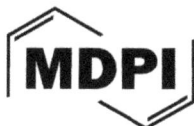

Editors

Takashi Hirai
Tokyo Medical and Dental University
Japan

Hiroaki Nakashima
Nagoya University
Japan

Masayuki Miyagi
Kitasato University
Japan

Shinji Takahashi
Osaka City University Graduate School of Medicine
Japan

Masashi Uehara
Shinshu University
Japan

Editorial Office
MDPI
St. Alban-Anlage 66
4052 Basel, Switzerland

This is a reprint of articles from the Special Issue published online in the open access journal *Journal of Clinical Medicine* (ISSN 2077-0383) (available at: http://www.mdpi.com).

For citation purposes, cite each article independently as indicated on the article page online and as indicated below:

LastName, A.A.; LastName, B.B.; LastName, C.C. Article Title. *Journal Name* **Year**, *Volume Number*, Page Range.

ISBN 978-3-0365-3899-0 (Hbk)
ISBN 978-3-0365-3900-3 (PDF)

© 2022 by the authors. Articles in this book are Open Access and distributed under the Creative Commons Attribution (CC BY) license, which allows users to download, copy and build upon published articles, as long as the author and publisher are properly credited, which ensures maximum dissemination and a wider impact of our publications.

The book as a whole is distributed by MDPI under the terms and conditions of the Creative Commons license CC BY-NC-ND.

Contents

Hyoungmin Kim, Sam Yeol Chang, Jongyeon Son, Sujung Mok, Sung Cheol Park and
Bong-Soon Chang
The Effect of Adding Biological Factors to the Decision-Making Process for Spinal Metastasis of
Non-Small Cell Lung Cancer
Reprinted from: *J. Clin. Med.* **2021**, *10*, 1119, doi:10.3390/jcm10051119 1

Hamidullah Salimi, Shoichiro Ohyama, Hidetomi Terai, Yusuke Hori, Shinji Takahashi,
Masatoshi Hoshino, Akito Yabu, Hasibullah Habibi, Akio Kobayashi, Tadao Tsujio,
Shiro Kotake and Hiroaki Nakamura
Trunk Muscle Mass Measured by Bioelectrical Impedance Analysis Reflecting the
Cross-Sectional Area of the Paravertebral Muscles and Back Muscle Strength: A Cross-Sectional
Analysis of a Prospective Cohort Study of Elderly Population
Reprinted from: *J. Clin. Med.* **2021**, *10*, 1187, doi:10.3390/jcm10061187 11

Ryuji Osawa, Shota Ikegami, Hiroshi Horiuchi, Ryosuke Tokida, Hiroyuki Kato
and Jun Takahashi
Osteoporosis Detection by Physical Function Tests in Resident Health Exams: A Japanese
Cohort Survey Randomly Sampled from a Basic Resident Registry
Reprinted from: *J. Clin. Med.* **2021**, *10*, 1896, doi:10.3390/jcm10091896 21

Kathryn Anne Jimenez, Ji-Won Kwon, Jayeong Yoon, Hwan-Mo Lee, Seong-Hwan Moon,
Kyung-Soo Suk, Hak-Sun Kim and Byung Ho Lee
Handgrip Strength Correlated with Falling Risk in Patients with Degenerative Cervical
Myelopathy
Reprinted from: *J. Clin. Med.* **2021**, *10*, 1980, doi:10.3390/jcm10091980 31

Sadayuki Ito, Hiroaki Nakashima, Kei Ando, Kazuyoshi Kobayashi, Masaaki Machino,
Taisuke Seki, Shinya Ishizuka, Shunsuke Kanbara, Taro Inoue, Hiroyuki Koshimizu,
Ryosuke Fujii, Hiroya Yamada, Yoshitaka Ando, Jun Ueyama, Takaaki Kondo, Koji Suzuki,
Yukiharu Hasegawa and Shiro Imagama
Human Nonmercaptalbumin Is a New Biomarker of Motor Function
Reprinted from: *J. Clin. Med.* **2021**, *10*, 2464, doi:10.3390/jcm10112464 43

Prevalence and Characteristics of Spinal Sagittal Malalignment in Patients with Osteoporosis
Reprinted from: *J. Clin. Med.* **2021**, *10*, 2827, doi:10.3390/jcm10132827 53

Hiroaki Nakashima, Keigo Ito, Yoshito Katayama, Mikito Tsushima, Kei Ando,
Kazuyoshi Kobayashi, Masaaki Machino, Sadayuki Ito, Hiroyuki Koshimizu,
Naoki Segi, Hiroyuki Tomita and Shiro Imagama
The Level of Conus Medullaris in 629 Healthy Japanese Individuals
Reprinted from: *J. Clin. Med.* **2021**, *10*, 3182, doi:10.3390/jcm10143182 61

Matthew T. Gulbrandsen, Nina Lara, James A. Beauchamp, Andrew Chung, Michael Chang
and Dennis Crandall
Early Gender Differences in Pain and Functional Recovery Following Thoracolumbar Spinal
Arthrodesis
Reprinted from: *J. Clin. Med.* **2021**, *10*, 3654, doi:10.3390/jcm10163654 67

Hidetomi Terai, Shinji Takahashi, Hiroyuki Yasuda, Sadahiko Konishi, Takafumi Maeno, Hiroshi Kono, Akira Matsumura, Takashi Namikawa, Minori Kato, Masatoshi Hoshino, Koji Tamai, Hiromitsu Toyoda, Akinobu Suzuki and Hiroaki Nakamura
Direct Lateral Corpectomy and Reconstruction Using an Expandable Cage Improves Local Kyphosis but Not Global Sagittal Alignment
Reprinted from: *J. Clin. Med.* 2021, 10, 4012, doi:10.3390/jcm10174012 . . . . **75**

Takashi Hirai, Soraya Nishimura, Toshitaka Yoshii, Narihito Nagoshi, Jun Hashimoto, Kanji Mori, Satoshi Maki, Keiichi Katsumi, Kazuhiro Takeuchi, Shuta Ushio, Takeo Furuya, Kei Watanabe, Norihiro Nishida, Kota Watanabe, Takashi Kaito, Satoshi Kato, Katsuya Nagashima, Masao Koda, Hiroaki Nakashima, Shiro Imagama, Kazuma Murata, Yuji Matsuoka, Kanichiro Wada, Atsushi Kimura, Tetsuro Ohba, Hiroyuki Katoh, Masahiko Watanabe, Yukihiro Matsuyama, Hiroshi Ozawa, Hirotaka Haro, Katsushi Takeshita, Morio Matsumoto, Masaya Nakamura, Masashi Yamazaki, Yu Matsukura, Hiroyuki Inose, Atsushi Okawa and Yoshiharu Kawaguchi
Associations between Clinical Findings and Severity of Diffuse Idiopathic Skeletal Hyperostosis in Patients with Ossification of the Posterior Longitudinal Ligament
Reprinted from: *J. Clin. Med.* , 10, 4137, doi:10.3390/jcm10184137 . . . . **85**

Masashi Uehara, Shota Ikegami, Hiroshi Horiuchi, Jun Takahashi and Hiroyuki Kato
Prevalence and Related Factors of Low Back Pain in the General Elderly Population: A Japanese Cross-Sectional Study Randomly Sampled from a Basic Resident Registry
Reprinted from: *J. Clin. Med.* 2021, 10, 4213, doi:10.3390/jcm10184213 . . . . **99**

Hong Jin Kim, Jae Hyuk Yang, Dong-Gune Chang, Seung Woo Suh, Hoon Jo, Sang-Il Kim, Kwang-Sup Song and Woojin Cho
Impact of Preoperative Total Knee Arthroplasty on Radiological and Clinical Outcomes of Spinal Fusion for Concurrent Knee Osteoarthritis and Degenerative Lumbar Spinal Diseases
Reprinted from: *J. Clin. Med.* 2021, 10, 4475, doi:10.3390/jcm10194475 . . . . **109**

Soraya Nishimura, Takashi Hirai, Narihito Nagoshi, Toshitaka Yoshii, Jun Hashimoto, Kanji Mori, Satoshi Maki, Keiichi Katsumi, Kazuhiro Takeuchi, Shuta Ushio, Takeo Furuya, Kei Watanabe, Norihiro Nishida, Takashi Kaito, Satoshi Kato, Katsuya Nagashima, Masao Koda, Hiroaki Nakashima, Shiro Imagama, Kazuma Murata, Yuji Matsuoka, Kanichiro Wada, Atsushi Kimura, Tetsuro Ohba, Hiroyuki Katoh, Masahiko Watanabe, Yukihiro Matsuyama, Hiroshi Ozawa, Hirotaka Haro, Katsushi Takeshita, Yu Matsukura, Hiroyuki Inose, Masashi Yamazaki, Kota Watanabe, Morio Matsumoto, Masaya Nakamura, Atsushi Okawa and Yoshiharu Kawaguchi
Association between Severity of Diffuse Idiopathic Skeletal Hyperostosis and Ossification of Other Spinal Ligaments in Patients with Ossification of the Posterior Longitudinal Ligament
Reprinted from: *J. Clin. Med.* 2021, 10, 4690, doi:10.3390/jcm10204690 . . . . **119**

Yu Matsukura, Toshitaka Yoshii, Shingo Morishita, Kenichiro Sakai, Takashi Hirai, Masato Yuasa, Hiroyuki Inose, Atsuyuki Kawabata, Kurando Utagawa, Jun Hashimoto, Masaki Tomori, Ichiro Torigoe, Tsuyoshi Yamada, Kazuo Kusano, Kazuyuki Otani, Satoshi Sumiya, Fujiki Numano, Kazuyuki Fukushima, Shoji Tomizawa, Satoru Egawa, Yoshiyasu Arai, Shigeo Shindo and Atsushi Okawa
Comparison of Lateral Lumbar Interbody Fusion and Posterior Lumbar Interbody Fusion as Corrective Surgery for Patients with Adult Spinal Deformity—A Propensity Score Matching Analysis
Reprinted from: *J. Clin. Med.* 2021, 10, 4737, doi:10.3390/jcm10204737 . . . . **131**

Takashi Hirai, Toshitaka Yoshii, Kenichiro Sakai, Hiroyuki Inose, Masato Yuasa, Tsuyoshi Yamada, Yu Matsukura, Shuta Ushio, Shingo Morishita, Satoru Egawa, Hiroaki Onuma, Yutaka Kobayashi, Kurando Utagawa, Jun Hashimoto, Atsuyuki Kawabata, Tomoyuki Tanaka, Takayuki Motoyoshi, Takuya Takahashi, Motonori Hashimoto, Kentaro Sakaeda, Tsuyoshi Kato, Yoshiyasu Arai, Shigenori Kawabata and Atsushi Okawa
Anterior Cervical Corpectomy with Fusion versus Anterior Hybrid Fusion Surgery for Patients with Severe Ossification of the Posterior Longitudinal Ligament Involving Three or More Levels: A Retrospective Comparative Study
Reprinted from: *J. Clin. Med.* **2021**, *10*, 5315, doi:10.3390/jcm10225315 . . . . **141**

Shota Ikegami, Masashi Uehara, Ryosuke Tokida, Hikaru Nishimura, Noriko Sakai, Hiroshi Horiuchi, Hiroyuki Kato and Jun Takahashi
Cervical Spinal Alignment Change Accompanying Spondylosis Exposes Harmonization Failure with Total Spinal Balance: A Japanese Cohort Survey Randomly Sampled from a Basic Resident Registry
Reprinted from: *J. Clin. Med.* **2021**, *10*, 5737, doi:10.3390/jcm10245737 . . . . **155**

Time Course of Acute Vertebral Fractures: A Prospective Multicenter Cohort Study
Reprinted from: *J. Clin. Med.* **2021**, *10*, 5961, doi:10.3390/jcm10245961 . . . . **165**

Alice Baroncini, Filippo Migliorini, Francesco Langella, Paolo Barletta, Per Trobisch, Riccardo Cecchinato, Marco Damilano, Emanuele Quarto, Claudio Lamartina and Pedro Berjano
Perioperative Predictive Factors for Positive Outcomes in Spine Fusion for Adult Deformity Correction
Reprinted from: *J. Clin. Med.* **2022**, *11*, 144, doi:10.3390/jcm11010144 . . . . **173**

Sadayuki Ito, Hiroaki Nakashima, Akiyuki Matsumoto, Kei Ando, Masaaki Machino, Naoki Segi, Hiroyuki Tomita, Hiroyuki Koshimizu and Shiro Imagama
Differences in Demographic and Radiographic Characteristics between Patients with Visible and Invisible T1 Slopes on Lateral Cervical Radiographic Images
Reprinted from: *J. Clin. Med.* **2022**, *11*, 411, doi:10.3390/jcm11020411 . . . . **181**

Franz Landauer and Klemens Trieb
An Indication-Based Concept for Stepwise Spinal Orthosis in Low Back Pain According to the Current Literature
Reprinted from: *J. Clin. Med.* **2022**, *13*, 510, doi:10.3390/jcm11030510 . . . . **191**

Hidetomi Terai, Shinji Takahashi, Koji Tamai, Yusuke Hori, Masayoshi Iwamae, Masatoshi Hoshino, Shoichiro Ohyama, Akito Yabu and Hiroaki Nakamura
Impact of the COVID-19 Pandemic on Elderly Patients with Spinal Disorders
Reprinted from: *J. Clin. Med.* **2022**, *11*, 602, doi:10.3390/jcm11030602 . . . . **203**

Sadayuki Ito, Hiroaki Nakashima, Kei Ando, Masaaki Machino, Taisuke Seki, Shinya Ishizuka, Yasuhiko Takegami, Kenji Wakai, Yukiharu Hasegawa and Shiro Imagama
Nutritional Influences on Locomotive Syndrome
Reprinted from: *J. Clin. Med.* , *11*, 610, doi:10.3390/jcm11030610 . . . . **213**

Koichiro Ono, Kazuo Ohmori, Reiko Yoneyama, Osamu Matsushige and Tokifumi Majima
Risk Factors and Surgical Management of Recurrent Herniation after Full-Endoscopic Lumbar Discectomy Using Interlaminar Approach
Reprinted from: *J. Clin. Med.* **2022**, *11*, 748, doi:10.3390/jcm11030748 . . . . **225**

Takashi Hirai, Masashi Uehara, Masayuki Miyagi, Shinji Takahashi and Hiroaki Nakashima
Current Advances in Spinal Diseases of the Elderly: Introduction to the Special Issue
Reprinted from: *J. Clin. Med.* **2021**, *10*, 3298, doi:10.3390/jcm10153298 . . . . **237**

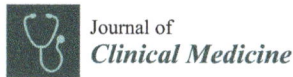 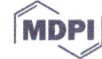

Article

The Effect of Adding Biological Factors to the Decision-Making Process for Spinal Metastasis of Non-Small Cell Lung Cancer

Hyoungmin Kim, Sam Yeol Chang *, Jongyeon Son, Sujung Mok, Sung Cheol Park and Bong-Soon Chang

Department of Orthopedic Surgery, Seoul National University Hospital, 101 Daehangno, Jongno-gu, Seoul 03080, Korea; hmkim21@gmail.com (H.K.); 2001jyson@hanmail.net (J.S.); charisma9025@naver.com (S.M.); neoz0708@gmail.com (S.C.P.); bschang@snu.ac.kr (B.-S.C.)
* Correspondence: hewl3102@gmail.com; Tel.: +82-2-2072-7607

Abstract: Molecular target therapies have markedly improved the survival of non-small cell lung cancer (NSCLC) patients, especially those with epidermal growth factor receptor (EGFR) mutations. A positive EGFR mutation is even more critical when the chronicity of spinal metastasis is considered. However, most prognostic models that estimate the life expectancy of spinal metastasis patients do not include these biological factors. We retrospectively reviewed 85 consecutive NSCLC patients who underwent palliative surgical treatment for spinal metastases to evaluate the following: (1) the prognostic value of positive EGFR mutation and the chronicity of spinal metastasis, and (2) the clinical significance of adding these two factors to an existing prognostic model, namely the New England Spinal Metastasis Score (NESMS). Among 85 patients, 38 (44.7%) were EGFR mutation-positive. Spinal metastasis presented as the initial manifestation of malignancy in 58 (68.2%) patients. The multivariate Cox proportional hazard model showed that the chronicity of spinal metastasis (hazard ratio (HR) = 1.88, $p = 0.015$) and EGFR mutation positivity (HR = 2.10, $p = 0.002$) were significantly associated with postoperative survival. The Uno's C-index and time-dependent AUC 6 months following surgery significantly increased when these factors were added to NESMS ($p = 0.004$ and $p = 0.022$, respectively). In conclusion, biological factors provide an additional prognostic value for NSCLC patients with spinal metastasis.

Keywords: spinal metastasis; non-small cell lung cancer; decompression; survival; prognosis; epidermal growth factor receptor; Uno's C-index; New England Spinal Metastasis Score

1. Introduction

Lung cancer is the most commonly diagnosed malignancy and accounts for approximately 25% of cancer deaths in men and women [1]. The spinal column is the most frequent site for the extrapulmonary metastasis of non-small cell lung cancer (NSCLC), which accounts for 80–85% of lung cancer cases [2]. The lung is also the most common location for primary cancer when a patient presents with spinal metastasis as an initial manifestation of the disease [3]. The incidence of spinal metastasis associated with NSCLC is increasing because of improved survival in these patients based on recent advancements in systemic treatment for NSCLC, such as tyrosine kinase inhibitors (TKIs) for epidermal growth factor receptor (EGFR) mutations [4,5]. Improved survival and increased incidence of spinal metastasis in NSCLC patients render surgical treatment and related decision-making processes for spinal metastasis more important.

Numerous decision-making systems or prognostic models have been introduced to estimate the remaining life expectancies and to suggest appropriate treatment options for patients with spinal metastasis [6]. Authors have used evolving methodologies, such as machine-learning algorithms, to develop a novel prognostic model for spinal metastasis [7]. These models are based on the prognostic factors significantly associated with patient survival in multivariate logistic or proportional hazards regression analyses [8]. Among these factors, the anatomical site for a primary cancer is the most significant prognostic factor,

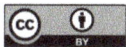

and is included in all models [9]. However, recent advances in tumor genetics suggest that a simple stratification of primary cancer by the anatomical site is insufficient [10]. Given the extensive evidence in the literature that molecular target therapies significantly improve survival in patients with certain mutations [11], genetic subtype analysis should also be considered when predicting survival in patients with spinal metastasis.

Another biological factor that should be considered in survival prediction is the chronicity of spinal metastasis. Several authors have reported that patients with spinal metastasis at the initial presentation of malignancy (synchronous metastasis) survive longer than those diagnosed with spinal metastasis later during treatment (metachronous metastasis) [3,12]. The development of resistance to previous systemic treatment and the availability of further systemic treatment options have been suggested as potential reasons for the difference in prognosis [13].

The New England Spinal Metastasis Score (NESMS) was recently introduced as a novel prognostic model for patients with spinal metastasis [14]. The NESMS consists of a modified Bauer score component, ambulatory function, and serum albumin (Table 1). The developers of NESMS prospectively validated the system in their following study [15]. However, even the recently developed NESMS system does not consider previously described biological factors when stratifying primary cancer and predicting survival. Therefore, we conducted this study to evaluate the effect of adding biological factors to a validated prognostic model for spinal metastasis—the NESMS. Although multiple prognostic models are available, from conventional scoring systems to novel machine-learning-based models, we chose NESMS because, to the best of our knowledge, it is thus far the only model validated using a well-designed prospective investigation with appropriate power [15].

Table 1. The New England Spinal Metastasis Score (NESMS).

Characteristics	Points Assigned
1. Modified Bauer Score	
No visceral metastasis (1 point)	-
Primary tumor is not lung cancer (1 point)	-
Primary tumor is breast, renal, lymphoma, or myeloma (1 point)	-
Single skeletal metastasis (1 point)	-
Score ≤ 2	0
Score ≥ 3	2
2. Ambulatory function	
Dependent ambulator/non-ambulator	0
Independent ambulator	1
3. Serum albumin	
<3.5 g/dL	0
$\geq$3.5 g/dL	1

2. Materials and Methods

Consecutive patients who underwent palliative surgical treatment for spinal metastasis of lung adenocarcinoma between March 2012 and October 2018 at the authors' institution were included in the current retrospective study. We included only patients who were biopsy-proven to have adenocarcinoma of the lung and underwent EGFR mutation analysis. Exclusion criteria were as follows: (1) missing data on EGFR mutation analysis results, (2) follow-up period of less than 12 months or unidentified survival period, and (3) patients who died within 2 weeks following surgery due to immediate postoperative complications (Figure 1). The current retrospective study obtained ethical approval and a waiver of informed consent from the institutional review board (IRB No. 2009-060-1155).

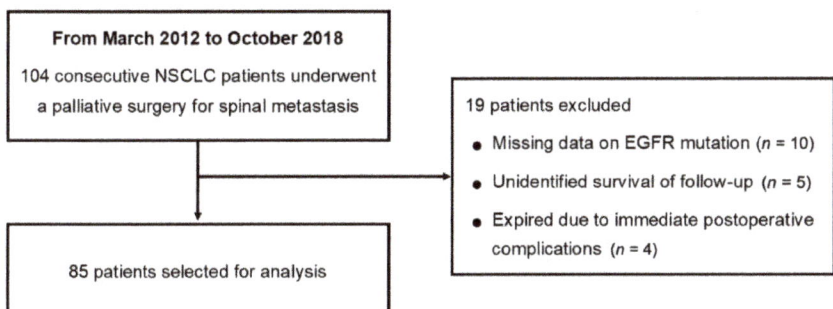

Figure 1. Flowchart for patient selection. (Abbreviations: NSCLC, non-small cell lung cancer; EGFR, epidermal growth factor receptor).

Surgeries for NSCLC patients with spinal metastasis were performed based on the decisions made during a weekly multidisciplinary tumor board meeting consisting of medical and radiation oncologists, orthopedic and neuro-surgeons, diagnostic radiologists, and pathologists. In general, surgical treatment was considered for patients who were anticipated to have a postoperative survival period longer than 6 months. Surgical indications included (1) metastatic spinal cord compression and (2) spinal instability causing pain that was uncontrolled by medications or radiotherapy. Three different surgeons from the Department of Orthopedic Surgery operated on these patients. We performed all surgeries for palliation.

Patient information was retrieved from electronic medical records and was retrospectively reviewed. Regarding NSCLC and spinal metastasis; we identified the chronicity of spinal metastasis and the positivity of EGFR mutation as primary dependent variables. Spinal metastasis diagnosed at the initial presentation of NSCLC was referred to as synchronous metastasis, and spinal metastasis diagnosed during the course of NSCLC treatment was referred to as metachronous metastasis. Analysis for EGFR mutation was performed using either direct DNA sequencing analysis or peptide nucleic acid (PNA)-mediated real-time polymerase chain reaction (PCR) clamping analysis [16]. Information on pre- and post-operative systemic treatment regimens, including conventional cytotoxic chemotherapy and target therapies, such as TKIs, were also collected. To evaluate the patients' preoperative status, we assessed the preoperative ambulatory status and serum albumin, and applied the NESMS using these variables (Table 1). Preoperative serum albumin within 1 week before surgery and preoperative ambulatory status, which was routinely recorded 1 day before surgery, were selected for the preoperative evaluation. Postoperative survival, defined as the time interval between spinal surgery and either death or the last follow-up, was identified as the primary outcome. Patients' survival beyond 6 months postoperatively was considered the secondary outcome.

Survival probability was estimated using the Kaplan–Meier method (product-limit estimator). The Cox proportional hazard model was applied to develop a prognostic model, and the proportion hazard assumption was checked using log–log plots and the time-by-covariate interaction for each predictor. The Uno's C-index and time-dependent area under the curve (AUC) 6 months postoperatively were utilized to evaluate the discrimination and prediction ability of the NESMS, and the effect of adding two biological factors (chronicity of spinal metastasis and EGFR mutation positivity) into the NESMS. p-values were adjusted using the Bonferroni method. All statistical analyses were performed using SAS system for Windows, version 9.4 (SAS Institute, Cary, NC, USA) and R software version 3.6.1 (R Foundation for Statistical Computing, Vienna, Austria). p-values less than 0.05 were considered statistically significant.

3. Results

Between March 2012 and October 2018, a total of 104 NSCLC patients received palliative surgery for spinal metastasis at the authors' institution. Among these patients, 19 were excluded from the analysis for the following reasons: (1) ten due to missing data on EGFR mutation analysis results, (2) five with an unidentified survival period or death, and (3) four who died within two weeks after surgery due to immediate postoperative complications (two pneumonia, one cardiac arrest, and one disseminated intravascular coagulation due to massive bleeding; Figure 1). As a result, 85 patients (58 males and 27 females) with a mean age of 60.9 (range, 32–81) years were analyzed in the current study. The characteristics of the study population are described in Table 2.

Table 2. Characteristics of the study cohort.

Categories	Variables	n (%)
Location of spinal metastasis	Cervical	16 (18.8%)
	Cervicothoracic	7 (8.2%)
	Thoracic	41 (48.2%)
	Thoracolumbar	3 (3.5%)
	Lumbar	18 (21.2%)
Chronicity of spinal metastasis	Synchronous	58 (68.2%)
	Metachronous	27 (31.8%)
EGFR mutation	Positive	38 (44.7%)
	Negative	47 (55.3%)
Ambulatory status	Independent ambulator	62 (72.9%)
	Dependent ambulator/non-ambulator	23 (27.1%)
Serum albumin	≥ 3.5 g/dL	67 (78.8%)
	<3.5 g/dL	18 (21.2%)
NESMS	0	8 (9.4%)
	1	25 (29.4%)
	2	52 (61.2%)

Seven patients were alive at the last follow-up, with a minimum follow-up period of 12 months, and the remaining 78 died during follow-up. The median postoperative survival period estimated by the Kaplan–Meier estimator was 6.4 months for the entire cohort ($n = 85$; Figure 2). Patients with a positive EGFR mutation had a significantly prolonged survival ($p = 0.007$), and those with synchronous metastasis tended to have longer survival ($p = 0.101$) than their counterparts in the log-rank test (Figure 3). According to the multivariate Cox proportional hazard model, the chronicity of spinal metastasis (hazard ratio (HR) = 1.88 (95% CI: 1.13. 3.12), $p = 0.015$), and EGFR mutation positivity (HR = 2.10 (95% CI: 1.30, 3.38), $p = 0.002$) were significantly associated with postoperative survival (Table 3). All predictors satisfied the proportional hazard assumption.

The Uno's C-index (discrimination ability) of NESMS was improved from 0.59 (95% CI: 0.54–0.65) to 0.62 (95% CI: 0.56–0.69), 0.64 (95% CI: 0.58–0.71), and 0.67 (95% CI: 0.61–0.74) when the chronicity of spinal metastasis, the EGFR mutation positivity, and both factors were added to the NESMS, respectively (Table 4). The improvement was statistically significant when the EGFR mutation positivity alone (adjusted $p = 0.019$) and both factors (adjusted $p = 0.004$) were added to the NESMS. The time-dependent AUC for predicting survival beyond 6 months postoperatively also increased from 0.63 (95% CI: 0.53–0.74) to 0.73 (95% CI: 0.64–0.82) when the two biological factors were added to the NESMS (adjusted $p = 0.022$; Table 5).

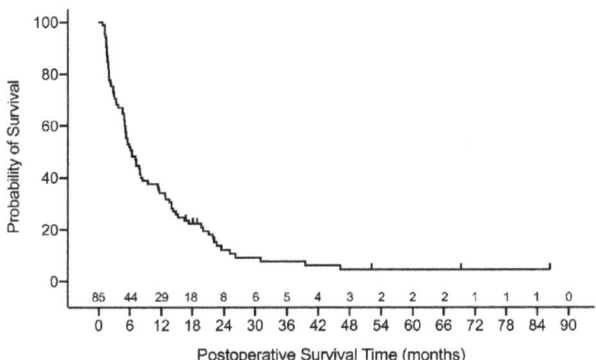

Figure 2. The Kaplan–Meier estimator graph for the total cohort.

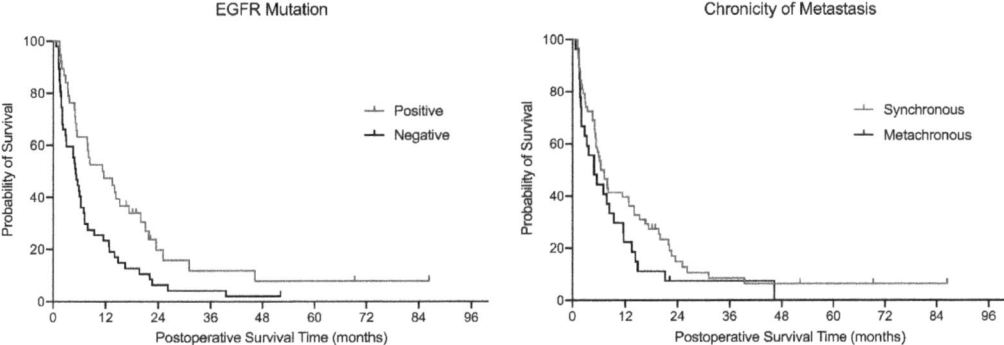

Figure 3. Comparison of the Kaplan–Meier curve stratified by the biological factors.

Table 3. Results of the multivariable Cox proportional hazards model.

Categories	Stratifications	Hazard Ratio (95% CI)	p-Value
NESMS	0	3.21 (1.44, 7.18)	0.0045
	1	2.57 (1.47, 4.50)	0.0010
	2	1	
Chronicity	Synchronous	1.88 (1.13, 3.12)	0.0149
	Metachronous	1	
EGFR mutation	Positive	2.10 (1.30, 3.38)	0.0024
	Negative	1	

Table 4. The changes in the discrimination ability (Uno's C-index) of prognostic models by adding biological factors.

Model	Uno's C-Index (95% CI)	p-Value	Adjusted p *
NESMS	0.59 (0.54, 0.65)		
NESMS + chronicity	0.62 (0.56, 0.69)	0.0760	0.2280
NESMS + EGFR	0.64 (0.58, 0.71)	0.0063	0.0189
NESMS + chronicity + EGFR	0.67 (0.61, 0.74)	0.0024	0.0042

* p-value adjusted using the Bonferroni method.

Table 5. The changes in the prediction ability (time-dependent area under curve (AUC)) of prognostic models by adding biological factors.

Model	Time-Dependent AUC at 6 Months (95% CI)	p-Value	Adjusted p *
NESMS	0.63 (0.53, 0.74)		
NESMS + chronicity	0.67 (0.55, 0.79)	0.1531	0.4593
NESMS + EGFR	0.69 (0.57, 0.81)	0.0320	0.0960
NESMS + chronicity + EGFR	0.73 (0.64, 0.82)	0.0073	0.0219

* p-value adjusted by Bonferroni method.

4. Discussion

In the late 1990s, gefitinib, an oral EGRF TKI, was introduced as a molecular target therapy for NSCLC patients. A few years later, researchers identified EGFR mutations in NSCLC patients sensitive to gefitinib. Since then, genetic mutation analyses and corresponding molecular target therapies have been game-changers in the management of NSCLC, improving the survival of patients with EGFR mutations [11]. Several previous studies have reported the clinical effects of EGFR mutation positivity and TKIs in NSCLC patients with skeletal [17] and spinal metastasis [18]. In the current study, patients with a positive EGFR mutation showed a significantly prolonged postoperative survival period compared to the EGFR mutation-negative group. The EGFR mutation positivity also significantly improved the discrimination (Uno's C-index) and prediction ability (time-dependent AUC at 6 months postoperatively) of a novel prognostic model—the NESMS. These results signify the importance of considering biological profiles in the decision-making process for spinal metastasis.

The timing of diagnosis of spinal metastasis, or the chronicity of spinal metastasis, was considered an additional biological factor in this study, which was significantly associated with postoperative survival. In previous studies, not only postoperative survival but also overall survival, was prolonged in patients with spinal metastasis as the initial manifestation of malignancy (synchronous metastasis) [3,12]. From the standpoint of tumor genetics, these findings can be related to the acquired resistance to first-line (first and second generation) TKIs. Common mechanisms for acquired resistance to TKIs, which usually develop within 12 months after TKI usage [13], are mutations in 20 exons (threonine-to-methionine substitution on codon 790, T790M) and MET oncogene amplification [19,20].

In our series, 7 (18.4%) of the 38 patients in the EGFR mutation-positive group showed a mutation in exon 20 (T790M) later in their disease course, which was not present in the initial molecular analysis. Five of these seven patients had metachronous spinal metastasis, and their exon 20 mutations were found in specimens obtained from the spine surgery. For these patients, third generation TKI (simertinib) or cytotoxic chemotherapy was considered after spinal surgery, and a shorter life expectancy was anticipated. This effect of acquired resistance to a TKI in metachronous metastasis patients was reflected in our finding that the time-dependent AUC 6 months postoperatively was significantly increased when both factors (EGFR mutation and chronicity) were added to the prognostic model ($p = 0.022$) and not when only EGFR mutation positivity was added ($p = 0.096$). As not all patients in our series underwent additional biopsies and molecular analyses during their disease course, the exact number of patients with acquired resistance to TKI in the metachronous metastasis group cannot be derived. Nevertheless, acquired resistance to TKIs can be associated with shortened survival in metachronous metastasis patients, and therefore, the chronicity of spinal metastasis should be considered as a significant biological factor (Figure 4).

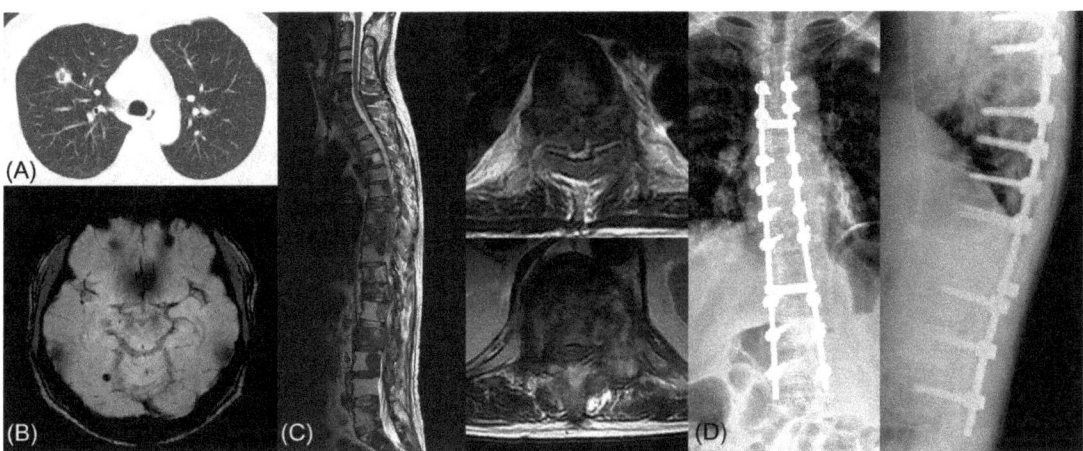

Figure 4. Comparison of Kaplan–Meier curve stratified by the biological factors. An illustrative case of acquired resistance to tyrosine kinase inhibitor (TKI) in an epidermal growth factor receptor (EGFR) mutation-positive non-small cell lung cancer (NSCLC) patient. (**A**,**B**) A 53 years-old male with lung adenocarcinoma in right upper lobe. EGFR mutation analysis from the lung specimen showed a microdeletion mutation in exon 19. (**C**) After 2 years of systemic treatment with multiple regimens including TKI (gefitinib), the patient was diagnosed with multiple spinal metastasis with spinal cord compression at T7 and T12. (**D**) The patient underwent a palliative decompression and stabilization, and EGFR mutation analysis from a spine specimen revealed a missense mutation of EGFR gene exon 20 (T790M). The patient expired 4 months postoperatively due to disease progression.

We examined the discrimination and prediction ability of the NESMS, a novel and prospectively validated prognostic model, in this study (Table 1). In this system, the primary tumor is stratified according to the modified Bauer score. As all patients in our series had lung adenocarcinoma, the modified Bauer score was 0 for all patients. Therefore, after eliminating the most significant factor from the NESMS, the remaining factors for the decision-making process are ambulatory function and serum albumin. In this setting, if there are two different NSCLC patients with ambulatory status and serum albumin falling into the same category, the decisions for two patients would be the same according to the NESMS, even if the two have significantly different biological profiles (e.g., synchronous metastasis with a positive EGFR mutation versus metachronous metastasis without EGFR mutation). This novel "classification-based" decision-making system, the NESMS, may be useful and straightforward when all spinal metastasis patients with diverse primary cancers are combined; however, its discrimination ability seems to be significantly limited for individual cancers.

We examined the discrimination and prediction ability of the NESMS, a novel and prospectively validated prognostic model, in this study (Table 1). In this system, the primary tumor is stratified according to the modified Bauer score. As all patients in our series had lung adenocarcinoma, the modified Bauer score was 0 for all patients. Therefore, after eliminating the most significant factor from the NESMS, the remaining factors for the decision-making process are ambulatory function and serum albumin. In this setting, if there are two different NSCLC patients with ambulatory status and serum albumin falling into the same category, decisions for two patients would be the same according to the NESMS, even if the two have significantly different biological profiles (e.g., synchronous metastasis with a positive EGFR mutation versus metachronous metastasis without EGFR mutation). This novel "classification-based" decision-making system, the NESMS, may be useful and straightforward when all spinal metastasis patients with diverse primary cancers are combined; however, its discrimination ability seems to be significantly limited for individual cancers.

It is obvious that a prognostic model's performance will improve if more prognostic factors are added to it. However, adding too many factors can make a prognostic model complicated and difficult to use in the clinical setting. Therefore, it is essential to prioritize prognostic factors according to their weights in multivariate logistic or proportional hazard regression analyses. Factors with higher odds or hazard ratios should be incorporated into the system. In our study, a multivariate Cox proportional hazard model (backward stepwise with likelihood ratio test) yielded a higher hazard ratio for EGFR mutation positivity (HR = 2.27 (95% CI: 1.41, 3.66), p = 0.001) than ambulatory status (HR = 2.26 (95% CI: 1.29, 3.95), p = 0.004) and serum albumin (HR = 1.71 (95% CI: 0.96, 3.02), p = 0.068), which are the main components of the NESMS. These results also emphasize the importance and necessity of adding biological factors as modifiers in the decision-making systems for spinal metastasis.

Among the various decision-making systems reported in the literature, there have been efforts to incorporate biological factors into these systems. In 2014, Katagiri et al. introduced a revised version of their prognostic system for spinal metastasis, in which the application of molecular target therapy was considered when stratifying the patient's primary tumor [10]. In their system, lung cancer treated with molecular target therapy was classified as a moderate-growth tumor, while lung cancer without available molecular target therapy was classified as a rapid-growth tumor. Efforts to incorporate biological factors into decision-making systems, as shown in the revised Katagiri system, are anticipated to be the future trends in the management of spinal metastases.

In this study, we stratified patients by EGFR mutation positivity rather than by the treatment they received (e.g., TKI versus platinum-based chemotherapy), as in a previous study [18]. The most important reason for choosing this categorization is that the EGFR mutation profile, rather than the type of postoperative systemic treatment the patient will receive after surgery, is more available at the time of decision-making for spinal metastasis surgeries. As the purpose of this study was to verify the prognostic value of biological factors and not to compare the treatment outcomes, our categorization seems to be more appropriate. Another reason is the diversity of systemic treatment that a patient with NSCLC receives after surgery, as well as the start point and duration of these treatments. In our series, 41 (48.2%) patients received a combination of molecular target therapy and cytotoxic chemotherapy, whereas only 14 (16.5%) received molecular target therapy alone postoperatively, regardless of EGFR mutation positivity. In addition, the molecular target therapies used in our study patients ranged from first to third generation EGFR TKIs (gefitinib, erlotinib, afatinib, and osimertinib), EGFR monoclonal antibody (cetuximab), anaplastic lymphoma kinase (ALT) inhibitors (crizotinib), mesenchymal-epithelial transition (MET) inhibitors (savolitinib, capmatinib), and PD-1 inhibitors (avelumab, nivolumab, and pembrolizumab). Therefore, it would be impossible and meaningless to stratify patients by postoperative systemic treatment, given the diversity of mechanisms and the treatment effects of these agents.

There are several limitations in the current study. First, because of its retrospective nature, selection bias regarding the inclusion and exclusion criteria cannot be ruled out. Second, there is a possibility that the differences in surgical aggressiveness between individual cases may have influenced the patients' prognosis and survival, such as the case described in Figure 4 [21,22]. However, this possible effect of surgical strategy on patients' outcomes was not considered in the analysis. Third, because this study included only lung adenocarcinoma patients, our results cannot be generalized to spinal metastases of various primary cancers. Finally, and most importantly, because we did not aim to develop a new prognostic model in this study and include all relevant prognostic factors in the analysis, we cannot perform any validations, including calibrations, on our results. We also cannot suggest how to incorporate biological factors into the decision-making systems as a modifier, which is well beyond the current study's scope. Despite these limitations, the results of this study provide valuable information for state-of-the-art care for patients with spinal metastasis, and suggest future directions for the development of decision-making systems for spinal metastasis.

5. Conclusions

EGFR mutation positivity and the chronicity of spinal metastasis provide additional prognostic value for NSCLC patients with spinal metastasis. These results signify the importance of considering biological profiles in the decision-making process for spinal metastasis.

Author Contributions: Conceptualization, H.K., S.Y.C., and B.-S.C.; methodology, H.K., S.Y.C., and J.S.; validation, H.K., S.M., and S.C.P.; formal analysis, S.Y.C., S.C.P., and B.-S.C.; investigation, H.K., S.Y.C., and J.S.; resources, S.M. and S.C.P.; data curation, H.K., S.M., and B.-S.C.; writing—original draft preparation, H.K., S.Y.C., and B.-S.C.; writing—review and editing, all authors; visualization, J.S., S.M., and S.C.P.; supervision, B.-S.C. All authors have read and agreed to the published version of the manuscript.

Funding: This research received no external funding.

Institutional Review Board Statement: The study was conducted according to the guidelines of the Declaration of Helsinki, and approved by the Institutional Review Board of Seoul National University Hospital. (IRB No. 2009-060-1155).

Informed Consent Statement: Patient consent was waived due to retrospective nature of the study.

Data Availability Statement: All relevant raw data from the data presented in the manuscript or the supplementary figures and tables are available from the authors of the study upon request.

Acknowledgments: The authors appreciate the statistical consultation provided by the Medical Research Collaborating Center at the Seoul National University College.

Conflicts of Interest: The authors declare no conflict of interest.

References

1. Siegel, R.L.; Miller, K.D.; Jemal, A. Cancer statistics, 2020. *CA Cancer J. Clin.* **2020**, *70*, 7–30. [CrossRef] [PubMed]
2. Chang, S.C.; Chang, C.Y.; Shih, J.Y. The role of epidermal growth factor receptor mutations and epidermal growth factor receptor-tyrosine kinase inhibitors in the treatment of lung cancer. *Cancers* **2011**, *3*, 2667–2678. [CrossRef]
3. Park, J.S.; Park, S.J.; Lee, C.S. Incidence and prognosis of patients with spinal metastasis as the initial manifestation of malignancy: Analysis of 338 patients undergoing surgical treatment. *Bone Jt. J.* **2019**, *101-b*, 1379–1384. [CrossRef]
4. Howlader, N.; Forjaz, G.; Mooradian, M.J.; Meza, R.; Kong, C.Y.; Cronin, K.A.; Mariotto, A.B.; Lowy, D.R.; Feuer, E.J. The Effect of Advances in Lung-Cancer Treatment on Population Mortality. *N. Engl. J. Med.* **2020**, *383*, 640–649. [CrossRef] [PubMed]
5. Xia, W.; Yu, X.; Mao, Q.; Xia, W.; Wang, A.; Dong, G.; Chen, B.; Ma, W.; Xu, L.; Jiang, F. Improvement of survival for non-small cell lung cancer over time. *Oncotargets Ther.* **2017**, *10*, 4295–4303. [CrossRef]
6. Ahmed, A.K.; Goodwin, C.R.; Heravi, A.; Kim, R.; Abu-Bonsrah, N.; Sankey, E.; Kerekes, D.; De la Garza Ramos, R.; Schwab, J.; Sciubba, D.M. Predicting survival for metastatic spine disease: A comparison of nine scoring systems. *Spine J.* **2018**, *18*, 1804–1814. [CrossRef] [PubMed]
7. Karhade, A.V.; Thio, Q.C.B.S.; Ogink, P.T.; Bono, C.M.; Ferrone, M.L.; Oh, K.S.; Saylor, P.J.; Schoenfeld, A.J.; Shin, J.H.; Harris, M.B.; et al. Predicting 90-Day and 1-Year Mortality in Spinal Metastatic Disease: Development and Internal Validation. *Neurosurgery* **2019**, *85*, E671–E681. [CrossRef]
8. Luksanapruksa, P.; Buchowski, J.M.; Hotchkiss, W.; Tongsai, S.; Wilartratsami, S.; Chotivichit, A. Prognostic factors in patients with spinal metastasis: A systematic review and meta-analysis. *Spine J.* **2017**, *17*, 689–708. [CrossRef] [PubMed]
9. Chang, S.Y.; Mok, S.; Park, S.C.; Kim, H.; Chang, B.S. Treatment Strategy for Metastatic Spinal Tumors: A Narrative Review. *Asian Spine J.* **2020**, *14*, 513–525. [CrossRef] [PubMed]
10. Katagiri, H.; Okada, R.; Takagi, T.; Takahashi, M.; Murata, H.; Harada, H.; Nishimura, T.; Asakura, H.; Ogawa, H. New prognostic factors and scoring system for patients with skeletal metastasis. *Cancer Med.* **2014**, *3*, 1359–1367. [CrossRef]
11. Herbst, R.S.; Morgensztern, D.; Boshoff, C. The biology and management of non-small cell lung cancer. *Nature* **2018**, *553*, 446–454. [CrossRef]
12. Chang, S.Y.; Chang, B.S.; Lee, C.K.; Kim, H. Remaining Systemic Treatment Options: A Valuable Predictor of Survival and Functional Outcomes after Surgical Treatment for Spinal Metastasis. *Orthop. Surg.* **2019**, *11*, 552–559. [CrossRef] [PubMed]
13. Cabanero, M.; Sangha, R.; Sheffield, B.S.; Sukhai, M.; Pakkal, M.; Kamel-Reid, S.; Karsan, A.; Ionescu, D.; Juergens, R.A.; Butts, C.; et al. Management of EGFR-mutated non-small-cell lung cancer: Practical implications from a clinical and pathology perspective. *Curr. Oncol.* **2017**, *24*, 111–119. [CrossRef]

14. Ghori, A.K.; Leonard, D.A.; Schoenfeld, A.J.; Saadat, E.; Scott, N.; Ferrone, M.L.; Pearson, A.M.; Harris, M.B. Modeling 1-year survival after surgery on the metastatic spine. *Spine J.* **2015**, *15*, 2345–2350. [CrossRef]
15. Schoenfeld, A.J.; Ferrone, M.L.; Schwab, J.H.; Blucher, J.A.; Barton, L.B.; Tobert, D.G.; Chi, J.H.; Shin, J.H.; Kang, J.D.; Harris, M.B. Prospective validation of a clinical prediction score for survival in patients with spinal metastases: The New England Spinal Metastasis Score. *Spine J.* **2020**. [CrossRef]
16. Kim, H.J.; Lee, K.Y.; Kim, Y.C.; Kim, K.S.; Lee, S.Y.; Jang, T.W.; Lee, M.K.; Shin, K.C.; Lee, G.H.; Lee, J.C.; et al. Detection and comparison of peptide nucleic acid-mediated real-time polymerase chain reaction clamping and direct gene sequencing for epidermal growth factor receptor mutations in patients with non-small cell lung cancer. *Lung Cancer* **2012**, *75*, 321–325. [CrossRef] [PubMed]
17. Kim, J.H.; Seo, S.W.; Chung, C.H. What Factors Are Associated With Early Mortality in Patients Undergoing Femur Surgery for Metastatic Lung Cancer? *Clin. Orthop. Relat. Res.* **2018**, *476*, 1815–1822. [CrossRef]
18. Lin, H.H.; Chiu, C.H.; Chou, P.H.; Ma, H.L.; Wang, J.P.; Wang, S.T.; Liu, C.L.; Chang, M.C. Functional outcomes and survival after surgical stabilization for inoperable non-small-cell lung cancer with spinal metastasis of the thoracic and lumbar spines: A retrospective comparison between epidermal growth factor receptor-tyrosine kinase inhibitor and platinum-based chemotherapy groups. *Spinal Cord* **2020**, *58*, 194–202. [CrossRef]
19. Wu, J.Y.; Wu, S.G.; Yang, C.H.; Gow, C.H.; Chang, Y.L.; Yu, C.J.; Shih, J.Y.; Yang, P.C. Lung cancer with epidermal growth factor receptor exon 20 mutations is associated with poor gefitinib treatment response. *Clin. Cancer Res. Off. J. Am. Assoc. Cancer Res.* **2008**, *14*, 4877–4882. [CrossRef] [PubMed]
20. Bean, J.; Brennan, C.; Shih, J.Y.; Riely, G.; Viale, A.; Wang, L.; Chitale, D.; Motoi, N.; Szoke, J.; Broderick, S.; et al. MET amplification occurs with or without T790M mutations in EGFR mutant lung tumors with acquired resistance to gefitinib or erlotinib. *Proc. Natl. Acad. Sci. USA* **2007**, *104*, 20932–20937. [CrossRef]
21. Horowitz, M.; Neeman, E.; Sharon, E.; Ben-Eliyahu, S. Exploiting the critical perioperative period to improve long-term cancer outcomes. *Nat. Rev. Clin. Oncol.* **2015**, *12*, 213–226. [CrossRef] [PubMed]
22. Kumar, N.; Patel, R.; Tan, J.H.; Song, J.; Pandita, N.; Hey, D.H.W.; Lau, L.L.; Liu, G.; Thambiah, J.; Wong, H.K. Symptomatic Construct Failure after Metastatic Spine Tumor Surgery. *Asian Spine J.* **2020**. [CrossRef] [PubMed]

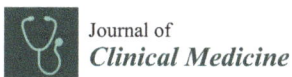

Article

Trunk Muscle Mass Measured by Bioelectrical Impedance Analysis Reflecting the Cross-Sectional Area of the Paravertebral Muscles and Back Muscle Strength: A Cross-Sectional Analysis of a Prospective Cohort Study of Elderly Population

Hamidullah Salimi [1], Shoichiro Ohyama [1], Hidetomi Terai [1,*], Yusuke Hori [1], Shinji Takahashi [1], Masatoshi Hoshino [1], Akito Yabu [1], Hasibullah Habibi [1], Akio Kobayashi [2], Tadao Tsujio [2], Shiro Kotake [3] and Hiroaki Nakamura [1]

[1] Department of Orthopaedic Surgery, Osaka City University Graduate School of Medicine, Osaka 545-8585, Japan; hamidullahsalimi@yahoo.com (H.S.); ohyama.shoichiro@med.osaka-cu.ac.jp (S.O.); yusukehori0702@gmail.com (Y.H.); shinji@med.osaka-cu.ac.jp (S.T.); hirotoy@msic.med.osaka-cu.ac.jp (M.H.); yabuakito@gmail.com (A.Y.); drhasibhabibi@gmail.com (H.H.); hnakamura@med.osaka-cu.ac.jp (H.N.)

[2] Department of Orthopaedic Surgery, Shiraniwa Hospital, Nara 630-0136, Japan; ak@med.osaka-cu.ac.jp (A.K.); t-tsujio@siren.ocn.ne.jp (T.T.)

[3] Kotake Orthopaedic Clinic, Nara 631-0003, Japan; kotakeseikei@gmail.com

* Correspondence: hterai@med.osaka-cu.ac.jp; Tel.: +81-6-6645-3851; Fax: +81-6-6646-6260

Abstract: Trunk muscles play an important role in supporting the spinal column. A decline in trunk muscle mass, as measured by bioelectrical impedance analysis (TMM–BIA), is associated with low back pain and poor quality of life. The purpose of this study was to determine whether TMM–BIA correlates with quantitative and functional assessments traditionally used for the trunk muscles. We included 380 participants (aged ≥ 65 years; 152 males, 228 females) from the Shiraniwa Elderly Cohort (Shiraniwa) study, for whom the following data were available: TMM–BIA, lumbar magnetic resonance imaging (MRI), and back muscle strength (BMS). We measured the cross-sectional area (CSA) and fat-free CSA of the paravertebral muscles (PVM), including the erector spinae (ES), multifidus (MF), and psoas major (PM), on an axial lumbar MRI at L3/4. The correlation between TMM–BIA and the CSA of PVM, fat-free CSA of PVM, and BMS was investigated. TMM–BIA correlated with the CSA of total PVM and each individual PVM. A stronger correlation between TMM–BIA and fat-free CSA of PVM was observed. The TMM–BIA also strongly correlated with BMS. TMM–BIA is an easy and reliable way to evaluate the trunk muscle mass in a clinical setting.

Keywords: trunk muscle; bioelectrical impedance analysis; MRI; back muscle strength

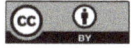

1. Introduction

Trunk muscles, especially the paravertebral muscles (PVM), play an important role in supporting the spinal column [1]. The trunk muscles, which include the erector spinae (ES), multifidus (MF), and psoas major (PM), are reported to provide spinal stability during both moving and static states [2]. A decrease in trunk muscle volume or quality, due to sarcopenia [3] and fatty infiltration, along with aging, leads to spinal problems such as low back pain [4] and spinal sagittal imbalance [5]. Therefore, the importance of assessing trunk muscles, especially for the elderly in clinical settings, has attracted attention in recent years.

Traditionally, the quantitative assessment of trunk muscles is performed by measuring the cross-sectional area (CSA) of PVM using magnetic resonance imaging (MRI) or computed tomography (CT) [6–9], and the functional assessment of trunk muscles is performed by measuring back muscle strength (BMS) [10,11]. However, quantitative assessment of trunk muscles using MRI or CT is not routinely performed owing to the high cost and time requirements [12].

Bioelectrical impedance analysis (BIA) is a non-invasive examination technique that determines body composition by measuring the electrical resistance (bioimpedance) of living tissues [13]. In recent years, it has frequently been used in clinical settings as a guiding tool for fluid management and identification of the optimal method for patients undergoing dialysis [14–16]. BIA has been widely used to determine appendicular skeletal muscle mass (ASM) for diagnosis of sarcopenia [17]. In the limbs, which are mainly composed of muscle, bone, and fat, the muscle mass calculated by BIA is considered to be reliable [18].

Moreover, BIA has been used to calculate trunk muscle mass (TMM–BIA) and, recently, a decline in TMM–BIA has been associated with low back pain and poor quality of life [12]. However, it has been unclear whether the TMM–BIA reflects actual muscle mass, since the trunk also contains organs. Only one study [19] has reported a correlation between TMM–BIA and the CSA of PVM on MRI; however, due to the small sample size in that study, the accuracy of TMM–BIA could not be adequately investigated. Thus, the purpose of this study was to verify whether TMM–BIA correlates with the quantitative and functional assessments traditionally used for trunk muscles.

2. Materials and Methods

2.1. Ethics Approval

This study used data obtained from the Shiraniwa Elderly Cohort (Shiraniwa) study [20]. The study protocol was approved by the Institutional Review Board of Osaka City University Graduate School of Medicine (No. 3484). All methods were performed in accordance with the Declaration of Helsinki and the Ethical Guidelines for Medical and Health Research Involving Human Subjects in Japan. Written informed consent was obtained from each participant.

2.2. Study Population

The Shiraniwa study is a prospective cohort study that investigates sarcopenia, locomotive syndrome, frailty, and spinal sagittal imbalance among elderly people (aged 65 years or more) living in suburban areas of Japan and recruited by community notices and bulletin boards within our hospital. The inclusion criteria of the subjects were as follows: able to visit the hospital for the survey, able to walk independently, and willing to participate in annual surveys for 5 years. In total, 458 people applied voluntarily and were sent consent forms and self-administered questionnaires. After written consent was obtained, 409 participants (164 males, 245 females; mean age, 73.5 years; SD, 5.4 years) were finally included in the Shiraniwa study. In this analysis, we obtained the data from the first-year survey of the Shiraniwa study and excluded participants who could not undergo MRI or who had metal implants for spinal fusion surgery in their trunk (Figure 1).

2.3. Measurements

All of the following measurements were performed on the same day for each participant.

2.3.1. Trunk Muscle Mass Measurement by BIA (TMM–BIA)

We measured the trunk muscle mass (kg) of participants using the BIA method with a body composition analyzer (MC-780A, Tanita Co., Tokyo, Japan). BIA is a non-invasive examination technique used to determine body composition by measuring the electrical resistance (bioimpedance) of living tissues [21]. The BIA device (MC-780A) measures bioimpedance using six electrical frequencies (1, 5, 50, 250, 500, and 1000 kHz). It can accurately identify bone and fat because it distinguishes tissues by their bioimpedance. Muscle mass (kg) was calculated by subtracting fat mass and bone mass from the total body weight (kg). Furthermore, trunk muscle mass (kg) was calculated by subtracting the ASM (kg) from the muscle mass of the whole body (kg).

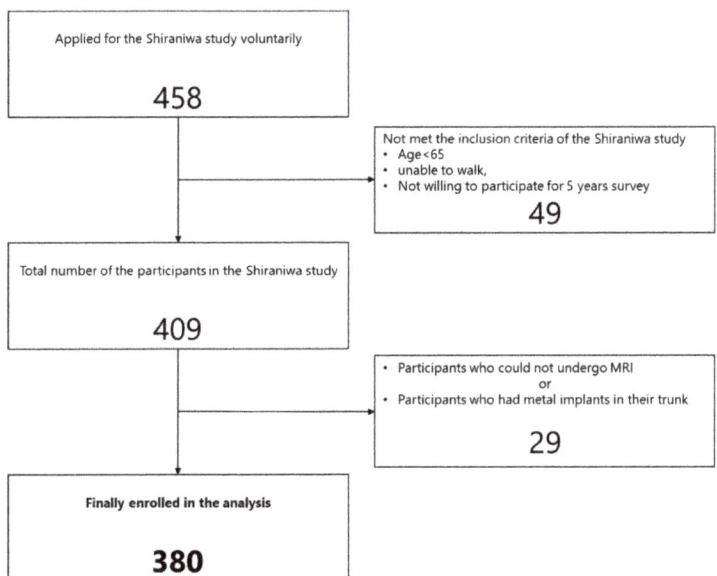

Figure 1. Flowchart of the included and excluded participants. A total of 380 participants were enrolled for this analysis.

2.3.2. Quantitative Evaluation of Trunk Muscle on MRI

In this study, MRI evaluations were performed using the Achieva 3.0 Quasar (Koninklijke Philips N.V., Amsterdam, Netherlands). A T2-weighted axial image (TR = 7670, TE = 90, FOV = 170 × 170 mm, slice = 5 mm) was used to measure the CSA of PVM, including ES, MF, and PM, at the L3/4 level, using the "pencil tool" from the 32-bit OsiriX software (version 3.8.1, Pixmeo, Geneva, Switzerland). The CSA including infiltrated fat was measured and determined, and then the intramuscular fat based on regions of interest (ROIs) with intensity changes was differentiated. The fat-free CSA for each PVM was then calculated as the difference between these two values [22].

2.3.3. Functional Evaluation of Trunk Muscles

The BMS of each participant was determined by measuring the maximal isometric strength of the trunk muscles in a standing position with 30° of lumbar flexion using a digital BMS meter (T.K.K.5402, TAKEI, Niigata, Japan) [10,11]. After performing warm-up exercises called "radio calisthenics", the participants underwent the BMS measurement twice. The average force from two trials was recorded. As the minimum measurable value of the digital BMS meter is 20 kg, in case the participant's BMS was too weak to be measured, it was not recorded and was excluded from the analysis of BMS.

2.4. Statistical Analysis

We investigated the correlation between TMM–BIA and the CSA of PVM and fat-free CSA of PVM using Spearman's rank correlation coefficient. The relationship between TMM–BIA and the CSA of each individual PVM (ES, MF, and PM) was also evaluated. Additionally, we examined the association between TMM–BIA and BMS. Patient demographics were compared using Student's t-tests. All statistical analyses were performed using Statistical Package for the Social Sciences (SPSS Inc., version 19.0, Chicago, IL, USA). Correlation strengths were categorized as very weak (<0.20), weak (0.20–0.39), moderate (0.40–0.59), strong (0.60–0.79), or very strong ($\geq$0.80). Statistical significance was set at $p < 0.05$.

3. Results

Data from 380 participants in the Shiraniwa study (152 males, 228 females; mean age, 73.4 years) who underwent TMM–BIA, lumbar MRI, and BMS measurements were analyzed in this study. The participants' characteristics are summarized in Table 1.

Table 1. Characteristics of the participants of the Shiraniwa study.

	Total	Male	Female	p-Value
Number of participants	380	152	228	
Age, years.	73.4 (5.3)	73.7 (5.2)	73.3 (5.5)	0.81
Height, cm	156.4 (9.1)	164.9 (5.9)	150.8 (6.0)	<0.01
Weight, kg	56.5 (10.6)	63.7 (8.7)	51.8 (8.9)	<0.01
BMI, kg/m^2	23.0 (3.3)	23.4 (2.8)	22.7 (3.6)	0.04
Back muscle strength, kg	60.0 (29.2)	84.2 (26.3)	47.3 (15.0)	<0.01
Number of participants whose BMS was too weak to be recorded	20 (5.3%)	1 (0.7%)	19 (8.3%)	<0.01
TMM–BIA, kg	21.95 (3.87)	25.94 (2.55)	19.28 (1.72)	<0.01
CSA of PVM, cm^2 (Total)	54.54 (11.56)	63.34 (9.40)	46.97 (7.52)	<0.01
CSA of Fat-free PVM, cm^2 (excluding intramuscular fat)	44.70 (11.95)	55.70 (9.15)	37.36 (6.89)	<0.01
Fat-free percentage of PVM, % (excluding intramuscular fat/Total)	83.0 (9.2)	87.9 (6.4)	79.7 (9.3)	<0.01

Data are presented as mean (standard deviation). BMI, body mass index; TMM–BIA, trunk muscle mass measured by bioelectrical impedance analysis; CSA, cross-sectional area; PVM, paravertebral muscles. Student's t-test was used to compare groups.

A significant and strong correlation was found between TMM–BIA and the CSA of PVM (r = 0.746, p < 0.01) (Figure 2), and between TMM–BIA and the fat-free CSA of PVM (r = 0.807; p < 0.01) (Figure 3). Similarly, TMM–BIA was significantly correlated with the CSA of each individual PVM (Figure 4). The CSA of PM was strongly correlated with the TMM–BIA (fat included, r = 0.752, p < 0.01; fat-free, r = 0.766, p < 0.01), whereas the CSA of MF, the smallest muscle of the PVM, was moderately correlated with TMM–BIA (fat included, r = 0.439, p < 0.01; fat-free, r = 0.571, p < 0.01). In addition, the CSA of ES was moderately correlated with TMM–BIA (fat included, r = 0.554, p < 0.01; fat-free, r = 0.658, p < 0.01) (Table 2). TMM–BIA and BMS were strongly correlated (r = 0.726, p < 0.001), although the strength of some participants could not be measured due to back pain (Figure 5).

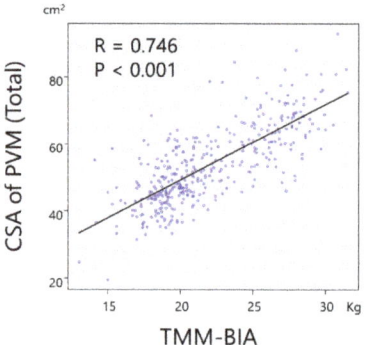

Figure 2. Correlation between TMM–BIA and the CSA of PVM. There was a significant correlation between TMM–BIA and the CSA of PVM with r = 0.746. TMM–BIA, trunk muscle mass measured by bioelectrical impedance analysis; CSA, cross-sectional area; PVM, paravertebral muscles.

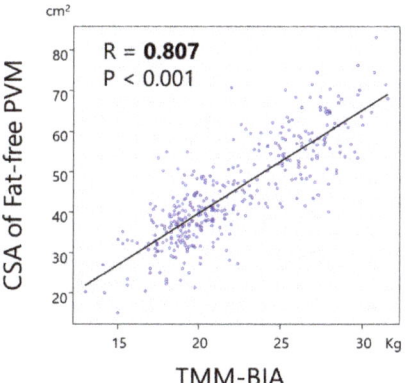

Figure 3. Correlation between TMM–BIA and the CSA of PVM without intramuscular fat. There was a significant correlation between TMM–BIA and the CSA of fat-free PVM with r = 0.807. TMM–BIA, trunk muscle mass measured by bioelectrical impedance analysis; CSA, cross-sectional area; PVM, paravertebral muscles.

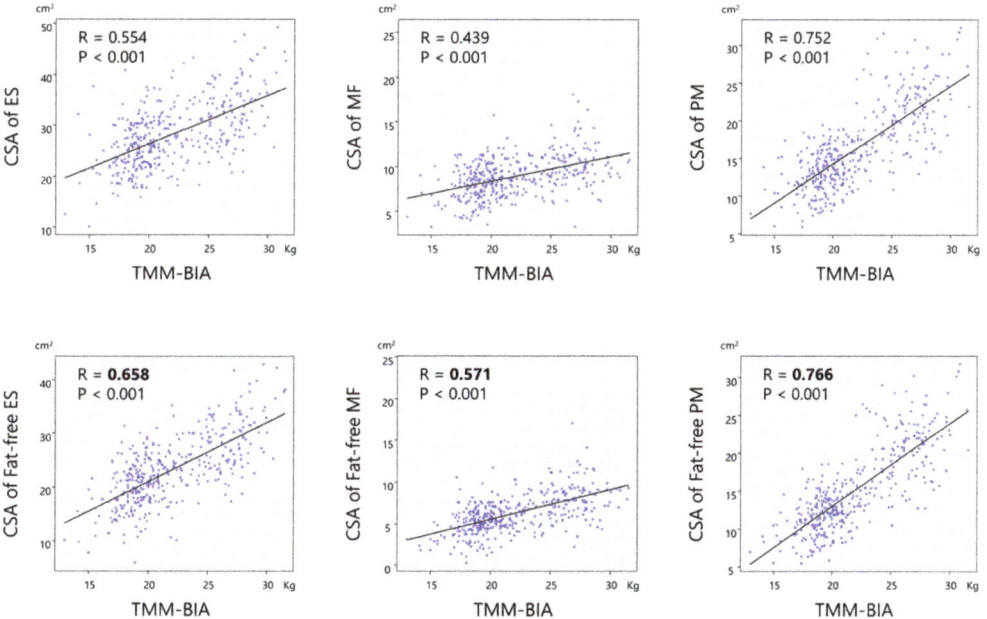

Figure 4. Correlations between TMM–BIA and the CSA of each individual PVM (upper row, total; lower row, excluding intramuscular fat). The CSA of the PM showed a strong correlation with the TMM–BIA (total, r = 0.752; fat-free, r = 0.766), whereas the CSA of MF, the smallest muscle of the PVM, showed a moderate correlation (total, r = 0.439; fat-free, r = 0.571). In addition, the CSA of ES had a moderate to strong correlation to the TMM–BIA (total, r = 0.554; fat-free, r = 0.658), respectively. TMM–BIA, trunk muscle mass measured by bioelectrical impedance analysis; CSA, cross-sectional area; PVM, paravertebral muscle; ES, erector spinae; MF, multifidus; PM, psoas major.

Table 2. Correlations between TMM–BIA and each PVM with and without intramuscular fat.

	CSA, cm^2	R with TMM–BIA	p-Value
ES	28.26 (6.36)	0.554	<0.01
ES (excluding intramuscular fat)	23.25 (6.22)	0.658	<0.01
MF	8.93 (2.40)	0.439	<0.01
MF (excluding intramuscular fat)	6.27 (2.48)	0.571	<0.01
PM	16.29 (5.38)	0.752	<0.01
PM (excluding intramuscular fat)	15.17 (5.39)	0.766	<0.01
Total PVM	54.54 (11.56)	0.746	<0.01
Total PVM (excluding intramuscular fat)	44.70 (11.95)	0.807	<0.01

Data are presented as mean (standard deviation). TMM–BIA, trunk muscle mass measured by bioelectrical impedance analysis; CSA, cross-sectional area; PVM, paravertebral muscles; R, correlation coefficient; ES, erector spinae; MF, multifidus; PM, psoas major.

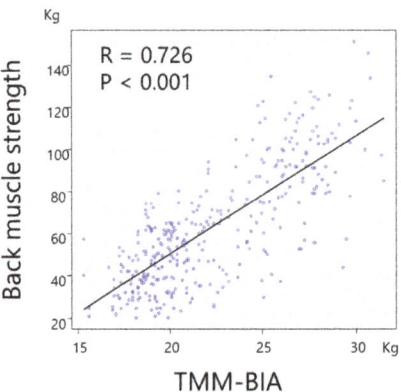

Figure 5. Correlation between TMM–BIA and back muscle strength. There was a strong correlation of r = 0.726, even though some of the participants exhibited minimum strength because of pain. TMM–BIA, trunk muscle mass measured by bioelectrical impedance analysis.

3.1. Case Presentation

3.1.1. Case 1

A 67-year-old male with a history of hepatitis and diabetes mellitus had a high TMM–BIA of 31.5 kg. The CSA of PVM on the MRI was 75.4 cm^2 (fat included) and 68.04 cm^2 (fat-free) (Figure 6). He reported his low back pain as 0 mm on a visual analog scale. His back muscle strength was 85.5 kg.

3.1.2. Case 2

A 70-year-old female with a history of diabetes mellitus and osteoporosis had a low TMM–BIA volume of 14.2 kg. MRI showed severe muscular atrophy and fatty degeneration in her PVM (Figure 7). The CSA was 36.59 cm^2 (fat included) and 20.02 cm^2 (fat-free). She reported severe low back pain as 76 mm on a visual analog scale. Her back muscle strength was too weak to be recorded (less than 20 kg).

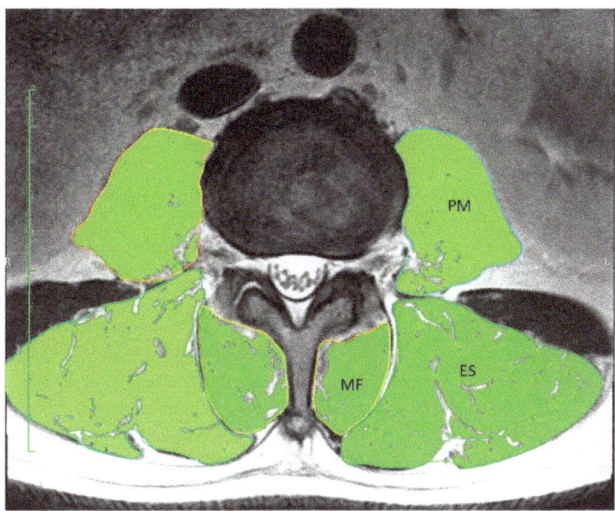

Figure 6. Case presentation 1. A 67-year-old male with no symptoms of low back pain had a CSA of PVM and fat-free PVM of 75.4 and 68.04 cm^2, respectively. The fat-free percentage of PVM was 90.2%. CSA, cross-sectional area; PVM, paravertebral muscles.

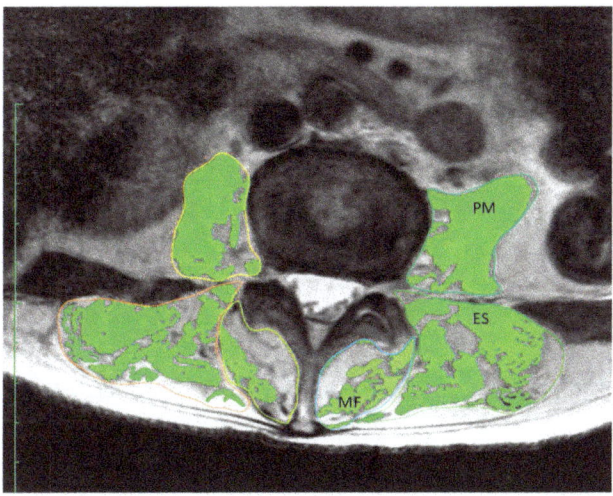

Figure 7. Case presentation 2. A 70-year-old female with severe low back pain. The patient's CSA of PVM and fat-free PVM was 36.59 and 20.02 cm^2, respectively. The fat-free percentage of PVM was 54.7%. TMM–BIA, trunk muscle mass measured by bioelectrical impedance analysis; CSA, cross-sectional area; PVM, paravertebral muscles.

4. Discussion

The clinical importance of TMM–BIA was first reported by Hori et al. [12]. They conducted a multicenter, cross-sectional study of 1738 patients (mean age, 70.2 ± 11.0 years; 781 males and 957 females) and found that TMM–BIA was significantly associated with various spinal pathologies, including low back pain, quality of life related to low back pain, and spinal sagittal imbalance, indicating that TMM–BIA is a useful indicator for understanding the pathology of the spine in clinical settings. However, only one study [19] has investigated the association between TMM–BIA and other pre-existing assessment methods for trunk muscles; therefore, the accuracy of TMM–BIA has yet to be validated.

The present study is the first validation study of TMM–BIA, and the results of this study indicate a strong correlation between TMM–BIA and the CSA of PVM. Furthermore, we clarified that TMM–BIA is more strongly correlated with the CSA of PVM, excluding fat infiltration, than the total PVM. Our results suggest that TMM–BIA is a valid index of trunk muscle mass.

The CSA of PVM and fat infiltration of the PVM measured via MRI or CT has been widely used for quantitative evaluation of the trunk muscles. Many studies have sought to investigate the association between the CSA, or fat infiltration, and spinal pathologies [2,23,24]. Takahashi et al. [24] reported that a decrease in PVM in patients with osteoporotic vertebral fractures was significantly related to low back pain and delayed union after fracture onset. Kjaer et al. determined that fat infiltration of the MF was associated with low back pain in adults [25]. Sasaki et al. [26] found that the fatty infiltration ratio of the ES in the upper lumbar spine was significantly associated with low back pain. However, the widespread use of MRI or CT for the evaluation of trunk muscle mass is impractical, as it is time-consuming and expensive, and CT exposes patients to radiation. In contrast, TMM–BIA is a straightforward, non-invasive, and reliable method for large-scale measurements.

Functional assessment of the trunk muscles was performed via BMS. Several studies have reported that BMS may be a useful index for spinal pathology and function, such as spinal sagittal alignment [27], thoracic kyphosis [28], and range of motion of the spine [29]. Despite its clinical importance, the measurement of BMS is difficult in patients with low back pain, and has the potential risk of vertebral fracture in patients with severe osteoporosis [30]. We found a strong correlation between TMM–BIA and BMS using a relatively large sample size, which indicates that TMM–BIA is an accurate tool for the functional assessment of trunk muscles without any risk of adverse effects.

Our study had several limitations. First, TMM–BIA includes the total volume of all trunk muscles (not only PVM); however, we could only measure the CSA of PVM. Therefore, other trunk muscles were not evaluated using TMM–BIA in this study. Second, in this study, we measured trunk muscle mass using only one type of BIA device. It has been reported that the ASM varies depending on the type and manufacturer of the BIA device [31]. Therefore, trunk muscle masses may differ when another BIA device is used. A conversion formula that shows the same ASM across BIA devices has been reported [32]. Future studies to develop a similar conversion formula for trunk muscle mass are needed. Third, we did not analyze the influence of sex or age in this study. There were significant differences in CSA, BMS, and TMM–BIA between male and female study participants (Table 1). As the purpose of this study was first to verify whether TMM–BIA correlates with the quantitative and functional assessments traditionally used for trunk muscles, an examination of the influence of sex or age on the relationship of TMM–BIA and the CSA of PVM will be the subject of our next research work. Last, this study was a cross-sectional analysis of the relationship between TMM–BIA and the CSA of PVM using data collected on the same day. Therefore, the relationship between changes in TMM–BIA and those in the CSA of PVM was not studied. Future studies should focus on analyzing the changes in these parameters via a longitudinal study design.

5. Conclusions

TMM–BIA is strongly correlated with the CSA of PVM, especially the fat-free CSA, as measured with MRI. Additionally, TMM–BIA is correlated with BMS. As CSA and BMS are gold standards for quantitative and functional assessments of trunk muscles, TMM–BIA can be considered a new method to measure these parameters. Our findings highlight the significance of TMM–BIA as a reliable, cost-effective, and efficient tool for the assessment of trunk muscles. Given its simplicity and reliability, BIA may be an alternative method for evaluating trunk muscles in clinical settings.

Author Contributions: Conceptualization, S.O., M.H., Y.H., S.T., and H.N.; methodology, A.Y., H.H., A.K., T.T., and S.K.; formal analysis, A.Y., H.S., A.K., T.T., and S.K.; data curation, H.T.; writing—original draft preparation, H.S.; writing—review and editing, S.O. All authors have read and agreed to the published version of the manuscript.

Funding: This research was funded by the Japanese Orthopaedic Association Research Grant, grant number 2017-1.

Institutional Review Board Statement: The study was conducted according to the guidelines of the Declaration of Helsinki and the Ethical Guidelines for Medical and Health Research involving Human Subjects in Japan and was approved by the Institutional Review Board of Osaka City University Graduate School of Medicine (No. 3484). All methods were performed in accordance with the Declaration of Helsinki.

Informed Consent Statement: Written informed consent for publication was obtained from the two participants whose information is presented in the case presentation sections and in Figures 6 and 7. They were informed that individual details and images would be published in our manuscript.

Data Availability Statement: Data available on request due to restrictions e.g. privacy or ethical. The data presented in this study are available on request from the corresponding author. The data are not publicly available due to patients privacy.

Acknowledgments: The authors thank Satomi Kawabata for her help in the collection of data and in interviews with the participants. The authors also express sincere thanks to the staff of Shiraniwa Hospital for their help in conducting the Shiraniwa study.

Conflicts of Interest: The authors declare no conflict of interest.

References

1. Shahidi, B.; Parra, C.L.; Berry, D.B.; Hubbard, J.C.; Gombatto, S.; Zlomislic, V.; Allen, R.T.; Hughes-Austin, J.; Garfin, S.; Ward, S.R. Contribution of Lumbar Spine Pathology and Age to Paraspinal Muscle Size and Fatty Infiltration. *Spine* **2017**, *42*, 616–623. [CrossRef] [PubMed]
2. Yagi, M.; Hosogane, N.; Watanabe, K.; Asazuma, T.; Matsumoto, M.; Keio Spine Research Group. The paravertebral muscle and psoas for the maintenance of global spinal alignment in patient with degenerative lumbar scoliosis. *Spine J.* **2016**, *16*, 451–458. [CrossRef] [PubMed]
3. Chen, L.K.; Liu, L.K.; Woo, J.; Assantachai, P.; Auyeung, T.W.; Bahyah, K.S.; Chou, M.Y.; Chen, L.Y.; Hsu, P.S.; Krairit, O.; et al. Sarcopenia in Asia: Consensus report of the Asian Working Group for Sarcopenia. *J. Am. Med. Dir. Assoc.* **2014**, *15*, 95–101. [CrossRef] [PubMed]
4. Kim, W.J.; Kim, K.J.; Song, D.G.; Lee, J.S.; Park, K.Y.; Lee, J.W.; Chang, S.H.; Choy, W.S. Sarcopenia and Back Muscle Degeneration as Risk Factors for Back Pain: A Comparative Study. *Asian Spine J.* **2020**, *14*, 364. [CrossRef] [PubMed]
5. Ohyama, S.; Hoshino, M.; Terai, H.; Toyoda, H.; Suzuki, A.; Takahashi, S.; Hayashi, K.; Tamai, K.; Hori, Y.; Nakamura, H. Sarcopenia is related to spinal sagittal imbalance in patients with spinopelvic mismatch. *Eur. Spine J.* **2019**, *28*, 1929–1936. [CrossRef]
6. Hyun, S.J.; Bae, C.W.; Lee, S.H.; Rhim, S.C. Fatty Degeneration of the Paraspinal Muscle in Patients With Degenerative Lumbar Kyphosis: A New Evaluation Method of Quantitative Digital Analysis Using MRI and CT Scan. *Clini. Spine Surg.* **2016**, *29*, 441–447. [CrossRef]
7. Ranger, T.A.; Cicuttini, F.M.; Jensen, T.S.; Peiris, W.L.; Hussain, S.M.; Fairley, J.; Urquhart, D.M. Are the size and composition of the paraspinal muscles associated with low back pain? A systematic review. *Spine J.* **2017**, *17*, 1729–1748. [CrossRef]
8. Goubert, D.; Oosterwijck, J.V.; Meeus, M.; Danneels, L. Structural Changes of Lumbar Muscles in Non-specific Low Back Pain: A Systematic Review. *Pain Physician* **2016**, *19*, E985–E1000.
9. Fortin, M.; Macedo, L.G. Multifidus and paraspinal muscle group cross-sectional areas of patients with low back pain and control patients: A systematic review with a focus on blinding. *Phys. Ther.* **2013**, *93*, 873–888. [CrossRef] [PubMed]
10. Imagama, S.; Matsuyama, Y.; Hasegawa, Y.; Sakai, Y.; Ito, Z.; Ishiguro, N.; Hamajima, N. Back muscle strength and spinal mobility are predictors of quality of life in middle-aged and elderly males. *Eur. Spine J.* **2011**, *20*, 954–961. [CrossRef]
11. Toyoda, H.; Hoshino, M.; Ohyama, S.; Terai, H.; Suzuki, A.; Yamada, K.; Takahashi, S.; Hayashi, K.; Tamai, K.; Hori, Y.; et al. The association of back muscle strength and sarcopenia-related parameters in the patients with spinal disorders. *Eur. Spine J.* **2019**, *28*, 241–249. [CrossRef]
12. Hori, Y.; Hoshino, M.; Inage, K.; Miyagi, M.; Takahashi, S.; Ohyama, S.; Suzuki, A.; Tsujio, T.; Terai, H.; Dohzono, S.; et al. ISSLS PRIZE IN CLINICAL SCIENCE 2019: Clinical importance of trunk muscle mass for low back pain, spinal balance, and quality of life-a multicenter cross-sectional study. *Eur. Spine J.* **2019**, *28*, 914–921. [CrossRef]

13. Janssen, I.; Heymsfield, S.B.; Ross, R. Low relative skeletal muscle mass (sarcopenia) in older persons is associated with functional impairment and physical disability. *J. Am. Geriatr. Soc.* **2002**, *50*, 889–896. [CrossRef]
14. Park, J.H.; Jo, Y.I.; Lee, J.H. Clinical usefulness of bioimpedance analysis for assessing volume status in patients receiving maintenance dialysis. *Korean J. Intern. Med.* **2018**, *33*, 660–669. [CrossRef]
15. Malbrain, M.L.; Huygh, J.; Dabrowski, W.; De Waele, J.J.; Staelens, A.; Wauters, J. The use of bio-electrical impedance analysis (BIA) to guide fluid management, resuscitation and deresuscitation in critically ill patients: A bench-to-bedside review. *Anaesthesiol. Intensive Ther.* **2014**, *46*, 381–391. [CrossRef]
16. Murakami, A.; Kobayashi, D.; Kubota, T.; Zukeyama, N.; Mukae, H.; Furusyo, N.; Kainuma, M.; Shimazoe, T. Bioelectrical Impedance Analysis (BIA) of the association of the Japanese Kampo concept "Suidoku" (fluid disturbance) and the body composition of women. *BMC Complement Altern. Med.* **2016**, *16*, 405. [CrossRef]
17. Chen, L.K.; Woo, J.; Assantachai, P.; Auyeung, T.W.; Chou, M.Y.; Iijima, K.; Jang, H.C.; Kang, L.; Kim, M.; Kim, S.; et al. Asian Working Group for Sarcopenia: 2019 Consensus Update on Sarcopenia Diagnosis and Treatment. *J. Am. Med. Dir. Assoc.* **2020**, *21*, 300–307. [CrossRef]
18. Kim, M.; Shinkai, S.; Murayama, H.; Mori, S. Comparison of segmental multifrequency bioelectrical impedance analysis with dual-energy X-ray absorptiometry for the assessment of body composition in a community-dwelling older population. *Geriatr. Gerontol. Int.* **2015**, *15*, 1013–1022. [CrossRef] [PubMed]
19. Fujimoto, K.; Inage, K.; Eguchi, Y.; Orita, S.; Toyoguchi, T.; Yamauchi, K.; Suzuki, M.; Kubota, G.; Sainoh, T.; Sato, J.; et al. Dual-Energy X-ray Absorptiometry and Bioelectrical Impedance Analysis are Beneficial Tools for Measuring the Trunk Muscle Mass of Patients with Low Back Pain. *Spine Surg. Relat. Res.* **2019**, *3*, 335–341. [CrossRef] [PubMed]
20. Ohyama, S.; Hoshino, M.; Takahashi, S.; Hori, Y.; Yabu, A.; Kobayashi, A.; Tsujio, T.; Kotake, S.; Nakamura, H. Predictors of dropout from cohort study due to deterioration in health status, with focus on sarcopenia, locomotive syndrome, and frailty: From the Shiraniwa Elderly Cohort (Shiraniwa) study. *J. Orthop. Sci.* **2021**, *26*, 167–172. [CrossRef] [PubMed]
21. Kyle, U.G.; Bosaeus, I.; De Lorenzo, A.D.; Deurenberg, P.; Elia, M.; Gomez, J.M.; Heitmann, B.L.; Kent-Smith, L.; Melchior, J.C.; Pirlich, M.; et al. Bioelectrical impedance analysis—Part I: Review of principles and methods. *Clin. Nutr.* **2004**, *23*, 1226–1243. [CrossRef] [PubMed]
22. Fortin, M.; Battie, M.C. Quantitative paraspinal muscle measurements: Inter-software reliability and agreement using OsiriX and ImageJ. *Phys. Ther.* **2012**, *92*, 853–864. [CrossRef] [PubMed]
23. Hebert, J.J.; Kjaer, P.; Fritz, J.M.; Walker, B.F. The Relationship of Lumbar Multifidus Muscle Morphology to Previous, Current, and Future Low Back Pain: A 9-Year Population-Based Prospective Cohort Study. *Spine* **2014**, *39*, 1417–1425. [CrossRef]
24. Takahashi, S.; Hoshino, M.; Takayama, K.; Sasaoka, R.; Tsujio, T.; Yasuda, H.; Kanematsu, F.; Kono, H.; Toyoda, H.; Ohyama, S.; et al. The natural course of the paravertebral muscles after the onset of osteoporotic vertebral fracture. *Osteoporos Int.* **2020**, *31*, 1089–1095. [CrossRef]
25. Kjaer, P.; Bendix, T.; Sorensen, J.S.; Korsholm, L.; Leboeuf-Yde, C. Are MRI-defined fat infiltrations in the multifidus muscles associated with low back pain? *BMC Med.* **2007**, *5*, 2. [CrossRef]
26. Sasaki, T.; Yoshimura, N.; Hashizume, H.; Yamada, H.; Oka, H.; Matsudaira, K.; Iwahashi, H.; Shinto, K.; Ishimoto, Y.; Nagata, K.; et al. MRI-defined paraspinal muscle morphology in Japanese population: The Wakayama Spine Study. *PloS ONE* **2017**, *12*, e0187765. [CrossRef]
27. Imagama, S.; Ito, Z.; Wakao, N.; Seki, T.; Hirano, K.; Muramoto, A.; Sakai, Y.; Matsuyama, Y.; Hamajima, N.; Ishiguro, N.; et al. Influence of spinal sagittal alignment, body balance, muscle strength, and physical ability on falling of middle-aged and elderly males. *Eur. Spine J.* **2013**, *22*, 1346–1353. [CrossRef] [PubMed]
28. Hongo, M.; Miyakoshi, N.; Shimada, Y.; Sinaki, M. Association of spinal curve deformity and back extensor strength in elderly women with osteoporosis in Japan and the United States. *Osteoporos Int.* **2012**, *23*, 1029–1034. [CrossRef] [PubMed]
29. Miyakoshi, N.; Hongo, M.; Maekawa, S.; Ishikawa, Y.; Shimada, Y.; Okada, K.; Itoi, E. Factors related to spinal mobility in patients with postmenopausal osteoporosis. *Osteoporos Int.* **2005**, *16*, 1871–1874. [CrossRef]
30. Fields, A.J.; Lee, G.L.; Liu, X.S.; Jekir, M.G.; Guo, X.E.; Keaveny, T.M. Influence of vertical trabeculae on the compressive strength of the human vertebra. *J. Bone Miner. Res.* **2011**, *26*, 263–269. [CrossRef]
31. Yamada, M.; Yamada, Y.; Arai, H. Comparability of two representative devices for bioelectrical impedance data acquisition. *Geriatr. Gerontol. Int.* **2016**, *16*, 1087–1088. [CrossRef] [PubMed]
32. Yoshida, D.; Shimada, H.; Park, H.; Anan, Y.; Ito, T.; Harada, A.; Suzuki, T. Development of an equation for estimating appendicular skeletal muscle mass in Japanese older adults using bioelectrical impedance analysis. *Geriatr. Gerontol. Int.* **2014**, *14*, 851–857. [CrossRef] [PubMed]

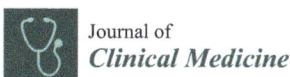
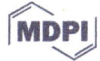

Article

Osteoporosis Detection by Physical Function Tests in Resident Health Exams: A Japanese Cohort Survey Randomly Sampled from a Basic Resident Registry

Ryuji Osawa [1], Shota Ikegami [1,2,*], Hiroshi Horiuchi [1,2], Ryosuke Tokida [1], Hiroyuki Kato [2] and Jun Takahashi [2]

1 Rehabilitation Center, Shinshu University Hospital, 3-1-1 Asahi, Matsumoto, Nagano 390-8621, Japan; ryuji-osawa@shinshu-u.ac.jp (R.O.); horiuchih@shinshu-u.ac.jp (H.H.); tryosuke@shinshu-u.ac.jp (R.T.)
2 Department of Orthopaedic Surgery, Shinshu University School of Medicine, 3-1-1 Asahi, Matsumoto, Nagano 390-8621, Japan; hirokato@shinshu-u.ac.jp (H.K.); jtaka@shinshu-u.ac.jp (J.T.)
* Correspondence: sh.ikegami@gmail.com; Tel.: +81-263-37-2659; Fax: +81-263-35-8844

Abstract: Osteoporosis may increase fracture risk and reduce healthy quality of life in older adults. This study aimed to identify an assessment method using physical performance tests to screen for osteoporosis in community dwelling individuals. A total of 168 women aged 50–89 years without diagnosed osteoporosis were randomly selected from the resident registry of a cooperating town for the evaluation of physical characteristics, muscle strength, and several physical performance tests. The most effective combinations of evaluation items to detect osteoporosis (i.e., T-score ≤ -2.5 at the spine or hip) were selected by multivariate analysis and cutoff values were determined by likelihood ratio matrices. Thirty-six women (21.4%) were classified as having osteoporosis. By analyzing combinations of two-step test (TST) score and body mass index (BMI), osteoporosis could be reliably suspected in individuals with TST ≤ 1.30 and BMI ≤ 23.4, TST ≤ 1.32 and BMI ≤ 22.4, TST ≤ 1.34 and BMI ≤ 21.6, or TST < 1.24 and any BMI. Setting cut-off values for TST in combination with BMI represents an easy and possibly effective screening tool for osteoporosis detection in resident health exams.

Keywords: epidemiological study; osteoporosis; osteopenia; locomotive syndrome; two-step test; frailty

1. Introduction

Osteoporosis is a disorder characterized by a diminution of bone mass and elevated fracture risk [1]. Fractures not only reduce mobility, living function, and quality of life, but also increase mortality and are directly related to life expectancy [2,3]. As the prevalence of older adults in Japan reached 28.1% in 2018 [4], early osteoporosis detection and prevention are important issues in terms of increasing healthy life expectancy and reducing medical costs [5].

Bone mass measurement is considered essential for precisely diagnosing osteoporosis [1]. However, it is difficult to detect bone loss at an early stage due to a lack of subjective symptoms. In their epidemiological study of healthy community members, Lo et al. witnessed that 25.7% of postmenopausal women had untreated osteoporosis [6]. If screening tests can be conducted for community dwelling residents simply and without expensive devices, the number of latent osteoporosis patients may become efficiently reduced by appropriate consultation and management.

Currently, several other simple tools have been established to test for osteoporosis (Female Osteoporosis Self-Assessment Tool for Asia; FOSTA) [7] and the risk of fractures caused by osteoporosis (Fracture Risk Assessment Tool; FRAX) [8].

The present study focused on physical performance as a possible index to easily understand the risk of osteoporosis since previous reports found levels of physical performance and daily activity to be related to bone mineral density (BMD). For instance, Miyakoshi described that women with sarcopenia associated with muscle aging had significantly higher

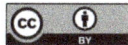

rates of complicating osteoporosis than those who did not [9], and Chan et al. reported that BMD in healthy adolescents had a high correlation with grip strength [10]. Indeed, the relationship between muscle and bone has attracted considerable attention, the mechanism of which is being gradually elucidated [11–13].

Several reports have investigated the relationship between physical performance and osteoporosis in the general population [14–18]. However, it remains uncertain which simple physical performance tests better reflect BMD and can be used for osteoporosis screening. Moreover, none have provided reference values for osteoporosis risk for such test items.

For several years, we have been conducting the "Obuse study", an epidemiology study on locomotor function in older community dwelling people that employs random sampling from the resident registry of a cooperating local government. The purpose of the present investigation is to establish a screening tool for identifying individuals in need of BMD measurement referral during simple physical health examinations.

2. Materials and Methods

2.1. Participants

The participants in this study were community dwelling women aged 50–89 years who had not been diagnosed as having postmenopausal osteoporosis. As described in a previous report [19], we randomly recruited participants from a local population between October 2014 and June 2017 to build a cohort for an epidemiology study on locomotor function termed the Obuse study. Briefly, we randomly selected men and women from among 11,326 citizens aged 50–89 years who were registered in a cooperating town office and asked them to participate in this study. Requests were made until the number of consenting participants reached approximately 50 for each age group and gender (8 groups: 50 s, 60 s, 70 s, and 80 s of male and female). The final Obuse study cohort contained 415 participants (212 women and 203 men). The participation rate was 32.0%. Of the 212 women, 168 were included in this study after excluding those taking osteoporosis drugs (28 women), receiving hormonal therapy (7 women), premenopausal (6 women), or unable to perform all of the physical performance tests (3 women) (Figure 1).

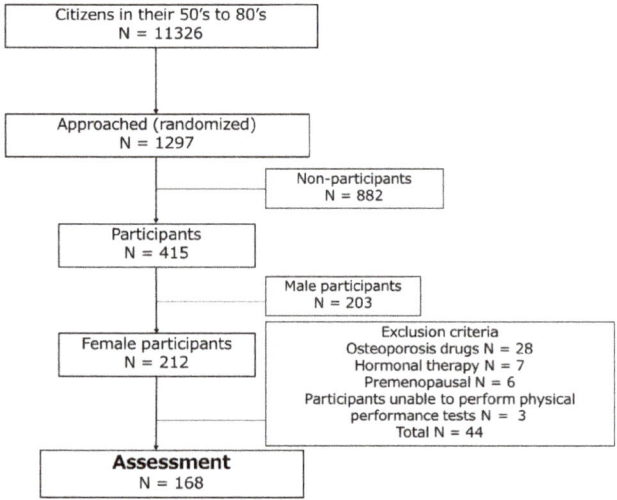

Figure 1. Participant selection flowchart.

All participants were surveyed after obtaining written consent based on the Helsinki declaration. This study was conducted after review by our ethics committee (approval number: 2729). The authors declare no conflict of interest of interest.

2.2. Osteoporosis Diagnosis

L2-L4 spine (L2-4), bilateral total hip, and bilateral femoral neck BMD were measured using dual-energy X-ray absorptiometry (Prodigy; GE Healthcare, Chicago, IL, USA). The T-scores for each site were calculated based on the manufacturer-provided reference [20]. The smallest T-score was treated as the representative value among the 5 measurement sites. Based on WHO diagnostic criteria, T-score ≥ -1 was classified as healthy, $-2.5 <$ T-score < -1 was classified as osteopenia, and T-score ≤ -2.5 was judged as osteoporosis [1]. FRAX scores were also calculated using patient information and T-scores.

2.3. Physical Performance Tests

We measured grip strength, knee extension muscle strength, and one-leg standing time with eyes open. As diagnostic criteria for the recently established locomotive syndrome, two-step test (TST), stand-up test, and Locomo25 scores were evaluated as well [21]. Grip strength in kilograms was determined using a Jamar Hydraulic Hand Dynamometer (Performance Health, Chicago, IL, USA) to obtain the mean values for each side. Knee extension strength was measured with the Leg Extension/Curl Rehab 5530 (HUR, Kokkola, Finland), with measurements taken for both lower limbs, averaged, and divided by body weight (% weight). One-leg standing time was assessed once for each side, with an upper limit of 60 s. The average value of the left and right sides (seconds) was used.

The TST, stand-up test, and Locomo25 are evaluation items for locomotive syndrome proposed by the Japanese Orthopaedic Association. The TST is performed by taking 2 maximum-stride steps and calculating the distance (centimeters) divided by body height (centimeters) [21]. The stand-up test consists of standing up from a sitting position. Participants progressively rise from boxes of 40, 30, 20, and 10 cm in height with both legs or one leg. The tasks were performed in the following order, from easiest to most difficult: both legs 40 cm→30 cm→20 cm→10 cm→one leg 40 cm→30 cm→20 cm→10 cm. The most difficult task completed was used as the subject's evaluation value. A score of 1 point was allotted for the first task, with 1 additional point given for each subsequent task [21]. Locomo25 is a questionnaire survey consisting of 25 items about pain and difficulties in daily life during the previous month. Each item is graded from 0 to 4 points for a total score of 100 points. A higher score indicates less activity [21]. The questionnaires were mailed to each participant's home before the screening and collected at the screening venue.

2.4. Statistical Analysis

Based on T-score, participants were classified as having healthy BMD, osteopenia, or osteoporosis. Fracture probabilities after 10 years were estimated based on the FRAX computer-based algorithm [8]. The clinical factors of FRAX included age, gender, height, weight, prior fragility fracture, parental history of hip fracture, current smoking habit, glucocorticoid use, rheumatoid arthritis, other causes of secondary osteoporosis, alcohol consumption of 3 units or more per day, and total hip T-score. Next, associations between each physical performance test and T-scores were evaluated by Spearman's correlation coefficient. Univariate logistic regression analysis was employed to detect physical performance tests related to low BMD. The objective variable was the presence of osteoporosis (i.e., T-score ≤ -2.5), and the explanatory variables were each physical performance test. Next, stepwise logistic regression analysis was performed using the explanatory variable items whose p-value was < 0.2 in univariate analysis. This analysis method was chosen to identify factors that were useful for simple screening by clinicians. The best model selected was evaluated by receiver operating characteristic (ROC) curve analysis. If the area under the ROC curve was ≥ 0.7, the combination of exams was considered appropriate for osteoporosis screening. Afterwards, matrices of positive/negative likelihood ratios were constructed for combinations of osteoporosis detection items, whereby a positive likelihood ratio of ≥ 5.0 was considered useful for a suspected diagnosis and a negative likelihood ratio of ≤ 0.2 was judged as useful for an exclusion diagnosis. Likelihood ratios between 0.2 and 5.0 were interpreted as having no screening value. We used R software version 3.6.1

(The R Foundation for Statistical Computing, Vienna, Austria) and EZR Version 2.4-0 [22] for statistical analyses. *p*-values of < 0.05 were considered statistically significant.

3. Results

3.1. Baseline Data and Osteoporosis Prevalence

Table 1 shows the baseline characteristics of the participants in this study. The mean ± standard deviation age of the cohort was 68.2 ± 10.6 (range: 51–88) years. Height and weight decreased with age, while BMI increased. L2-4 BMD dropped remarkably from the 60 s, and femoral neck BMD was notably low in the 80 s. Table 2 presents the prevalence of osteoporosis by age group. Of the 168 participants, 46 (27.4%) had healthy BMD, 86 (51.2%) had osteopenia, and 36 (21.4%) had osteoporosis. According to FRAX, the incidence of osteoporosis after 10 years by FRAX and the risk of fractures due to falls both increased with age.

Table 1. Baseline characteristics of study subjects.

Age Stratum (Years)	N	Height (cm)	Weight (kg)	BMI (kg/m^2)	L2-4 T-Score	Femoral Neck T-Score	Total Hip T-Score
50–59	42	158.1 ± 5.1	55.0 ± 8.8	22.0 ± 3.9	−0.2 ± 1.5	−0.9 ± 0.9	−0.6 ± 1.1
60–69	58	153.0 ± 5.1	52.4 ± 7.6	22.4 ± 2.8	−0.8 ± 1.5	−1.3 ± 0.9	−1.0 ± 0.9
70–79	39	150.3 ± 5.5	51.6 ± 7.6	22.8 ± 3.1	−0.9 ± 1.6	−1.6 ± 0.9	−1.1 ± 1.0
80–89	29	145.4 ± 5.8	50.4 ± 7.6	23.8 ± 3.1	−0.7 ± 1.8	−2.0 ± 0.7	−1.9 ± 0.8
Total	168	152.3 ± 6.8	52.3 ± 8.0	22.6 ± 3.2	−0.6 ± 1.6	−1.4 ± 0.9	−1.1 ± 1.0

Note: Values are presented as the mean ± standard deviation. Abbreviation: BMI, body mass index.

Table 2. Prevalence of osteoporosis and osteopenia and 10 year probability of fractures calculated by FRAX.

Age Stratum (Years)	Normal	Osteopenia	Osteoporosis	FRAX Major Osteoporotic [†]	FRAX Hip Fracture [†]
50–59	22 (52.3%)	16 (38.0%)	4 (9.5%)	4.3 ± 1.4	0.5 ± 0.7
60–69	13 (22.4%)	34 (58.6%)	11 (19.0%)	6.9 ± 1.7	0.9 ± 0.7
70–79	9 (23.0%)	19 (48.7%)	11 (28.2%)	9.4 ± 3.7	2.2 ± 2.1
80–89	2 (6.9%)	17 (58.6%)	10 (34.5%)	14.7 ± 4.0	5.8 ± 2.9
Total	46 (27.4%)	86 (51.2%)	36 (21.4%)	8.2 ± 4.4	1.9 ± 2.5

Notes: Values are presented as the number (prevalence). [†] The 10 year probability of fracture (%) is expressed as the mean ± standard deviation.

3.2. Physical Performance Test Results and Correlations with BMD

Physical performance diminished with age, especially in women aged 70 years and above (Table 3). L2-4 T-score had a significant but weak positive correlation with grip strength (Table 4). Femoral neck BMD was significantly correlated with all physical performance tests apart from the stand-up test. Total hip BMD was significantly correlated with all physical performance tests. Both types of femoral BMD exhibited moderate positive correlations with grip strength and TST, while displaying moderate negative associations with age.

Table 3. Results of physical performance tests by age stratum.

Age Stratum (Years)	Grip Strength (kg)	Knee Extension (%Weight)	One-Leg Standing (Sec)	Two-Step Test (No Unit)	Stand-Up Test (Points)	Locomo25 (Points)
50–59	25.1 ± 4.7	1.37 ± 0.36	47.6 ± 15.8	1.54 ± 0.13	4.4 ± 0.9	5.0 ± 4.6
60–69	21.8 ± 3.7	1.22 ± 0.36	44.2 ± 16.7	1.45 ± 0.14	4.4 ± 0.8	4.4 ± 4.6
70–79	20.7 ± 4.2	0.94 ± 0.34	24.6 ± 15.6	1.36 ± 0.19	3.5 ± 1.0	9.9 ± 10.2
80–89	16.9 ± 3.9	0.73 ± 0.36	9.1 ± 9.1	1.05 ± 0.25	3.0 ± 1.0	20.4 ± 15.3
Total	21.5 ± 4.9	1.10 ± 0.42	34.4 ± 20.9	1.38 ± 0.24	4.0 ± 1.1	8.6 ± 10.4

Note: Values are presented as the mean ± standard deviation.

Table 4. Correlations between bone mineral density and physical performance.

	L2-4 T-Score		Femoral Neck T-Score		Total Hip T-Score	
	rho	p-Value	rho	p-Value	rho	p-Value
Grip strength	0.24	<0.01 *	0.38	<0.01 *	0.37	<0.01 *
Knee extension	0.03	0.73	0.25	<0.01 *	0.23	<0.01 *
One-leg standing	0.02	0.81	0.31	<0.01 *	0.25	<0.01 *
Two-step test	0.01	0.92	0.39	<0.01 *	0.43	<0.01 *
Stand-up test	−0.11	0.17	0.12	0.10	0.17	0.02 *
Locomo25	0.10	0.18	−0.19	0.01 *	−0.22	<0.01 *
Age	−0.10	0.17	−0.40	<0.01 *	−0.41	<0.01 *
BMI	0.19	0.01 *	0.11	0.17	0.17	0.02 *

Notes: Values represent Spearman's rho (correlation coefficient). * $p < 0.05$. Abbreviation: BMI, body mass index.

3.3. Physical Performance Tests Associated with Osteoporosis

Age, BMI, grip strength, one-leg standing, and TST were significantly related factors to osteoporosis in univariate analysis (Table 5). Multivariate analysis revealed significant associations for BMI and TST with osteoporosis (both $p < 0.01$).

Table 5. Physical performance tests related to osteoporosis.

Candidate	Univariate Analysis		Multivariate Analysis	
	Odds Ratio	p-Value	Odds Ratio	p-Value
Grip strength (−1 kg)	1.09 (1.01–1.19)	0.03 *		
Knee extension (−1%weight)	1.31 (0.53–3.18)	0.55		
One-leg standing (−1 sec)	1.02 (1.01–1.04)	0.01 *		
Two-step test (−1)	10.4 (2.30–46.7)	<0.01 *	31.5 (5.29–188.0)	<0.01 *
Stand-up test (−1 point)	1.12 (0.79–1.59)	0.50		
Locomo25 (+1 point)	1.02 (0.98–1.05)	0.21		
Age (+1 year)	1.06 (1.02–1.10)	<0.01 *		
BMI (−1 kg/m^2)	1.18 (1.02–1.34)	0.01 *	1.3 (1.11–1.53)	<0.01 *

Notes: Values are presented as the odds ratio (95% confidence interval). * $p < 0.05$. Abbreviation: BMI, body mass index.

3.4. Osteoporosis Screening by Physical Performance Tests

Screening for osteoporosis using the combination of BMI and TST was judged as valid by ROC analysis, with an area under the curve of 0.73 (95% confidence interval 0.64–0.82) (Figure 2). Table 6 displays a positive likelihood ratio matrix with incremental values of BMI and TST. For cases of TST ≤ 1.30 and BMI ≤ 23.4, TST ≤ 1.32 and BMI ≤ 22.4, TST ≤ 1.34 and BMI ≤ 21.6, or TST < 1.24 and any BMI, the positive likelihood ratio exceeded 5.0 and osteoporosis could therefore be suspected. On the other hand, no negative likelihood ratios of < 0.2 were detected (Table 7).

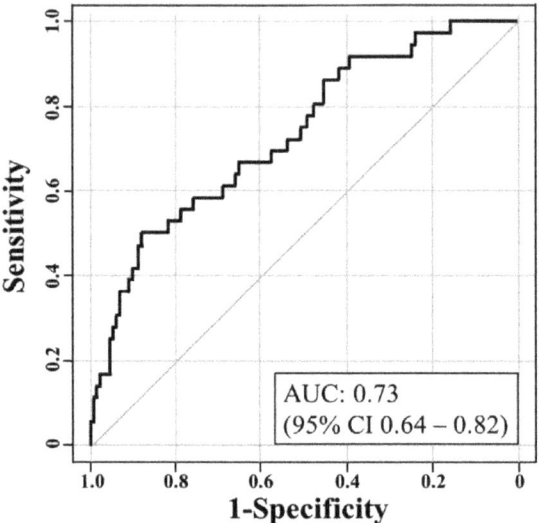

Figure 2. Receiver operating characteristic curve for detecting osteoporosis with the combination of body mass index and two-step test.

Table 6. Calculations of positive likelihood ratios for combinations of body mass index and two-step test.

BMI/TST Score	1.24	1.26	1.28	1.3	1.32	1.34	1.36	1.38
21.0	22.0	7.3	8.6	7.3	7.3	6.1	5.8	4.5
21.6	12.8	6.4	7.3	6.6	6.7	5.8	5.5	4.4
22.2	9.8	5.9	5.5	5.2	5.5	4.4	4.0	3.7
22.4	11.0	6.6	6.1	5.8	5.3	4.3	3.7	3.4
23.0	9.2	6.1	5.8	5.5	4.3	3.4	3.1	2.9
23.4	10.1	6.7	6.3	6.0	4.6	3.7	3.1	3.0
23.8	5.0	4.0	4.0	4.0	3.4	2.8	2.4	2.4
24.0	5.0	4.0	4.0	4.0	3.4	2.8	2.4	2.4

Notes: Leftmost column shows BMI values and top row shows two-step test scores. Values represent positive likelihood ratios. Shaded values indicate ratio $\geq$ 5.0. Abbreviations: BMI, body mass index; TST, two-step test.

Table 7. Calculations of negative likelihood ratios for combinations of body mass index and two-step test.

BMI/TST Score	1.24	1.26	1.28	1.3	1.32	1.34	1.36	1.38
21.0	0.8	0.7	0.7	0.7	0.8	0.8	0.7	0.7
21.6	0.7	0.7	0.7	0.7	0.7	0.8	0.7	0.6
22.2	0.7	0.7	0.7	0.7	0.7	0.7	0.7	0.6
22.4	0.7	0.7	0.7	0.7	0.7	0.7	0.6	0.5
23.0	0.7	0.7	0.7	0.7	0.7	0.6	0.6	0.5
23.4	0.7	0.6	0.6	0.6	0.7	0.6	0.6	0.5
23.8	0.7	0.7	0.7	0.7	0.7	0.6	0.6	0.5
24.0	0.7	0.7	0.7	0.7	0.7	0.6	0.6	0.5

Notes: Leftmost column shows BMI values and top row shows two-step test scores. Values represent negative likelihood ratios. Abbreviations: BMI, body mass index; TST, two-step test.

4. Discussion

According to the results of this study of postmenopausal women aged 50–89 years not treated for bone loss, 21.4% had latent osteoporosis and 51.2% had osteopenia. After adjustment for the age distribution in Japan, the rates of osteopenia and osteoporosis were estimated as 50.5% and 21.9%, respectively. L2-4 BMD correlated significantly with grip strength, while total femur and femoral neck BMD correlated with almost all physical performance tests. The combination of BMI and TST appeared useful to identify possible osteoporosis; this condition may be suspected for TST $\leq$ 1.30 and BMI $\leq$ 23.4, TST $\leq$ 1.32 and BMI $\leq$ 22.4, TST $\leq$ 1.34 and BMI $\leq$ 21.6, or TST < 1.24 regardless of BMI.

We observed that aging affected not only BMD, but also physical performance. Each physical performance test result decreased with age, with marked declines from the age of 70 years. Many studies have described the relationship between muscle and bone [9,10,16,18]. Furthermore, Tachiki et al. [23] reported that maximal muscle strength related to BMD more strongly than did muscle mass because it was an index including stimulation of bone. Similarly in this study, the correlations between many physical performance tests and BMD were considered the result of interactions involving muscle and bone.

Interestingly, TST and Locomo25, which have been used to diagnose locomotive syndrome, showed significant associations with femoral BMD. Locomotive syndrome is a concept defined as a decrease in movement capabilities as proposed by the Japanese Orthopaedic Association [21]. One cause of locomotive syndrome is osteoporosis. No reports have shown a significant association between locomotive syndrome diagnosis and BMD to date. However, lower limb function was found to significantly correlate with locomotion ability, and the amount of activity in daily life was related to BMD [24–26]. The present study also supports a relationship between locomotive syndrome and osteoporosis.

Lastly, TST appeared useful as a screening tool for osteoporosis. TST is an examination in which the subject takes two steps at maximum width without losing balance. Earlier studies revealed that TST correlated significantly with such lower limb functions as 6 min walking distance and maximum 10 m walking speed [27] as well as with the ability to perform activities of daily living [28]. Ashe et al. [29] also described that muscle power correlated more strongly with bone density than did maximum muscle tension or muscle mass. Our results suggest that TST may be an indicator of osteoporosis since it can reflect lower limb power more directly than can maximum knee extensor strength or balance of standing on one leg. The influence of TST increased considerably after multivariate analysis, such that the effect of age might have been absorbed. It was also relevant that the cohort's age range was 50–89 years and did not include young adults with less frequent osteoporosis.

We witnessed that the combination of BMI and TST provided a clinically effective combination of values for osteoporosis screening. Based on the findings in Table 6, there was no single combination of note. However, BMI was a unique value for each participant, with only 1 TST threshold for each participant. TST and BMI can be easily and inexpensively tested anywhere. Using them, it may be possible to encourage residents to undergo osteoporosis testing before symptom onset. On the other hand, no clinically effective negative likelihood ratios were detected in the cohort, indicating that the possibility of osteoporosis in postmenopausal women cannot be excluded by any particular body function test. In the osteoporosis high-risk group with a FOSTA score of less than −4, the positive likelihood ratio was 2.2 and the negative likelihood ratio was 0.5, indicating an inadequacy in detecting osteoporosis.

This study had several limitations. First, there was a deviation in participant selection. Random sampling from a resident registry was presumed as an effective way to construct a study population that faithfully reproduced the target cohort. However, the process of passive participation may have contributed to a high non-participation rate and incomplete removal of extraction bias. Nonetheless, our passive participation method that randomly selected subjects from the general population could create a study group that was more reflective of the actual conditions of community dwelling residents than could an active participation method, by which volunteers were recruited. Another limitation was the existence of regional characteristics. As the local government in our study was located in a suburban area in Japan, which likely differed from the environment of urban areas, our target population might not be qualitatively representative of the general Japanese population and the cut-off range for detecting osteoporosis could be slightly wider. Such regional differences may become more pronounced when race is taken into consideration. The physical characteristics of the cohort could also have limited the study. The small number of patients with very low BMI might have influenced the results; thus, if BMI is higher than 21, it should be assessed in combination with TST for osteoporosis screening. Furthermore, smoking was excluded from the list of factors associated with osteoporosis because few participants smoked. Lastly, this was a small study due to human resource and financial constraints. Larger scale, multiregional surveys are needed.

5. Conclusions

In conclusion, in post-menopausal women aged 50–89 years without a diagnosis of osteoporosis, an estimated 21.4% had osteoporosis and 51.2% had osteopenia. More precise BMD measurements are recommended in individuals exhibiting TST $\leq$ 1.30 and BMI $\leq$ 23.4, TST $\leq$ 1.32 and BMI $\leq$ 22.4, TST $\leq$ 1.34 and BMI $\leq$ 21.6, or TST < 1.24 and any BMI in general health exams towards improving healthy life expectancy in community dwelling older adults.

Author Contributions: S.I. and J.T. designed the study and wrote the manuscript. R.O. and S.I. performed the data analysis and wrote the manuscript. H.H. and R.T. provided clinical experience and wrote the manuscript. H.K. and J.T. supervised the whole study. All authors have read and agreed to the published version of the manuscript.

Funding: This work was supported by a grant from the Japan Orthopaedics and Traumatology Research Foundation, Inc. (number: 339) as well as research funds from the Promotion Project of Education, Research, and Medical Care from Shinshu University Hospital, the Japanese Orthopaedic Association, the Japanese Society for Musculoskeletal Medicine, the Shinshu Public Utility Foundation for Promotion of Medical Sciences, and The Nakatomi Foundation.

Institutional Review Board Statement: This study was approved by the investigational review board of our hospital (approval number: 2792). Written consent was obtained from all participants. All research was conducted in accordance with the STROBE guidelines for observational research.

Informed Consent Statement: Informed consent was obtained from all subjects involved in the study. Written informed consent has been obtained from the patients to publish this paper.

Data Availability Statement: The complete database of the cohort can be accessed at the Zenodo repository (doi.org/10.5281/zenodo.4722536).

Acknowledgments: We thank Hironobu Sato of the Obuse Town Institute for Community Health Promotion, Takashi Igarashi of the Center for Clinical Research at Shinshu University Hospital, and the Obuse town office for sample selection in this study.

Conflicts of Interest: The authors declared no potential conflicts of interest with respect to the research, authorship, and/or publication of this article.

References

1. Assessment of fracture risk and its application to screening for postmenopausal osteoporosis. Report of a WHO Study Group. *World Health Organ Tech. Rep. Ser.* **1994**, *843*, 1–129.
2. Nguyen, N.D.; Center, J.R.; Eisman, J.A.; Nguyen, T.V. Bone loss, weight loss, and weight fluctuation predict mortality risk in elderly men and women. *J. Bone Miner. Res.* **2007**, *22*, 1147–1154. [CrossRef] [PubMed]
3. Suzuki, T.; Yoshida, H. Low bone mineral density at femoral neck is a predictor of increased mortality in elderly Japanese women. *Osteoporos. Int.* **2010**, *21*, 71–79. [CrossRef] [PubMed]
4. Portal Site of Official Statistics of Japan Website. Statistics Dashboard. Available online: https://dashboard.e-stat.go.jp/dataSearch (accessed on 25 November 2020).

5. Goeree, R.; Blackhouse, G.; Adachi, J. Cost-effectiveness of alternative treatments for women with osteoporosis in Canada. *Curr. Med. Res. Opin.* **2006**, *22*, 1425–1436. [CrossRef]
6. Lo, S.S. Bone health status of postmenopausal Chinese women. *Hong Kong Med. J.* **2015**, *21*, 536–541. [CrossRef]
7. Tong, H.; Zong, H.; Xu, S.Q.; Wang, X.R.; Gong, X.; Xu, J.H.; Cheng, M. Osteoporosis Self-Assessment Tool as a Screening Tool for Predicting Osteoporosis in Elderly Chinese Patients With Established Rheumatoid Arthritis. *J. Clin. Densitom.* **2019**, *22*, 321–328. [CrossRef]
8. Kanis, J.A.; Oden, A.; Johansson, H.; Borgström, F.; Ström, O.; McCloskey, E. FRAX and its applications to clinical practice. *Bone* **2009**, *44*, 734–743. [CrossRef]
9. Miyakoshi, N.; Hongo, M.; Mizutani, Y.; Shimada, Y. Prevalence of sarcopenia in Japanese women with osteopenia and osteoporosis. *J. Bone Miner. Metab.* **2013**, *31*, 556–561. [CrossRef]
10. Chan, D.C.; Lee, W.T.; Lo, D.H.; Leung, J.C.; Kwok, A.W.; Leung, P.C. Relationship between grip strength and bone mineral density in healthy Hong Kong adolescents. *Osteoporos. Int.* **2008**, *19*, 1485–1495. [CrossRef]
11. Bettis, T.; Kim, B.J.; Hamrick, M.W. Impact of muscle atrophy on bone metabolism and bone strength: Implications for muscle-bone crosstalk with aging and disuse. *Osteoporos. Int.* **2018**, *29*, 1713–1720. [CrossRef]
12. Brotto, M.; Bonewald, L. Bone and muscle: Interactions beyond mechanical. *Bone* **2015**, *80*, 109–114. [CrossRef]
13. Brotto, M.; Johnson, M.L. Endocrine crosstalk between muscle and bone. *Curr. Osteoporos. Rep.* **2014**, *12*, 135–141. [CrossRef]
14. Coupland, C.A.; Cliffe, S.J.; Bassey, E.J.; Grainge, M.J.; Hosking, D.J.; Chilvers, C.E. Habitual physical activity and bone mineral density in postmenopausal women in England. *Int. J. Epidemiol.* **1999**, *28*, 241–246. [CrossRef]
15. Cousins, J.M.; Petit, M.A.; Paudel, M.L.; Taylor, B.C.; Hughes, J.M.; Cauley, J.A.; Zmuda, J.M.; Cawthon, P.M.; Ensrud, K.E.; Osteoporotic Fractures in Men (MrOS) Study Group. Muscle power and physical activity are associated with bone strength in older men: The osteoporotic fractures in men study. *Bone* **2010**, *47*, 205–211. [CrossRef]
16. Kitamura, K.; Nakamura, K.; Kobayashi, R.; Oshiki, R.; Saito, T.; Oyama, M.; Takahashi, S.; Nishiwaki, T.; Iwasaki, M.; Yoshihara, A. Physical activity and 5-year changes in physical performance tests and bone mineral density in postmenopausal women: The Yokogoshi Study. *Maturitas* **2011**, *70*, 80–84. [CrossRef]
17. Locquet, M.; Beaudart, C.; Bruyere, O.; Kanis, J.A.; Delandsheere, L.; Reginster, J.Y. Bone health assessment in older people with or without muscle health impairment. *Osteoporos. Int.* **2018**, *29*, 1057–1067. [CrossRef]
18. Ikegami, S.; Uchiyama, S.; Nakamura, Y.; Mukaiyama, K.; Hirabayashi, H.; Kamimura, M.; Nonaka, K.; Kato, H. Factors that characterize bone health with aging in healthy postmenopausal women. *J. Bone Miner. Metab.* **2015**, *33*, 440–447. [CrossRef]
19. Tokida, R.; Uehara, M.; Ikegami, S.; Takahashi, J.; Nishimura, H.; Sakai, N.; Kato, H. Association Between Sagittal Spinal Alignment and Physical Function in the Japanese General Elderly Population: A Japanese Cohort Survey Randomly Sampled from a Basic Resident Registry. *J. Bone Joint Surg. Am.* **2019**, *101*, 1698–1706. [CrossRef]
20. Orimo, H.; Hayashi, Y.; Fukunaga, M.; Sone, T.; Fujiwara, S.; Shiraki, M.; Hagino, H.; Hosoi, T.; Ohta, H.; Yoneda, T.; et al. Diagnostic criteria for primary osteoporosis: Year 2000 revision. *J. Bone Miner. Metab.* **2001**, *19*, 331–337. [CrossRef]
21. Nakamura, K.; Ogata, T. Locomotive Syndrome: Definition and Management. *Clin. Rev. Bone Miner. Metab.* **2016**, *14*, 56–67. [CrossRef]
22. Kanda, Y. Investigation of the freely available easy-to-use software 'EZR' for medical statistics. *Bone Marrow Transplant.* **2013**, *48*, 252–258. [CrossRef] [PubMed]
23. Tachiki, T.; Kouda, K.; Dongmei, N.; Tamaki, J.; Iki, M.; Kitagawa, J.; Takahira, N.; Sato, Y.; Kajita, E.; Fujita, Y.; et al. Muscle strength is associated with bone health independently of muscle mass in postmenopausal women: The Japanese population-based osteoporosis study. *J. Bone Miner. Metab.* **2019**, *37*, 53–59. [CrossRef] [PubMed]
24. Elhakeem, A.; Hartley, A.; Luo, Y.; Goertzen, A.L.; Hannam, K.; Clark, E.M.; Leslie, W.D.; Tobias, J.H. Lean mass and lower limb muscle function in relation to hip strength, geometry and fracture risk indices in community-dwelling older women. *Osteoporos. Int.* **2019**, *30*, 211–220. [CrossRef] [PubMed]
25. Johansson, J.; Nordstrom, A.; Nordstrom, P. Objectively measured physical activity is associated with parameters of bone in 70-year-old men and women. *Bone* **2015**, *81*, 72–79. [CrossRef]
26. Reid, K.F.; Naumova, E.N.; Carabello, R.J.; Phillips, E.M.; Fielding, R.A. Lower extremity muscle mass predicts functional performance in mobility-limited elders. *J. Nutr. Health Aging* **2008**, *12*, 493–498. [CrossRef]
27. Muranaga, S.; Hirano, K. Development of a convenient way to predict ability to walk, using a two-step test. *J. Showa Med. Assoc.* **2003**, *63*, 301–308.
28. Demura, S.; Yamada, T. The maximal double step length test can evaluate more adequately the decrease of physical function with age, than the maximal single step length test. *Arch. Gerontol. Geriatr.* **2010**, *53*, 21–24. [CrossRef]
29. Ashe, M.; Liu-Ambrose, T.; Cooper, D.; Khan, K.; McKay, H. Muscle power is related to tibial bone strength in older women. *Osteoporos. Int.* **2008**, *19*, 1725–1732. [CrossRef]

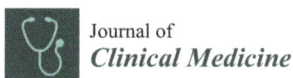

Article

Handgrip Strength Correlated with Falling Risk in Patients with Degenerative Cervical Myelopathy

Kathryn Anne Jimenez, Ji-Won Kwon, Jayeong Yoon, Hwan-Mo Lee, Seong-Hwan Moon, Kyung-Soo Suk, Hak-Sun Kim and Byung Ho Lee *

Orthopedic Department, College of Medicine, Yonsei University, Seoul 03722, Korea; kathrynjimenez@yahoo.com (K.A.J.); KWONJJANNG@yuhs.ac (J.-W.K.); COFFEESOUND2@yuhs.ac (J.Y.); hwanlee@yuhs.ac (H.-M.L.); shmoon@yuhs.ac (S.-H.M.); sks111@yuhs.ac (K.-S.S.); haksunkim@yuhs.ac (H.-S.K.)
* Correspondence: bhlee96@yuhs.ac; Tel.: +82-2-2228-2180

Abstract: Background: Few studies have investigated associations between hand grip strength (HGS) and the surgical outcomes of degenerative cervical myelopathy (DCM). Methods: This study was designed as a prospective observational study of 203 patients who had undergone fusion surgery for DCM. We divided the patients according to sex and HGS differences. Clinical outcome parameters, including HGS, a fall diary and four functional mobility tests (alternative step test, six-meter walk test, timed up and go test, and sit-to-stand test) were measured preoperatively, at 3 months and 1 year after surgery. Results: Mean patient ages were 59.93 years in the male group and 67.33 years in the female group ($p = 0.000$; independent t-test). The mean HGS of both hands improved significantly at postoperative 3 months and 1 year in all patients ($p = 0.000$ for both; ANOVA). In male patients, preoperative risk of falls was negatively correlated with HGS ($p = 0.000$). In female patients, pre- and postoperative risk of falls were correlated negatively with HGS ($p = 0.000$). The postoperative incidence of falls decreased in both groups ($p = 0.000$) Conclusions: Postoperative HGS in patients with DCM is correlated with postoperative falls and functional outcome differently, when comparing male and female patients, for predicting favorable outcomes and neurologic deficit recovery after surgery in DCM patients.

Keywords: cervical myelopathy; hand grip strength; falls; postoperative

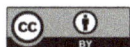

1. Introduction

Patients with spinal stenosis, either cervical and/or lumbar, are at an increased risk of falling [1,2]. Surgical treatment for both cervical and lumbar stenosis have been shown to decrease the risk of falling by improving physical performance, including walking and balancing [1–5]. There are many reported studies on prevalence, results of conservative or surgical treatment, gait patterns, hand dexterity–functional impairment and predictors of degenerative cervical myelopathy (DCM) [6–18]. A recent study reported that hand grip strength (HGS) might be a useful surrogate marker with which to predict the risk of falls and clinical outcomes in patients with lumbar stenosis [19].

Compared to lumbar stenosis, patients with DCM could have higher correlation between increased risk of falling and weakened HGS [20–24]. We also suspected that any observed correlations would differ according to sex. Our objectives in this investigation were to assess correlations for HGS with postoperative changes in the risk of falling and QoL in patients with DCM, separately for both men and women.

2. Materials and Methods

2.1. Subjects

This study was approved by the Institutional Review Board of the authors' hospital (IRB No. 4-2020-1162). From March 2017 to August 2019, 203 patients who had undergone cervical spine surgery, including decompression and fusion procedure(s), for the treatment of DCM were included prospectively. All included patients had completed postoperative follow up for 1 year. All of the patients exhibited myelopathic symptoms, including clumsiness of the hand, poor hand coordination (e.g., difficulty with handwriting and using chopsticks), and walking difficulty, and had been recommended for surgical intervention by the management guidelines of DCM [25].

The exclusion criteria were as follows: comorbidity impairing physical function (e.g., history of cerebral infarction, cerebral palsy, Parkinson's disease, spine surgery, head trauma, current/old cerebrovascular events (cerebral hemorrhage and cerebral infarct), and other neurodegenerative conditions or severe rheumatoid arthritis); bedridden status or full dependence on a wheelchair before surgery because of severe cervical myelopathy; and difficulty completing the questionnaire because of cognitive impairment. Furthermore, patients with severe osteo-arthropathic conditions that could cause knee and hip joint contracture affecting whole spinal sagittal balance were also excluded from the patient pool [26]. No patients were diagnosed with hand- or wrist-related diseases, such as carpal tunnel syndrome and tardy ulnar nerve palsy.

The major included diagnoses were cervical stenosis with myelopathy (DCM) (135 patients), ossified posterior longitudinal ligament (44 patients), and herniated cervical disc with myelopathy (24 patients).

Patients were treated with decompression and instrumented fusion (anterior plate-screw system; ZEVO™ plate and screw system; Medtronic Sofamor Danek, Memphis, TN, USA) for anterior surgery or a posterior screw-rod system (Poseidon, Medyssey, Jecheon, Korea) for combined anterior-posterior surgery. Cervical allograft allospacers (Cornerstone™; ASR Medtronic Sofamor Danek, Memphis, TN, USA) were utilized for anterior fusion surgery. For posterior surgery, local autologous and demineralized bone matrix grafts (Bongener™; CG-BIO, Seoul, Korea) were used. The surgically treated level and other demographic data, including the presence of spinal cord signal changes on MRI scans, are presented in Table 1.

Table 1. Demographic parameters of the enrolled patients.

	All (N = 203)	Male (N = 98)	Female (N = 105)	p Value
Age (years)	63.76 ± 10.56	59.93 ± 10.26	67.33 ± 9.56	0.000
Symptom duration (months)	37.17 ± 40.87	29.92 ± 33.22	46.73 ± 44.98	0.000
Body mass index (kg/m^2)	24.30 ± 3.82	23.69 ± 2.45	24.86 ± 4.71	0.026
Waist circumference (cm)	89.43 ± 10.0	88.82 ± 9.30	90.00 ± 1.04	N.S
Modified frailty index	1.37 ± 1.27	1.14 ± 1.13	1.60 ± 1.36	0.010
Smoker:non-smoker *	42:161	35:63	7:98	0.000
Spinal cord signal change (+):(−) *	133:70	77:21	56:49	0.000
Operation length (fusion level) *	2.96 ± 0.93	2.85 ± 0.91	3.06 ± 0.93	
1 level	7 (3.4%)	0	7 (6.7%)	
2 level	63 (31%)	42 (42.9%)	21 (20%)	
3 level	70 (34.5%)	35 (35.7%)	35 (33.3%)	0.000
4 level	56 (27.6%)	14 (14.3%)	42 (40.0%)	
5 level	7 (3.4%)	7 (7.1%)	0	
Surgery type *				
Anterior	91 (44.8%)	56 (57.1%)	35 (33.3%)	
Posterior	42 (20.7%)	14 (14.3%)	28 (26.7%)	0.002
Combined anterior-posterior	70 (34.5%)	28 (28.6%)	42 (40.0%)	

Statistical analyses were performed by independent t-test and * chi-squared test.

2.2. Outcome Measures

For all enrolled patients, the Neck Disability Index (NDI, higher scores reflecting worse functional status), Euro-QoL Visual Analog Scale (VAS, higher scores indicating better QoL), modified Japanese Orthopedic Association (JOA) score (higher scores representing better functional status), modified JOA grade (16~17 = Grade 0; 12~15 = Grade 1; 8~11 = Grade 2;

0~7 = Grade 3, with higher grades reflecting worse functional status), modified frailty index (mFi) (higher index scores indicating greater frailty), and HGS of both hands were measured and recorded preoperatively and at 3 months and 1 year after surgery [27–31].

2.3. HGS Measurement

HGS was measured using a Jamar Plus+ hand grip dynamometer (Global Medical Devices, Maharashtra, India). Patients were instructed to squeeze the handle as hard as possible for 3 s, and the maximum contractile force (lbs.) was recorded. The tests were performed three times on both hands. The highest value of the three repeated measurements was used for analysis [30]. The HGS of patients was measured preoperatively and at 3 months and 1 year after surgery. Considering basic physical differences, the patient groups were divided into male and female groups and compared.

2.4. Assessment of the Risk of Falling Using Four Functional Mobility Tests and an Actual Fall Diary

To evaluate the risk of falling, four functional mobility tests were used: the alternate-step test (AST), the six-meter-walk test (SMT), the sit-to-stand test (STS), and the timed up and go test (TUGT). These four tests have been validated in previous studies [2]. Additionally, a fall diary was given to patients or caregivers who were encouraged to record every fall and fall-related neurologic deficit and to report it to the clinical research coordinator when they visited the outpatient clinic for regular follow up at 3 months and 1 year postoperatively [4].

2.5. Statistical Analysis

Basic statistical tests, independent t-test, analysis of variance (ANOVA), and chi-squared test were used to evaluate whether the differences between the male and female surgery groups in terms of QoL, the four functional mobility tests, and other demographic data were statistically significant. Multiple linear regression analyses among measured HGS, falls, signal changes of the spinal cord, NDI, EQ-VAS, fall-related functional mobility tests, and other values were performed. All statistical analyses were performed using the SPSS 22.0 statistics package (SPSS, Inc., Chicago, IL, USA). p values < 0.05 were considered statistically significant.

3. Results

Mean patient ages were 59.93 years in the male group (range, 52–85 years) and 67.33 years in the female group (range, 52–86 years) ($p = 0.000$; independent t-test). Other demographic comparisons, including sex and body mass index (BMI), are shown in Table 1. All parameters differed significantly between the male and female groups.

3.1. Functional Mobility Test Results and Actual Falls

The pre- and postoperative values of the four functional tests in the male and female groups are presented in Table 2. In both groups, preoperative measures improved significantly at postoperative 3 months and 1 year, except STS ($p = 0.000, 0.000,$ and 0.000 for AST, SMT, and TUGT, respectively; ANOVA; Figure 1). All measures were significantly different between the male and female groups, except preoperative falls and AST, at postoperative 1 year.

Table 2. Comparison of functional test results between male and female patients.

	All	Males	Females	p Value
Preoperative (unit: seconds)				
Alternate-Step Test	15.74 ± 4.38	13.71 ± 3.2	17.78 ± 4.46	0.000
Six-Meter-Walk Test	6.91 ± 2.82	5.74 ± 2.52	8.08 ± 2.61	0.000
Sit-to-Stand test	12.78 ± 3.82	11.18 ± 3.46	14.38 ± 3.49	0.000
Time Up and Go Test	20.66 ± 5.12	18.47 ± 5.18	23.02 ± 3.87	0.000
Actual fall *				
No fall:fall	168:35	84:14	84:21	NS
Single:multiple	20:15	8:6	12:9	NS
Postoperative 3 months (unit: seconds)				
Alternate-Step Test	14.12 ± 3.52	13.06 ± 3.72	15.04 ± 3.07	0.000
Six-Meter-Walk Test	5.84 ± 1.96	5.19 ± 0.85	6.40 ± 2.42	0.000
Sit-to-Stand test	12.24 ± 3.55	10.63 ± 2.10	13.64 ± 3.94	0.000
Time Up and Go Test	19.22 ± 7.70	15.92 ± 2.97	22.29 ± 9.32	0.000
Actual fall *				
No fall:fall	189:14	98:0	91:14	0.000
Single:multiple	10:4	0	10:4	0.000
Postoperative 1 year (unit: seconds)				
Alternate-Step Test	14.05 ± 3.35	13.69 ± 3.08	14.65 ± 3.71	NS
Six-Meter-Walk Test	6.02 ± 1.98	5.42 ± 1.23	7.02 ± 2.53	0.000
Sit-to-Stand test	12.57 ± 5.03	10.87 ± 1.95	15.42 ± 7.00	0.000
Time Up and Go Test	17.23 ± 4.77	16.21 ± 5.06	19.27 ± 3.33	0.000
Actual fall *				
No fall:fall	189:14	96:2	93:12	0.000
Single:multiple	12:2	1:1	11:1	0.000

Statistical analyses were performed by independent *t*-test and * chi-squared test. NS, not significant.

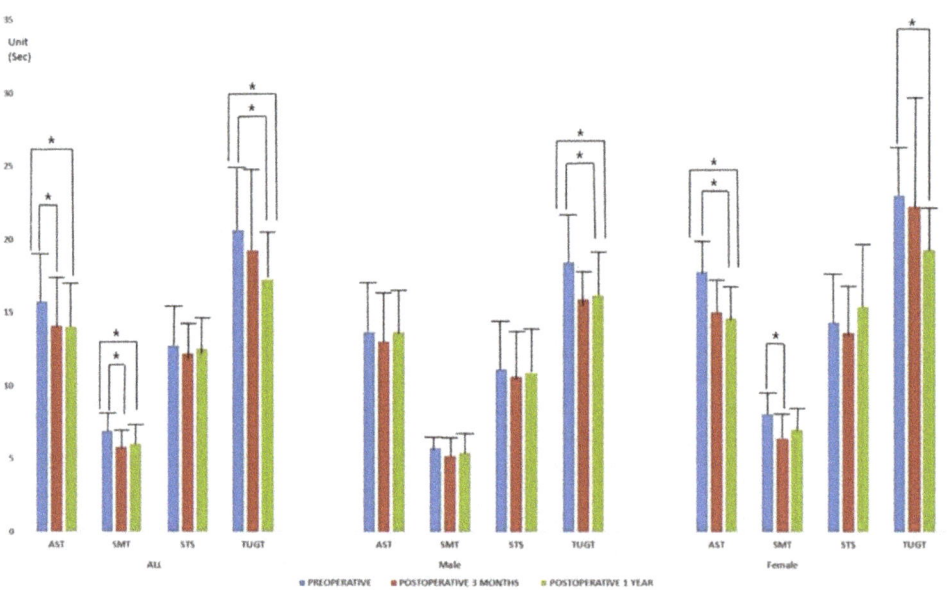

Figure 1. The pre- and postoperative values of the four functional tests depending on the patient groups. Preoperative measures were improved significantly at postoperative 3 months and 1 year in the male and female patient groups ($p = 0.000$ for all; ANOVA). * indicates the statistical difference between measures.

The average number of actual falls per patient among all patients during follow up was 0.48 ± 1.82 in the preoperative group, 0.09 ± 0.37 at postoperative 3 months, and 0.09 ± 0.43 at postoperative 1 year ($p = 0.000$; ANOVA). A significant difference was found in the distribution of non-fallers and fallers (single-time and multiple fallers) between preoperative and postoperative follow up among all patients ($p = 0.005$; chi-squared test). During follow up, no neurology deterioration related to falls was recorded.

3.2. QoL Outcomes: EQ-VAS, NDI, and mJOA Score and Grade

Mean EQ-VAS scores were 48.62 ± 23.79 preoperatively, 58.55 ± 22.48 at 3 months postoperatively, and 60.31 ± 17.88 at 1 year postoperatively in all patients ($p = 0.000$; ANOVA). Mean NDI values in all patients were 17.31 ± 7.77 preoperatively, 14.82 ± 5.73 at 3 months postoperatively, and 12.68 ± 9.06 at 1 year postoperatively ($p = 0.000$; ANOVA). Other mJOA scores and grade measures also improved after surgery in all patients ($p = 0.013$ and 0.010, respectively; ANOVA). The results are presented in Table 3.

Table 3. Comparison of functional test results between male and female patients.

	All	Males	Females	*p* Value
Preoperative				
Modified JOA score	9.51 ± 3.04	10.92 ± 3.00	8.20 ± 2.41	0.000
Modified JOA grade *				
Grade 0:1:2:3	7:49:98:49	7:35:42:14	0:14:58:35	0.000
Neck Disability Index	17.31 ± 7.77	14.85 ± 6.67	19.60 ± 8.05	0.000
Euro-QoL Visual Analog Scale	48.62 ± 23.79	50.71 ± 18.40	46.66 ± 27.86	NS
Postoperative 3 months				
Modified JOA score	11.58 ± 3.14	12.35 ± 3.1	10.86 ± 3.02	0.001
Modified JOA grade *				
Grade 0:1:2:3	28:77:63:35	21:35:35:7	7:42:28:28	0.001
Neck Disability Index	14.82 ± 5.73	14.21 ± 7.13	15.40 ± 3.96	NS
Euro-QoL Visual Analog Scale	58.55 ± 22.48	62.71 ± 25.68	54.66 ± 18.29	0.011
Postoperative 1 year				
Modified JOA score	12.61 ± 3.50	12.444 ± 2.38	12.71 ± 3.61	NS
Modified JOA grade *				
Grade 0:1:2:3	30:79:64:30	22:34:35:7	8:45:29:23	0.001
Neck Disability Index	12.68 ± 9.06	12.66 ± 10.80	12.71 ± 6.26	NS
Euro-QoL Visual Analog Scale	60.31 ± 17.88	62.22 ± 16.13	57.85 ± 19.81	NS

Statistical analyses were performed by independent *t*-test and * chi-squared test between the male and female groups. NS, not significant.

3.3. HGS

The mean HGS of both hands improved significantly at postoperative 3 months and 1 year, compared with the preoperative measures, in all patients ($p = 0.000$ for both; ANOVA) (Figure 2 and Table 4). A significant difference was found between the male and female groups for every measure ($p = 0.000$; independent *t*-test).

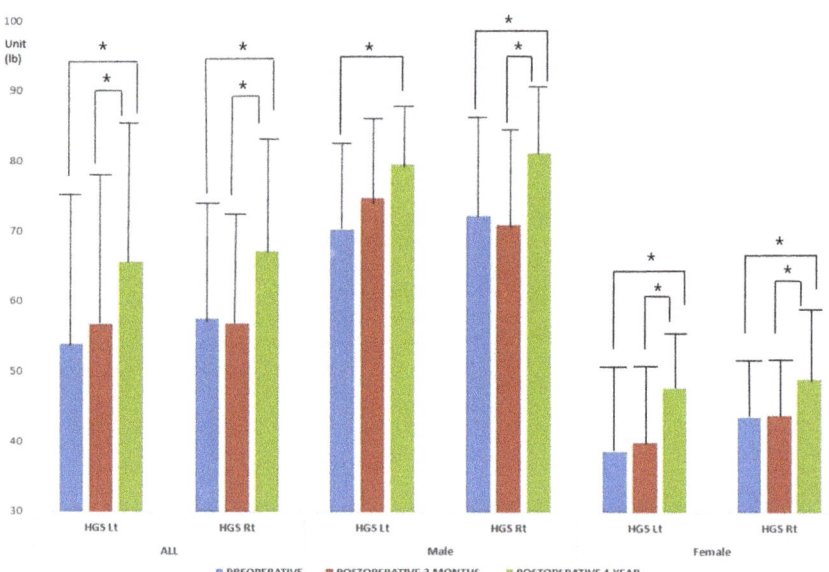

Figure 2. The mean HGS of both hands improved significantly at postoperative 3 months and 1 year compared with the preoperative measures in all patient groups ($p = 0.000$ for all; ANOVA). * indicates the statistical difference between measures.

Table 4. Hand grip strength measurements.

(Unit: lbs.)	All	Males	Females	*p* Value
Preoperative				
HGS Lt	53.90 ± 23.83	70.30 ± 19.46	38.59 ± 16.11	0.000
HGS Rt	57.51 ± 22.43	72.35 ± 21.96	43.66 ± 11.26	0.000
Postoperative 3 months				
HGS Lt	56.78 ± 24.47	74.79 ± 21.39	39.97 ± 12.07	0.000
HGS Rt	56.97 ± 21.42	71.01 ± 20.48	43.86 ± 11.88	0.000
Postoperative 1 year				
HGS Lt	65.72 ± 21.50	79.60 ± 16.93	47.86 ± 10.95	0.000
HGS Rt	67.23 ± 23.21	81.32 ± 18.75	49.12 ± 14.02	0.000

Statistical analyses were performed by independent *t*-test comparing the male and female groups.

3.4. Multiple Regression Analyses of Parameters Associated with Falls and Fall-Related Mobility Tests

In male patients, preoperative falls were correlated positively with symptom duration (beta ± standard error = 0.003 ± 0.001, $p = 0.000$) and mFi (beta ± standard error = 0.362 ± 0.043, $p = 0.000$) and negatively with EQ-VAS (−0.002 ± 0.001) and HGS (beta ± standard error = −0.004 ± 0.001, $p = 0.000$). Falls at postoperative 3 months and 1 year were not correlated with any parameter.

In female patients, preoperative falls were correlated negatively with mJOA score (beta ± standard error = −0.057 ± 0.015, $p = 0.000$) and HGS (beta ± standard error = −0.035 ± 0.005, $p = 0.000$). At postoperative 3 months, number of falls was positively correlated with mFi (beta ± standard error = 0.246 ± 0.017, $p = 0.000$) and NDI (beta ± standard error = 0.050 ± 0.006, $p = 0.000$). Fall measures at 12 months were positively correlated with NDI (beta ± standard error = 0.066 ± 0.000, $p = 0.000$) and WC (beta ± standard error = 0.046 ± 0.000, $p = 0.000$) and negatively with HGS (beta ± standard error = −0.049 ± 0.000, $p = 0.000$). Other correlations with functional mobility tests are listed in Table 5: Correlations between parameters not presented in Table 5 lacked statistical significance. Additionally, univariate linear regression analyses were presented in the Table S1.

Table 5. Multiple regression analyses of fall-related functional mobility tests.

Males								
Variables	AST		SMT		STS		TUGT	
	Beta ± S.E	p Value	Beta ± S.E	p Value	Beta ± S.E	p Value	Beta ± S.E	p Value
Preoperative								
NDI	0.330 ± 0.016	0.000	0.325 ± 0.001	0.000	0.460 ± 0.000	0.000	0.545 ± 0.014	0.000
AGE	0.168 ± 0.010	0.000	−0.084 ± 0.001	0.000	0.023 ± 0.000	0.000		
mFI	1.988 ± 0.145	0.000	1.605 ± 0.008	0.000	−0.386 ± 0.003	0.000	2.370 ± 0.143	0.000
BMI	0.681 ± 0.063	0.000	0.989 ± 0.003	0.000	1.299 ± 0.001	0.000	2.029 ± 0.048	0.000
Operation length	0.955 ± 0.095	0.000	1.153 ± 0.006	0.000	4.326 ± 0.002	0.000	3.998 ± 0.128	0.000
* Modified JOA grade			−0.711 ± 0.015	0.000	4.467 ± 0.006	0.000	3098 ± 0.278	0.000
Postoperative 3 months								
NDI	−0.387 ± 0.024	0.000	0.190 ± 0.016	0.000			−0.127 ± 0.007	0.000
AGE	0.326 ± 0.007	0.000			0.224 ± 0.002	0.000	0.227 ± 0.004	0.000
mFI			0.438 ± 0.173	0.013	−2.639 ± 0.024	0.000	1.164 ± 0.055	0.000
Smoking	1.199 ± 0.115	0.000	1.647 ± 0.068	0.000	4.264 ± 0.023	0.000	−4.956 ± 0.041	0.000
BMI	2.280 ± 0.051	0.000			0.053 ± 0.005	0.000	2.003 ± 0.021	0.000
Operation length	3.169 ± 0.152	0.000			0.672 ± 0.008	0.000	1.452 ± 0.036	0.000
* Modified JOA grade	6.866 ± 0.256	0.000	1.309 ± 0.209	0.000	9.980 ± 0.045	0.000		
Postoperative 1 year								
mFI	3.040 ± 0.004	0.000			2.156 ± 0.022	0.000		
Smoking	0.275 ± 0.009	0.000	−0.079 ± 0.000	0.000	1.331 ± 0.031	0.000		
HGS	−0.051 ± 0.000	0.000			−0.129 ± 0.001	0.000	−0.024 ± 0.001	0.000
Symptom duration	0.063 ± 0.000	0.000	0.006 ± 0.000	0.000	0.042 ± 0.000	0.000	0.074 ± 0.00	0.000
* Modified JOA grade			1.836 ± 0.000	0.000	.		7.679 ± 0.055	0.000

Females								
Variables	AST		SMT		STS		TUGT	
	Beta ± S.E	p Value	Beta ± S.E	p Value	Beta ± S.E	p Value	Beta ± S.E	p Value
Preoperative								
NDI	0.539 ± 0.018	0.000	0.791 ± 0.010	0.000	0.890 ± 0.004	0.000	−0.275 ± 0.026	0.000
AGE	0.812 ± 0.034	0.000	1.162 ± 0.018	0.000	0.899 ± 0.005	0.000	−0.620 ± 0.044	0.000
WC	0.271 ± 0.018	0.000	0.387 ± 0.010	0.000		0.000		
Cord signal change	2.674 ± 0.251	0.000	−2.885 ± 0.136	0.000	5.966 ± 0.042		6.574 ± 0.184	0.000
* Modified JOA score	−2.500 ± 0.051	0.000	−2.578 ± 0.028	0.000	−1.309 ± 0.011	0.000	0.498 ± 0.086	0.000
HGS			−0.725 ± 0.014	0.000	−0.035 ± 0.003	0.000	−0.300 ± 0.018	0.000
Operation length	4.793 ± 0.075	0.000	2.934 ± 0.041	0.000	3.301 ± 0.013	0.000	−0.825 ± 0.149	0.000
Postoperative 3 months								
NDI	−1.414 ± 0.080	0.000	−0.079 ± 0.034	0.022	0.412 ± 0.038	0.000	0.831 ± 0.278	0.004
AGE	0.036 ± 0.013	0.006	0.132 ± 0.015	0.000	0.141 ± 0.006	0.000	0.654 ± 0.055	0.000
WC	0.425 ± 0.031	0.000	0.177 ± 0.028	0.000	0.612 ± 0.017	0.000	1.132 ± 0.100	0.000
* Modified JOA score	−1.528 ± 0.118		−0.725 ± 0.163	0.000	−2.569 ± 0.070	0.000	−2.606 ± 0.553	0.000
HGS	−0.335 ± 0.052	0.000			−0.168 ± 0.012	0.000		
BMI		0.000	−0.066 ± 0.063	0.000	−0.989 ± 0.029	0.000	−1.954 ± 0.227	0.000
Postoperative 1 year								
* Modified JOA score	−1.474 ± 0.055	0.000	−1.616 ± 0.000	0.000	−3.734 ± 0.050	0.000	0.837 ± 0.008	0.000
HGS	−0.269 ± 0.016	0.000	0.010 ± 0.000	0.000				
Operation length			−0.974 ± 0.001	0.000	−5.774 ± 0.170	0.000	−1.758 ± 0.017	0.000
* Modified JOA grade	−6.145 ± 0.232	0.000	−6.533 ± 0.002	0.000	−13.403 ± 0.277	0.000		

* modified JOA grade (16~17 = Grade 0, 12~15 = Grade 1, 8~11 = Grad 2, 0~7 = Grade 3, higher grades reflect worse functional status); Neck Disability Index (NDI) (=higher scores indicate worse functional status), Euro-QoL Visual Analog Scale (VAS) (=higher scores represent better QoL status), modified Japanese orthopedic association (JOA) score (=higher scores reflect better functional status).

4. Discussion

Surgical treatment for DCM is associated with improvements in functional, disability-related, and QoL outcomes and reduced incidences of both falls and fall-related deterioration of subjective symptoms [5,32,33]. Compared with lumbar stenosis, the lack of data on DCM patients and the related risk of falls therein makes it difficult to predict surgical outcomes and postoperative rates of improvement in preoperative neurologic deficits. Additionally, prior studies that have characterized grip strength in association with myelopathic symptoms have presented mixed evidence with postoperative improvement, or no difference [34–36].

Compared with a recently published lumbar stenosis study, the present study confirmed differences in correlations between male and female sex and the postoperative risk of falling [19]. The previous study excluded cervical stenosis patients with upper-extremity motor deficits to focus on the sarcopenic conditions of the patients [37]. The present study focused on cervical myelopathy-related HGS weakness and postoperative functional changes according to sex. As expected, differences between the male and female groups were observable. Meanwhile, different from other available studies, all of the enrolled patients developed cervical myelopathic symptoms, and more than half also showed spinal cord signal changes (65.5%; 133/203). We confirmed that the spinal cord signal changes were not necessarily correlated with actual falls and other outcomes, such as functional mobility tests and QoL (Table 5), and the direction of correlations varied from positive to negative depending on the measured time and the sex, a finding that is consistent with the literature [38]. Healing of the spinal cord after surgical decompression is based on the intrinsic ability of the spinal cord to heal itself. Thus, the pre-operative health of the cord is paramount to post-operative improvement [39]. For the enrolled male and female patients in the present study, preoperative status, including the general condition and duration of symptoms (Table 1), could differ, and these could affect the observed variations in correlations with fall and fall-related parameters. Although there was a negative correlation between postoperative fall-related functional tests and HGS in female patients, it was smaller than that in the male patients in this study.

Along with HGS, the present study demonstrated sex differences in the recovery of QoL reflected in the outcomes and related functional mobility results. For male patients, because baseline HGS and muscle strength are much greater than those in female patients, a higher increase in HGS was expected postoperatively. Although a lesser amount of recovery of HGS and related function was observed in the female group by postoperative 3 months, the larger delayed recovery between postoperative 3 months and 1 year (Table 4) could lead the patients and medical team to encourage functional rehabilitation to improve muscle strength and lower the risk of falling up to postoperative 1 year. [40].

In a study by Kalsi-Ryan et al., [14,15] a more specific hand assessment study was suggested. Unfortunately, in this study, the patients were enrolled from March 2017 to August 2019, and therefore the specific test was not yet available. The authors believe that the hand assessment study would be better to describe upper extremity function in DCM patients in future studies.

The surgical effect of decompression in patients with DCM could differ in relation to a variety of factors. Since HGS improved after surgical decompression, the recovery of HGS was not only related to preoperative HGS but also to the overall functional outcome originating from compressive myelopathy-related pyramidal tract dysfunction [36]. Improved concordant motor function and muscle coordination with the resolution of myelopathy symptoms postoperatively elicited better functional mobility tests related to the risk of falling and actual falls [5,32].

The key findings of the present study are the following: postoperative HGS may be correlated with postoperative falling and functional outcomes differently in male and female patients. Meanwhile, surgical intervention for DCM significantly reduced the incidence rate of falls to less than 40% of the preoperative rate. The incidence of falls decreased significantly from 17.2% (35/203) to 6.8% (14/203) after surgery. Frequent falling is one of the most common symptoms in patients with DCM, and our analysis revealed that the incidence of both actual falls and multiple falls decreased significantly during postoperative follow up (Table 2). The decrease in actual falls during follow-up, however, made multiple regression analyses thereof in relation to other parameters impossible.

In another study, the incidence of postoperative falls peaked at 5 to 6 months after surgery, likely because many patients may have increased their daily walking activity during this period, leading to a transiently increased fall rate [5]. However, only a limited number of patients fell during follow up and no aggravation of symptoms and related fractures were reported in the present study. This finding could be explained by the peri- and postoperative fall prevention education program provided by our institution to emphasize the risk and caution of postoperative falls to patients and caregivers during admission and at every outpatient clinic follow up, based on previous publications [2–4,19].

Another possible reason for the decreased number of falls during follow-up could be the low BMI (mean: 24.30 ± 3.82 kg/m^2) of the enrolled patients. A higher BMI is an independent risk factor for falls, and an association between increasing BMI (ranging from 25.0 to 29.9 kg/m^2 and 30.0 kg/m^2 and higher) and the risk of falls has been reported [41]. However, no significant association was found between increasing BMI and fall-related injury in the present study: correlations between functional mobility tests and BMI are presented in Table 5.

Our study had several strong points compared with previous studies. We evaluated a comprehensive range of risk factors, including the duration of symptoms and comorbidity. As the general condition of the patients is related to the preoperative and postoperative recovery of function, the overall condition of the patients is an important factor [42,43]. Additionally, we included more severe spondylotic myeloradiculopathic cases that had undergone combined anterior–posterior surgery [44–46], and as such the rate of combined anterior–posterior surgeries was much higher than that in another study [5]. Moreover, we report not only actual falls but also the objective measures of functional mobility tests and HGS, which all affect patient subjective symptoms.

A limitation of the present study was that the radiologic factors for the risk of falling were not reported at the same time. However, regarding the functional evaluation in the present study, all parameters, including mFi and HGS, would help clarify the postoperative recovery patterns of DCM patients. The results concerning radiologic evaluation and analyses are now being prepared for a future study. Despite these limitations, this is the first study to analyze correlations between HGS and the risk of falls in relation to functional tests and actual falls, as well as QoL, in DCM.

5. Conclusions

Postoperative HGS in patients with DCM is correlated with postoperative falls and functional outcome differently in male and female patients. Altogether, our results suggest that postoperative HGS could be used as a surrogate marker for predicting favorable outcomes and neurologic deficit recovery after surgery in DCM patients, provided careful consideration in given to sexual differences therein.

Supplementary Materials: The following are available online at https://www.mdpi.com/article/10.3390/jcm10091980/s1, Table S1: Pearson correlation analysis of HGS.

Author Contributions: Conceptualization, K.A.J., J.-W.K., J.Y., H.-M.L., S.-H.M., K.-S.S., H.-S.K. and B.H.L.; methodology, K.A.J. and B.H.L.; software, B.H.L.; validation, K.A.J. and B.H.L.; formal analysis, K.A.J., J.-W.K., J.Y., H.-M.L., S.-H.M., K.-S.S., H.-S.K. and B.H.L.; investigation, K.A.J. and B.H.L.; resources, K.-S.S., and B.H.L.; data curation, K.A.J. and B.H.L.; writing—original draft preparation, K.A.J. and B.H.L.; writing—review and editing, K.A.J. and B.H.L.; visualization, K.A.J., J.-W.K., J.Y., H.-M.L., S.-H.M., K.-S.S., H.-S.K. and B.H.L.; supervision, K.A.J., J.-W.K., J.Y., H.-M.L., S.-H.M., K.-S.S., H.-S.K. and B.H.L.; project administration, B.H.L. All authors have read and agreed to the published version of the manuscript.

Funding: This research received no external funding.

Institutional Review Board Statement: The study was conducted according to the guidelines of the Declaration of Helsinki, and approved by the Institutional Review Board (or Ethics Committee) of Severance hospital, college of medicine, Yonsei university (IRB No. 4-2020-1162 and 7 December 2020).

Informed Consent Statement: Patient consent was waived due to retrospective design of study.

Data Availability Statement: Not applicable.

Conflicts of Interest: The authors declare no conflict of interest.

References

1. Kimura, A.; Seichi, A.; Takeshita, K.; Inoue, H.; Kato, T.; Yoshii, T.; Furuya, T.; Koda, M.; Takeuchi, K.; Matsunaga, S. Fall-related deterioration of subjective symptoms in patients with cervical myelopathy. *Spine* **2017**, *42*, E398–E403. [CrossRef] [PubMed]
2. Lee, B.H.; Kim, T.-H.; Park, M.-S.; Lim, S.; Park, J.-O.; Kim, H.-S.; Kim, H.-J.; Lee, H.-M.; Moon, S.-H. Comparison of effects of nonoperative treatment and decompression surgery on risk of patients with lumbar spinal stenosis falling: Evaluation with functional mobility tests. *J. Bone Jt. Surg.* **2014**, *96*, e110. [CrossRef] [PubMed]
3. Lee, B.H.; Yang, J.-H.; Kim, H.-S.; Suk, K.-S.; Lee, H.-M.; Park, J.-O.; Moon, S.-H. Effect of sagittal balance on risk of falling after lateral lumbar interbody fusion surgery combined with posterior surgery. *Yonsei Med J.* **2017**, *58*, 1177–1185. [CrossRef] [PubMed]
4. Lee, B.H.; Park, J.-O.; Kim, H.-S.; Suk, K.-S.; Lee, S.-Y.; Lee, H.-M.; Yang, J.-H.; Moon, S.-H. Spinal sagittal balance status affects postoperative actual falls and quality of life after decompression and fusion in-situ surgery in patients with lumbar spinal stenosis. *Clin. Neurol. Neurosurg.* **2016**, *148*, 52–59. [CrossRef] [PubMed]
5. Kimura, A.; Takeshita, K.; Shiraishi, Y.; Inose, H.; Yoshii, T.; Maekawa, A.; Endo, K.; Miyamoto, T.; Furuya, T.; Nakamura, A.; et al. Effectiveness of surgical treatment for degenerative cervical myelopathy in preventing falls and fall-related neurological deterioration: A prospective multi-institutional study. *Spine* **2020**, *45*, E631–E638. [CrossRef] [PubMed]
6. Bednarik, J.; Kadanka, Z.; Dusek, L.; Kerkovsky, M.; Vohanka, S.; Novotny, O.; Urbanek, I.; Kratochvilova, D. Presymptomatic spondylotic cervical myelopathy: An updated predictive model. *Eur. Spine J.* **2008**, *17*, 421–431. [CrossRef] [PubMed]
7. Bednarik, J.; Kadanka, Z.; Dusek, L.; Novotny, O.; Surelova, D.; Urbanek, I.; Prokes, B. Presymptomatic spondylotic cervical cord compression. *Spine* **2004**, *29*, 2260–2269. [CrossRef] [PubMed]
8. Bednařík, J.; Sládková, D.; Kadaňka, Z.; Dušek, L.; Keřkovský, M.; Voháňka, S.; Novotný, O.; Urbánek, I.; Němec, M. Are subjects with spondylotic cervical cord encroachment at increased risk of cervical spinal cord injury after minor trauma? *J. Neurol. Neurosurg. Psychiatry* **2011**, *82*, 779–781. [CrossRef] [PubMed]
9. Kadaňka Jr, Z.; Adamova, B.; Kerkovsky, M.; Kadanka, Z.; Dusek, L.; Jurova, B.; Vlckova, E.; Bednarik, J. Predictors of symptomatic myelopathy in degenerative cervical spinal cord compression. *Brain Behav.* **2017**, *7*, e00797. [CrossRef] [PubMed]
10. Kadaňka, Z.; Bednařík, J.; Novotný, O.; Urbánek, I.; Dušek, L. Cervical spondylotic myelopathy: Conservative versus surgical treatment after 10 years. *Eur. Spine J.* **2011**, *20*, 1533–1538. [CrossRef]
11. Kadaňka, Z.; Bednařík, J.; Voháňka, S.; Vlach, O.; Stejskal, L.; Chaloupka, R.; Filipovičová, D.; Šurelová, D.; Adamová, B.; Novotný, O. Conservative treatment versus surgery in spondylotic cervical myelopathy: A prospective randomised study. *Eur. Spine J.* **2000**, *9*, 538–544. [CrossRef]
12. Kadaňka, Z.; Mareš, M.; Bednařík, J.; Smrčka, V.; Krbec, M.; Chaloupka, R.; Dušek, L. Predictive factors for mild forms of spondylotic cervical myelopathy treated conservatively or surgically. *Eur. J. Neurol.* **2005**, *12*, 16–24. [CrossRef]
13. Kadanka, Z.; Mareš, M.; Bednarík, J.; Smrcka, V.; Krbec, M.; Stejskal, L.; Chaloupka, R.; Dagmar, S.; Novotný, O.; Urbánek, I. Approaches to spondylotic cervical myelopathy: Conservative versus surgical results in a 3-year follow-up study. *Spine* **2002**, *27*, 2205–2210. [CrossRef]
14. Kalsi-Ryan, S.; Riehm, L.E.; Tetreault, L.; Martin, A.R.; Teoderascu, F.; Massicotte, E.; Curt, A.; Verrier, M.C.; Velstra, I.-M.; Fehlings, M.G. Characteristics of upper limb impairment related to degenerative cervical myelopathy: Development of a sensitive hand assessment (graded redefined assessment of strength, sensibility, and prehension version myelopathy). *Neurosurgery* **2019**, *86*, E292–E299. [CrossRef]
15. Kalsi-Ryan, S.; Rienmueller, A.C.; Riehm, L.; Chan, C.; Jin, D.; Martin, A.R.; Badhiwala, J.H.; Akbar, M.A.; Massicotte, E.M.; Fehlings, M.G. Quantitative assessment of gait characteristics in degenerative cervical myelopathy: A prospective clinical study. *J. Clin. Med.* **2020**, *9*, 752. [CrossRef]
16. Kerkovský, M.; Bednařík, J.; Dušek, L.; Šprláková-Puková, A.; Urbánek, I.; Mechl, M.; Válek, V.; Kadanka, Z. Magnetic resonance diffusion tensor imaging in patients with cervical spondylotic spinal cord compression: Correlations between clinical and electrophysiological findings. *Spine* **2012**, *37*, 48–56. [CrossRef]
17. Kovalova, I.; Kerkovsky, M.; Kadanka, Z.; Kadanka Jr, Z.; Nemec, M.; Jurova, B.; Dusek, L.; Jarkovsky, J.; Bednarik, J. Prevalence and imaging characteristics of nonmyelopathic and myelopathic spondylotic cervical cord compression. *Spine* **2016**, *41*, 1908–1916. [CrossRef]
18. Martin, A.R.; De Leener, B.; Cohen-Adad, J.; Kalsi-Ryan, S.; Cadotte, D.W.; Wilson, J.R.; Tetreault, L.; Nouri, A.; Crawley, A.; Mikulis, D.J. Monitoring for myelopathic progression with multiparametric quantitative mri. *PLoS ONE* **2018**, *13*, e0195733.
19. Kwon, J.-W.; Lee, B.H.; Lee, S.-B.; Sung, S.; Lee, C.-U.; Yang, J.-H.; Park, M.-S.; Byun, J.; Lee, H.-M.; Moon, S.-H. Hand grip strength can predict clinical outcomes and risk of falls after decompression and instrumented posterolateral fusion for lumbar spinal stenosis. *Spine J.* **2020**, *20*, 1960–1967. [CrossRef]
20. Foster, J. Handbook of clinical neurology, vol. 26 (injuries of the spine and spinal cord, part ii): By pj vinken and gw bruyn (eds.), in collaboration with r. Braakman, associate editor hl klawans, jr., xii+ 550 pages, 310 illustrations, 71 tables, north-holland publishing company, amsterdam, 1976, US $78.75, dfl 205.00, subscription price us $66.95, dfl 174.25. *J. Neurol. Sci.* **1977**, *34*, 299.

21. Nardone, R.; Höller, Y.; Brigo, F.; Frey, V.; Lochner, P.; Leis, S.; Golaszewski, S.; Trinka, E. The contribution of neurophysiology in the diagnosis and management of cervical spondylotic myelopathy: A review. *Spinal Cord* **2016**, *54*, 756–766. [CrossRef] [PubMed]
22. Cole, T.S.; Almefty, K.K.; Godzik, J.; Muma, A.H.; Hlubek, R.J.; Martinez-del-Campo, E.; Theodore, N.; Kakarla, U.K.; Turner, J.D. Functional improvement in hand strength and dexterity after surgical treatment of cervical spondylotic myelopathy: A prospective quantitative study. *J. Neurosurg. Spine* **2020**, *32*, 907–913. [CrossRef] [PubMed]
23. Al-Mefty, O.; Harkey, L.H.; Middleton, T.H.; Smith, R.R.; Fox, J.L. Myelopathic cervical spondylotic lesions demonstrated by magnetic resonance imaging. *J. Neurosurg.* **1988**, *68*, 217–222. [CrossRef] [PubMed]
24. Choi, S.H.; Kang, C.-N. Degenerative cervical myelopathy: Pathophysiology and current treatment strategies. *Asian Spine J.* **2020**, *14*, 710–720. [CrossRef]
25. Fehlings, M.G.; Tetreault, L.A.; Riew, K.D.; Middleton, J.W.; Aarabi, B.; Arnold, P.M.; Brodke, D.S.; Burns, A.S.; Carette, S.; Chen, R.; et al. A clinical practice guideline for the management of patients with degenerative cervical myelopathy: Recommendations for patients with mild, moderate, and severe disease and nonmyelopathic patients with evidence of cord compression. *Glob. Spine J.* **2017**, *7*, 70S–83S. [CrossRef]
26. Kim, H.-J.; Chun, H.-J.; Han, C.-D.; Moon, S.-H.; Kang, K.-T.; Kim, H.-S.; Park, J.-O.; Moon, E.-S.; Kim, B.-R.; Sohn, J.-S. The risk assessment of a fall in patients with lumbar spinal stenosis. *Spine* **2011**, *36*, E588–E592. [CrossRef]
27. Bohannon, R.W. Hand-grip dynamometry predicts future outcomes in aging adults. *J. Geriatr. Phys. Ther.* **2008**, *31*, 3–10. [CrossRef]
28. Vernon, H.; Mior, S. The neck disability index: A study of reliability and validity. *J. Manip. Physiol. Ther.* **1991**, *14*, 409–415.
29. Kato, S.; Oshima, Y.; Oka, H.; Chikuda, H.; Takeshita, Y.; Miyoshi, K.; Kawamura, N.; Masuda, K.; Kunogi, J.; Okazaki, R. Comparison of the japanese orthopaedic association (joa) score and modified joa (mjoa) score for the assessment of cervical myelopathy: A multicenter observational study. *PLoS ONE* **2015**, *10*, e0123022. [CrossRef]
30. Whynes, D.K.; Group, T. Correspondence between eq-5d health state classifications and eq vas scores. *Health Qual. Life Outcomes* **2008**, *6*, 94. [CrossRef]
31. Ali, R.; Schwalb, J.M.; Nerenz, D.R.; Antoine, H.J.; Rubinfeld, I. Use of the modified frailty index to predict 30-day morbidity and mortality from spine surgery. *J. Neurosurg. Spine* **2016**, *25*, 537–541. [CrossRef]
32. Fehlings, M.G.; Wilson, J.R.; Kopjar, B.; Yoon, S.T.; Arnold, P.M.; Massicotte, E.M.; Vaccaro, A.R.; Brodke, D.S.; Shaffrey, C.I.; Smith, J.S. Efficacy and safety of surgical decompression in patients with cervical spondylotic myelopathy: Results of the aospine north america prospective multi-center study. *J. Bone Jt. Surg.* **2013**, *95*, 1651–1658. [CrossRef]
33. Cheung, J.P.Y.; Cheung, P.W.H.; Chiu, C.K.; Chan, C.Y.W.; Kwan, M.K. Variations in practice among asia–pacific surgeons and recommendations for managing cervical myelopathy: The first asia–pacific spine society collaborative study. *Asian Spine J.* **2019**, *13*, 45. [CrossRef]
34. Omori, M.; Shibuya, S.; Nakajima, T.; Endoh, T.; Suzuki, S.; Irie, S.; Ariyasu, R.; Unenaka, S.; Sano, H.; Igarashi, K. Hand dexterity impairment in patients with cervical myelopathy: A new quantitative assessment using a natural prehension movement. *Behav. Neurol.* **2018**. [CrossRef]
35. Doita, M.; Sakai, H.; Harada, Y.; Nishida, K.; Miyamoto, H.; Kaneko, T.; Kurosaka, M. Evaluation of impairment of hand function in patients with cervical myelopathy. *Clin. Spine Surg.* **2006**, *19*, 276–280. [CrossRef]
36. Yoo, J.S.; Ahn, J.; Mayo, B.C.; Bohl, D.D.; Ahn, J.; Hrynewycz, N.M.; Brundage, T.S.; Park, D.D.; Colman, M.W.; Phillips, F.M. Improvements in grip and pinch strength and patient-reported outcomes after anterior cervical discectomy and fusion. *Clin. Spine Surg.* **2019**, *32*, 403–408. [CrossRef]
37. Chen, L.-K.; Liu, L.-K.; Woo, J.; Assantachai, P.; Auyeung, T.-W.; Bahyah, K.S.; Chou, M.-Y.; Chen, L.-Y.; Hsu, P.-S.; Krairit, O. Sarcopenia in asia: Consensus report of the asian working group for sarcopenia. *J. Am. Med. Dir. Assoc.* **2014**, *15*, 95–101. [CrossRef]
38. Matsumoto, M.; Toyama, Y.; Ishikawa, M.; Chiba, K.; Suzuki, N.; Fujimura, Y. Increased signal intensity of the spinal cord on magnetic resonance images in cervical compressive myelopathy: Does it predict the outcome of conservative treatment? *Spine* **2000**, *25*, 677–682. [CrossRef]
39. Dolan, R.T.; Butler, J.S.; O'Byrne, J.M.; Poynton, A.R. Mechanical and cellular processes driving cervical myelopathy. *World J. Orthop.* **2016**, *7*, 20. [CrossRef]
40. Pandita, N.; Gupta, S.; Raina, P.; Srivastava, A.; Hakak, A.Y.; Singh, O. Neurological recovery pattern in cervical spondylotic myelopathy after anterior surgery: A prospective study with literature review. *Asian Spine J.* **2019**, *13*, 423. [CrossRef]
41. Mitchell, R.J.; Watson, W.L.; Milat, A.; Chung, A.Z.; Lord, S. Health and lifestyle risk factors for falls in a large population-based sample of older people in australia. *J. Saf. Res.* **2013**, *45*, 7–13. [CrossRef]
42. Leven, D.M.; Lee, N.J.; Kothari, P.; Steinberger, J.; Guzman, J.; Skovrlj, B.; Shin, J.I.; Caridi, J.M.; Cho, S.K. Frailty index is a significant predictor of complications and mortality after surgery for adult spinal deformity. *Spine* **2016**, *41*, E1394–E1401. [CrossRef]
43. Shin, J.I.; Kothari, P.; Phan, K.; Kim, J.S.; Leven, D.; Lee, N.J.; Cho, S.K. Frailty index as a predictor of adverse postoperative outcomes in patients undergoing cervical spinal fusion. *Spine* **2017**, *42*, 304–310. [CrossRef]
44. Fiore, S.; Labiak, J.J.; Davis, R.P. Combined anterior-posterior decompression and fusion for cervical spondylotic myelopathy. *Am. J. Orthop.* **2017**, *46*, E97–E104.

45. Kang, K.-C.; Lee, H.S.; Lee, J.-H. Cervical radiculopathy focus on characteristics and differential diagnosis. *Asian Spine J.* **2020**, *14*, 921–930. [CrossRef]
46. Suk, K.-S.; Jimenez, K.A.; Jo, J.H.; Kim, H.-S.; Lee, H.-M.; Moon, S.-H.; Lee, B.H. Anterior plate-screws and lower postoperative t1 slope affect cervical allospacer failures in multi-level acdf surgery: Anterior versus posterior fixation. *Glob. Spine J.* **2021**, 2192568221991515. [CrossRef]

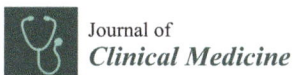

Article

Human Nonmercaptalbumin Is a New Biomarker of Motor Function

Sadayuki Ito [1], Hiroaki Nakashima [1,*], Kei Ando [1], Kazuyoshi Kobayashi [1], Masaaki Machino [1], Taisuke Seki [1], Shinya Ishizuka [1], Shunsuke Kanbara [1], Taro Inoue [1], Hiroyuki Koshimizu [1], Ryosuke Fujii [2], Hiroya Yamada [3], Yoshitaka Ando [4], Jun Ueyama [5], Takaaki Kondo [5], Koji Suzuki [2], Yukiharu Hasegawa [6] and Shiro Imagama [1]

[1] Department of Orthopaedic Surgery, Graduate School of Medicine, Nagoya University, Nagoya 466-8560, Japan; sadaito@med.nagoya-u.ac.jp (S.I.); andokei@med.nagoya-u.ac.jp (K.A.); k_koba1@f2.dion.ne.jp (K.K.); masaaki_machino_5445_2@yahoo.co.jp (M.M.); taiseki@med.nagoya-u.ac.jp (T.S.); shinyai@med.nagoya-u.ac.jp (S.I.); shunaly0108@gmail.com (S.K.); bluesdrivemonster@hotmail.com (T.I.); love_derika@yahoo.co.jp (H.K.); imagama@med.nagoya-u.ac.jp (S.I.)
[2] Department of Preventive Medical Sciences, School of Medical Sciences, Fujita Health University, Toyoake 470-1192, Japan; rfujii@fujita-hu.ac.jp (R.F.); ksuzuki@fujita-hu.ac.jp (K.S.)
[3] Department of Hygiene, School of Medicine, Fujita Health University, Toyoake 470-1192, Japan; hyamada@fujita-hu.ac.jp
[4] Department of Biomedical and Analytical Sciences, School of Medical Sciences, Fujita Health University, Toyoake 470-1192, Japan; yando@fujita-hu.ac.jp
[5] Department of Pathophysiological Laboratory Sciences, Graduate School of Medicine, Nagoya University, Nagoya 466-8560, Japan; ueyama@met.nagoya-u.ac.jp (J.U.); taka@met.nagoya-u.ac.jp (T.K.)
[6] Department of Rehabilitation, Kansai University of Welfare Science, Osaka 582-0026, Japan; hasegawa@tamateyama.ac.jp
* Correspondence: hirospine@med.nagoya-u.ac.jp

Abstract: The ratio of human nonmercaptalbumin (HNA) and reduced albumin (HMA) may be a new marker for oxidative stress. Locomotive syndrome (LS) is reduced mobility due to impairment of locomotive organs. We investigated whether the HNA/HMA ratio could be a new biomarker of LS. This study included 306 subjects (mean age 64.24 ± 10.4 years) who underwent LS tests, grip strength, walking speed, and tests for HNA and HMA. Oxidative stress was measured by the ratio of HMA (f(HMA) = (HMA/(HMA + HNA) × 100)), and the subjects were divided into normal (N group; f[HMA] ≥ 70%) and low (L group; f[HMA] < 70%) groups. There were 124 non-elderly (<65 years) and 182 elderly subjects (≥65 years). There were no significant differences in LS, grip strength, and walking speed between the L and N groups in the non-elderly subjects. However, significant differences were found in the elderly subjects. In logistic regression analysis, there was an association between f(HMA) and the LS severity at older ages. LS in the elderly is associated with a decline in HMA and, thus, an increase in oxidative stress. Thus, f(HMA) is a new biomarker of LS.

Keywords: human nonmercaptalbumin; reduced albumin; oxidative stress; locomotive syndrome

1. Introduction

The majority of developed countries have an aging population [1], and the number of people requiring support and care in their daily lives due to musculoskeletal disorders is increasing [2]. Locomotive syndrome (LS), which is a condition of reduced mobility due to impairment of locomotive organs, was proposed by the Japanese Orthopedic Association (JOA) as an overarching term for this condition [2,3]. LS has received worldwide attention for an assessment of the motor function in motor diseases [4]. LS is associated with a significantly lower quality of life (QOL) [5] and a shorter life expectancy. Prevention of LS has long been advocated for maintaining and improving physical function in middle-aged and elderly people [6].

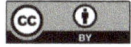

Oxidative stress reflects the imbalance of reactive oxidative species and antioxidant defenses and plays an important role in the decline of body functions in old age [7–9]. Elevated oxidative stress induces apoptosis of skeletal muscle [10], abnormality in neuromuscular junctions [11] and impaired mitochondrial function [12], resulting in decreased muscle performance, one of the major determinants of exercise capacity [13]. A recent systematic review of older adults has shown an association between increased oxidative stress and physical frailty [14]. Given that oxidative stress is one of the origins of age-related decline in functional reserve, the use of biomarkers that reflect the redox status of the body may allow early identification of individuals at risk of functional decline due to musculoskeletal disease. The human serum albumin (HSA) cysteine-34 accounts for about 80% of the extracellular free thiols and is a major extracellular antioxidant [15]. Thus, HSA has been considered an important scavenger of reactive oxidative species, for example hydroxyl radical and hydrogen peroxide [16], but there are reports of differing antioxidative effects of HSA depending on its chemical structure. For example, Cys-34 residue functions as a universal antioxidant residue with excellent scavenging ability against a variety of reactive oxygen species, while Met residue may play an auxiliary role [17,18].

HSAs have been chemically classified into two major categories based on their redox status: human non-mercaptalbumin (HNA: oxidized form) and human mercaptalbumin (HMA: reduced form) [19]. Under oxidative stress, HMA changes to reversibly oxidized HNA-1 and highly oxidized HNA-2. Under oxidative stress, HMA buffers reactive oxidized species and turns them into HNAs; therefore, the proportion of HMA in HSA (f(HMA)) has been considered a biomarker reflecting the redox status of the human body [20]. Although the proportion of each HSA form is generally age- and disease-dependent, studies have shown that HMA, HNA-1, and HNA-2 account for 70–80%, 20–30%, and 2–5%, respectively, of the total albumin in healthy young adults [21].

Several clinical studies have examined the relationship between the redox status of HSA and the severity and progression of hypertension [22,23], obesity [24], liver injury [25], renal function [26,27], anemia [28], and cardiovascular complications in patients on dialysis [29,30]. It is also associated with Diabetes Mellitus [31] and Alzheimer's disease [32].

Although limited epidemiological studies have analyzed the association between HSA redox status and motor function [33], this redox status might be a biomarker for LS. The purpose of this study was to evaluate the redox status of albumin in a middle-aged and elderly Japanese population, and to investigate its correlation with motor function, including LS.

2. Materials and Methods

2.1. Study Participants

The individuals surveyed were volunteers who underwent a municipal-supported health checkup in the town of Yakumo in 2016. The town of Yakumo has a population of about 17,000 of whom 28% are over 65 years old. More people are engaged in agriculture and fishing than in urban areas. This town has been conducting annual health checkups since 1982. Physical examinations include voluntary orthopedic and physical function tests, internal examinations, and psychological examinations, as well as a health-related QOL survey (SF-36) [34,35]. This study included all participants who completed an assessment of the LS risk stage. The exclusion criteria were: a history of spine or joint surgery, severe knee injury, severe hip osteoarthritis, history of hip or spine fractures, neuropathy, severe mental illness, diabetes, kidney or heart disease, non-fasting, severe impairment of walking or standing, and impairment of the central or peripheral nervous system.

Of the 555 participants who underwent health checks, 306 (128 men and 178 women) met the inclusion criteria. The research protocol was approved by the Human Research Ethics Committee and the University's Institutional Review Board (No. 2014-0207). All participants gave written informed consent prior to participation. The research procedure was carried out in accordance with the principles of the Declaration of Helsinki.

2.2. Examination of Motor Function

Grip strength in the standing position was measured once for each hand with a hand-grip dynamometer (Toei Light Co., Ltd., Saitama, Japan), and the mean value was used [36]. Subjects walked a straight 10 m course once at their fastest pace, and the time required to complete the course was recorded as the 10 m gait time [37].

2.3. LS Stage Tests

To evaluate the risk of LS, the JOA has proposed three tests: the two-step test, the stand-up test, and the 25-question geriatric locomotive function scale (GLFS-25) [2]. LS is categorized into stages 1 and 2, and these tests assess the degree of motor function and define the stages of LS. Stage 1 indicates that movement function has begun to decline, and stage 2 indicates that movement function has progressed towards a decline in mobility.

Three tests were conducted according to the JOA guidelines [2].

In the stand-up test, the ability to stand with a single- or double-leg stance from stools of heights, 40, 30, 20, and 10 cm, is evaluated. The grading of difficulty, from easy to difficult, is in the order of double-leg stance with 40, 30, 20, and 10 cm stools, followed by single-leg stance with 40, 30, 20, and 10 cm. The test result is expressed as the minimum height of the stool that the subject was able to stand up from.

In the two-step test, a physical therapist measured the length of two steps from the starting line to the tip of the toe. Scores were calculated by normalizing the maximum length of two steps by height.

The GLFS-25 is a self-reported comprehensive survey that refers to the previous month [38]. The scale consists of four questions about pain, 16 questions about Activities of Daily Living (ADL), three questions about social functioning, and two questions about mental status. Each item was graded from no disability (0 points) to severe disability (4 points).

We defined LS0, 1, 2 as follows:

LS0

The subject is categorized as Stage 0 if all three of the conditions are met as follows:

1. Stand-up test, ability to stand on one-leg from a 40-cm-high seat (both legs).
2. Two-step test, >1.3.
3. 25-question GLFS score, <7.

LS1

The subject is categorized as Stage 1 if any of the three conditions are met as follows:

1. Stand-up test, difficulty in one-leg standing from a 40-cm-high seat (either leg).
2. Two-step test, <1.3.
3. 25-question GLFS score, ≥7.

LS2

The subject is categorized as Stage 2 if any of the three conditions are met as follows:

1. Stand-up test, difficulty in standing from a 20-cm-high seat using both legs.
2. Two-step test, <1.1.
3. 25-question GLFS score, ≥16.

2.4. Measurements of HSA

During the checkup, fasting blood samples were collected through venipuncture and centrifuged within 1 h of sampling. Serum samples were stored at $-80\ °C$ until the assay was performed. Routine biochemical analyses were performed in the laboratory of the Yakumo Town Hospital. Interpersonal measurements of height and weight were taken to calculate the body mass index (BMI, kg/m^2).

The determination of HSA, HNA, and HMA using high performance liquid chromatography (HPLC) with an ultraviolet detector has been reported by Sogami et al. [39]. In this study, the HPLC-post-column bromocresol green (BCG) method was used, which was engineered to ensure that serum uric acid and bilirubin did not interfere with chromatographic peaks [40]. Frozen serum samples were thawed at room temperature and filtered through a Mini-UniPrep syringe-less filter (Agilent, Tokyo, Japan); HPLC was performed and reacted with BCG reagents to separate HMA and HNA detected at a 620 nm wavelength. The sample volume injected into the HPLC was 5 μL. The mobile phase reagent consisted of N-methylpiperazine-HCl buffer (pH 4.5), 40 mM Na_2SO_4, and 3% ethanol; the BCG reagent consisted of 150 mM citric acid, 3% Brigi 35, and 0.3 mM BCG. For all experiments, distilled water deionized to 18 mΩ using the Millipore Milli-Q System (Millipore Co., Bedford, MA, USA) was used.

The HPLC system used in this study was the Hitachi Lacrom Ice System (Hitachi, Tokyo, Japan), which consisted of an isocratic pump (L-2130), an auto-injector (L-2200), and a column oven (L-2300). Chromatograms were obtained using a photodiode array detection system (model L-2455). A Shodex Asahipak GS-570 GS column (100 mm × 7.5 mm ID) was used to separate the HSA components before sample injection.

In the present experiment, the peak of HNA-2 was not sufficiently quantified, and its peak area was not considered in subsequent analyses. To numerically assess the redox state of HSA from the HPLC profile, f(HMA), which represents the ratio of the peak area of HMA to the peak area of HSA, has been used in previous similar studies [41]. Hence, we followed these reports for the present study.

The f(HMA) was calculated using the following equation: f(HMA) = HMA area/(HMA area + HNA area) × 100.

Previous studies have demonstrated that f(HMA) accounts for 70–80% of the total albumin in a healthy young adult [42]. Therefore, the cut-off value of f(HMA) was determined to be 70%. We divided the participants into the normal (N, f(HMA) ≥ 70%) and lower (L, f(HMA) < 70%) oxidative stress groups.

2.5. Statistical Analysis

Continuous variables were expressed as mean ± standard deviation (SD). We compared continuous variables of the L group to those of the N group using the student t-test, and categorical variables of the L group to those of the N group using the Chi-squared test. Logistic regression analysis was performed to evaluate important risk factors of elevated oxidative stress, as defined by f(HMA) < 70%: L group. The dependent variable was N versus L groups. Following univariable analysis, variables that yielded a p-value < 0.20 were included in the multivariable analysis.

Each analysis was done separately for the under-65 (non-elderly) and the over-65 (elderly) groups.

All statistical analyses were performed using SPSS Statistics v.22.0 software for Mac (IBM Corp., Armonk, NY, USA). A p-value < 0.05 was considered significant in all analyses.

3. Results

Table 1 shows the participant characteristics. The participants had an average age of 64.24 ± 10.4 years; 128 were male and 178 were female. The mean albumin serum level was 4.39 ± 0.25 (g/dL); The mean f(HMA) was 69.49 ± 7.02%; there were 151 and 155 participants in the N and L groups, respectively. With respect to the severity of LS, 118 participants (38.6%) were at no risk (stage 0), 116 (37.9%) were stage 1, and 72 (23.5%) were stage 2 [43].

Table 1. Demographics and clinical characteristics.

Characteristics	Total (n = 306)	Non-Elderly (n = 124)	Elderly (n = 182)
male/female	128/178	40/84	88/94
Age (years old)	64.24 ± 10.4	54.19 ± 7.34	71.19 ± 5.24
Height (cm)	157.88 ± 8.15	159.56 ± 8.16	156.71 ± 7.97
Weight (kg)	58.84 ± 11.35	60.04 ± 12.61	58.02 ± 10.36
BMI (kg/cm^2)	23.5 ± 3.48	23.44 ± 3.73	23.54 ± 3.31
grip strength (kg)	27.06 ± 8.88	27.28 ± 9.47	26.9 ± 8.46
gait speed (m/s)	1.88 ± 0.29	1.94 ± 0.28	1.84 ± 0.29
Albumin (g/dL)	4.39 ± 0.25	4.42 ± 0.25	4.36 ± 0.26
f(HMA) (%)	69.49 ± 7.02	72.96 ± 5.86	67.09 ± 6.76
N/L	151/155	84/40	67/115
Stage of LS (0/1/2)	118/116/72	52/50/22	66/66/50

BMI: body mass index; f(HMA): fraction of human mercaptalbumin; f(HMA) = HMA area/(HMA area + HNA area); HMA: human mercaptalbumin; N: participants with f(HMA) of 70% or more; L: participants with f(HMA) less than 70%; LS: locomotive syndrome. Values are mean ± SD for each group.

3.1. Non-Elderly Participants

The average age was 54.19 ± 7.34 years, and the mean f(HMA) was 72.96 ± 5.86%. Eighty-four (67.7%) and 40 (32.3%) subjects were considered to be in the N and L oxidative stress groups, respectively. In terms of LS, 52 (41.9%), 50 (40.3%), and 22 participants (17.8%) were grouped into no risk (stage 0), stage 1, and stage 2, respectively (Table 1). The average age was significantly higher in the L group (N: 53.42 ± 7.5, L: 56.89 ± 6.15, $p < 0.001$). Gender, height, weight, BMI, grip strength, and gait speed were not significantly different between the groups. There was no significant difference in the severity of LS between the N and L oxidative stress groups (stage 0: 41.7 and 42.5%, stage 1: 40.5 and 40.0%, and stage 2: 17.8 and 17.5% in the N and L groups, $p = 0.90$) (Table 2).

Table 2. The comparison of each parameter between the N and L groups in non-elderly participants.

Non-Elderly (n = 124)	N Group (n = 84)	L Group (n = 40)	p
male/female	32/52	16/24	0.304
Age (years)	53.42 ± 7.5	56.89 ± 6.15	<0.001
Height (cm)	160.76 ± 7.87	159.47 ± 8.45	0.579
Weight (kg)	59.28 ± 11.48	61.8 ± 12.28	0.283
BMI (kg/cm^2)	22.9 ± 3.52	24.27 ± 3.84	0.69
grip strength (kg)	28.44 ± 9.55	27.57 ± 9.63	0.639
gait speed (m/s)	1.95 ± 0.27	1.92 ± 0.31	0.623
Stage of LS (0/1/2)	35/34/15	17/16/7	0.904

BMI: body mass index; N group: participants with f(HMA) of 70% or more; L group: participants with f(HMA) less than 70%; LS: locomotive syndrome. Values are mean ± SD for each group.

3.2. Elderly Participants

The average age was 71.19 ± 5.24 years, and the mean f(HMA) was 67.09 ± 6.76%. Sixty-seven (36.8%) and 115 (63.2%) subjects were categorized in the N and L oxidative stress groups, respectively. In terms of LS, 66 (36.3%), 66 (36.3%), and 50 (27.4%) participants were grouped into stage 0, stage 1, and stage 2, respectively (Table 1).

Age and BMI were not significantly different between the N and L oxidative stress groups. There were significant differences in the percentage of LS in elderly participants (N: stage 0: 33 (49.3%), stage 1: 21 (31.3%), stage 2: 13 (19.4%); L: stage 0: 33 (28.7%), stage 1: 45 (39.1%), stage 2: 37 (32.2%); $p = 0.004$). There were significant differences in gender, height, weight, grip strength, and gait speed in elderly participants ($p < 0.001$, $p < 0.001$, $p = 0.018$, $p < 0.001$, $p = 0.002$, respectively) (Table 3).

Table 3. The comparison of each parameter between the N and L groups in elderly participants.

Elderly (n = 182)	N Group (n = 67)	L Group (n = 115)	p
male/female	40/27	47/68	<0.001
Age (years)	69.95 ± 4.41	71.55 ± 5.63	0.057
Height (cm)	159.13 ± 7.94	155.32 ± 7.81	<0.001
Weight (kg)	59.11 ± 10.2	57.37 ± 10.43	0.018
BMI (kg/cm^2)	23.25 ± 3	23.69 ± 3.42	0.930
grip strength (kg)	28.35 ± 8.51	25.8 ± 8.39	<0.001
gait speed (m/s)	1.92 ± 0.24	1.78 ± 0.3	0.002
Stage of LS (0/1/2)	33/21/13	33/45/37	0.004

BMI: body mass index; N group: participants with f(HMA) of 70% or more; L group: participants with f(HMA) less than 70%; LS: locomotive syndrome. Values are mean ± SD for each group.

Since there were several factors with significant differences, they were examined as covariates for risk factors for elevated oxidative stress, as defined by f(HMA) > 70%: L group in logistic regression analysis, which found only LS as a risk factor for elevated oxidative stress (OR 0.515, 95% confidence interval, 95% CI: 0.281–0.943, p = 0.032) (Table 4). As the LS stage increased by 1, the risk of becoming L increased by 0.515 times.

Table 4. Logistic regression analysis for risk factors of the elevation of oxidative stress (L group) in elderly participants.

Elderly	B	SE	Wald	df	p	OR	95% CI
male/female	0.031	0.709	0.002	1	0.966	1.031	0.257–4.136
Age (years)	−0.05	0.042	1.412	1	0.235	0.951	0.876–1.033
Height (cm)	0.079	0.042	3.482	1	0.062	1.082	0.996–1.175
Weight (kg)	−0.005	0.025	0.043	1	0.836	0.995	0.947–1.045
grip strength (kg)	−0.08	0.755	0.011	1	0.915	0.923	0.21–4.054
gait speed (m/s)	−0.003	0.039	0.007	1	0.932	0.997	0.924–1.075
Stage of LS (0/1/2)	−0.663	0.309	4.62	1	0.032	0.515	0.281–0.943

OR: odds ratio; CI: confidence interval; L group: participants with f(HMA) less than 70%; LS: locomotive syndrome.

4. Discussion

There have been several reports of the association between f(HMA), a marker of oxidative stress, and chronic diseases [16]. However, few reports have indicated its association with motor function [33]. Furthermore, to our knowledge, this is the first study to report on the association between f(HMA) and LS. The present study indicated that subjects with more severe LS stages had higher oxidative stress as assessed by f(HMA) levels in the elderly group, where oxidative stress was associated with a decline in locomotive function. The f(HMA) ratio could be a new biomarker associated with LS in elderly subjects.

Oxidative stress reflects the imbalance of reactive oxidative species and antioxidant defenses, and it plays an important role in the decline of body functions [7]. It has been reported that oxidative stress is associated with chronic diseases, including hypertension, obesity, liver injury, renal function, anemia, and cardiovascular complications [30]. Furthermore, increased oxidative stress in the elderly might be associated with a deterioration in motor function as increased oxidative stress reduces walking speed in elderly women [33]. This study concurred, showing increased oxidative stress and reduced motor functions, such as grip strength and walking speed, in elderly people, which worsened the degree of impairment of locomotion.

There are several possible mechanisms to explain the association between f(HMA) levels and motor performance in LS. Oxidative stress is associated with muscle function through several pathways, including changes in neuromuscular junctions, reduced muscle energy metabolism, and reduced calcium release from the endoplasmic reticulum [11]. Another possible mechanism is muscle atrophy from increased proteolysis and decreased protein synthesis due to increased oxidative stress [11]. Oxidative stress has been reported to impair skeletal muscle as well as cardiovascular energy metabolism [11]. The association between f(HMA) and exercise capacity may be explained by the effect of oxidative stress on these systemic factors that determine exercise capacity.

In multivariate analysis, f(HMA) was associated with locomotion rather than simple motor functions, such as grip strength and gait, in the elderly group. LS is the concept of functional decline due to problems in bone, cartilage, muscle, and nerves [44], and f(HMA) may be related to abnormalities in these motor organs. However, an association between f(HMA) and decline in motor function or LS was not found in the non-elderly. The simple increase in oxidative stress does not affect motor function, but long-term exposure to oxidative stress, such as with age-related chronic inflammation, may be associated with a functional decline [45].

LS is a condition that requires nursing care. As it is a motor disease that is expected to improve with locomotion training, early detection leads to the preclusion of unnecessary nursing care [44]. In the current study, the oxidative stress marker f(HMA) was found to be associated with the degree of LS, and it may therefore be a new biomarker for the early detection of LS. If this is confirmed, it will be possible to intervene in LS from an early stage, resulting in nursing care being unnecessary. Furthermore, as exercise testing to diagnose LS is difficult in the limited time in an outpatient setting, if f(HMA) becomes a biomarker for suspected LS, it could provide a simple objective diagnostic modality for LS.

The modifiability of f(HMA) by intervention, and its responsiveness to changes in motor performance, need to be investigated in future studies. Supplementation with branched-chain amino acids is a potential intervention to increase f(HMA) levels. A previous study in patients with cirrhosis showed that administration of branched-chain amino acids increased f(HMA) [19]. LS may be improved by nutritional therapies that improve f(HMA), which may be a potential new treatment other than exercise therapy. There is scope to consider the link between LS, f(HMA), and nutritional status.

It may also be possible that the exercise regimens reported so far to improve LS may improve f(HMA) and reduce oxidative stress. Therefore, the results of this study may provide a basis for the hypothesis that exercise therapy, as previously described, improves systemic diseases caused by oxidative stress [46].

This study has several potential limitations. First, the participants were middle-aged and elderly people who lived in a relatively rural area, where many had jobs in agriculture or fishing. Thus, the lifestyle of these subjects differed from that of people in an urban environment. Furthermore, the participants attended for annual health examinations, which suggests that they may be more health conscious than other people. Second, this was a cross-sectional, single-center study. In the future, longitudinal and multicenter collaborative research will be needed to verify our findings. Finally, the specificity of f(HMA) as a biomarker of LS could not be discussed, because other biomarkers related to oxidative stress were not measured. Nevertheless, the present study still has a clinical application, by indicating that the redox state of HSA might serve as a biomarker for LS.

5. Conclusions

In conclusion, this study demonstrated that f(HMA), a marker for the redox state of HSA, correlated with the severity of LS in elderly people. Thus, we suggest that f(HMA) could be a novel biomarker of LS.

Author Contributions: Conceptualization, S.I. (Sadayuki Ito); methodology, S.I. (Sadayuki Ito); software, R.F.; validation, R.F., H.Y., Y.A., J.U., T.K., K.S.; formal analysis, S.I. (Sadayuki Ito); investigation, S.I. (Sadayuki Ito), H.N., K.A., K.K., T.S., S.I. (Shinya Ishizuka), M.M., S.K., T.I., H.K., R.F., H.Y., Y.A., J.U., T.K., K.S., Y.H. and S.I. (Shiro Imagama); resources, S.I. (Sadayuki Ito), H.N., K.A., K.K., T.S., S.I. (Shinya Ishizuka), M.M., S.K., T.I., H.K., R.F., H.Y., Y.A., J.U., T.K., K.S., Y.H. and S.I. (Shiro Imagama); data curation, S.I. (Sadayuki Ito); writing—original draft preparation, S.I. (Sadayuki Ito);

writing—review and editing, S.I. (Sadayuki Ito) and H.N.; supervision, S.I. (Shiro Imagama); project administration, H.N. All authors have read and agreed to the published version of the manuscript.

Funding: This research did not receive any specific grant from funding agencies in the public, commercial, or not-for-profit sectors.

Institutional Review Board Statement: The research protocol was approved by the Human Research Ethics Committee and the University's Institutional Review Board (No. 2014-0207). All participants gave written informed consent prior to participation. The research procedure was carried out in accordance with the principles of the Declaration of Helsinki.

Informed Consent Statement: All participants gave written informed consent prior to participation.

Data Availability Statement: The data of health checkups used to support the findings of this study are available from the corresponding author upon request.

Acknowledgments: We are grateful to the staff of the Comprehensive Health Care Program held in Yakumo, Hokkaido, and Aya Henmi and Hiroko Ino of Nagoya University for their assistance throughout this study.

Conflicts of Interest: The authors declare that there is no conflict of interest regarding the publication of this paper.

References

1. Preston, S.H.; Stokes, A. Sources of population aging in more and less developed countries. *Popul. Dev Rev.* **2012**, *38*, 221–236. [CrossRef] [PubMed]
2. Nakamura, K.; Ogata, T. Locomotive Syndrome: Definition and Management. *Clin. Rev. Bone Miner. Metab.* **2016**, *14*, 56–67. [CrossRef]
3. Nakamura, K. The concept and treatment of locomotive syndrome: Its acceptance and spread in Japan. *J. Orthop. Sci.* **2011**, *16*, 489–491. [CrossRef] [PubMed]
4. Yi, H.-S.; Lee, S. Overcoming osteoporosis and beyond: Locomotive syndrome or dysmobility syndrome. *Osteoporos. Sarcopenia* **2018**, *4*, 77–78. [CrossRef] [PubMed]
5. Hirano, K.; Imagama, S.; Hasegawa, Y.; Ito, Z.; Muramoto, A.; Ishiguro, N. The influence of locomotive syndrome on health-related quality of life in a community-living population. *Mod. Rheumatol* **2013**, *23*, 939–944. [CrossRef] [PubMed]
6. Muramoto, A.; Imagama, S.; Ito, Z.; Hirano, K.; Ishiguro, N.; Hasegawa, Y. Spinal sagittal balance substantially influences locomotive syndrome and physical performance in community-living middle-aged and elderly women. *J. Orthop. Sci.* **2016**, *21*, 216–221. [CrossRef] [PubMed]
7. Saum, K.U.; Dieffenbach, A.K.; Jansen, E.H.; Schottker, B.; Holleczek, B.; Hauer, K.; Brenner, H. Association between oxidative stress and frailty in an elderly german population: Results from the ESTHER cohort study. *Gerontology* **2015**, *61*, 407–415. [CrossRef] [PubMed]
8. Venkataraman, K.; Khurana, S.; Tai, T.C. Oxidative stress in aging-matters of the heart and mind. *Int. J. Mol. Sci.* **2013**, *14*, 17897–17925. [CrossRef]
9. Jenny, N.S. Inflammation in aging: Cause, effect, or both? *Discov. Med.* **2012**, *13*, 451–460.
10. Wang, D.; Yang, Y.; Zou, X.; Zhang, J.; Zheng, Z.; Wang, Z. Antioxidant apigenin relieves age-related muscle atrophy by inhibiting oxidative stress and hyperactive mitophagy and apoptosis in skeletal muscle of mice. *J. Gerontol. A Biol. Sci. Med. Sci.* **2020**, *75*, 2081–2088. [CrossRef]
11. Baumann, C.W.; Kwak, D.; Liu, H.M.; Thompson, L.V. Age-induced oxidative stress: How does it influence skeletal muscle quantity and quality? *J. Appl Physiol (1985)* **2016**, *121*, 1047–1052. [CrossRef]
12. Liguori, I.; Russo, G.; Curcio, F.; Bulli, G.; Aran, L.; Della-Morte, D.; Gargiulo, G.; Testa, G.; Cacciatore, F.; Bonaduce, D.; et al. Oxidative stress, aging and diseases. *Clin. Interv. Aging* **2018**, *13*, 757–772. [CrossRef]
13. Gomes, M.J.; Martinez, P.F.; Pagan, L.U.; Damatto, R.L.; Cezar, M.D.M.; Lima, A.R.R.; Okoshi, K.; Okoshi, M.P. Skeletal muscle aging: Influence of oxidative stress and physical exercise. *Oncotarget* **2017**, *8*, 20428–20440. [CrossRef]
14. Soysal, P.; Isik, A.T.; Carvalho, A.F.; Fernandes, B.S.; Solmi, M.; Schofield, P.; Veronese, N.; Stubbs, B. Oxidative stress and frailty: A systematic review and synthesis of the best evidence. *Maturitas* **2017**, *99*, 66–72. [CrossRef]
15. Oettl, K.; Stauber, R.E. Physiological and pathological changes in the redox state of human serum albumin critically influence its binding properties. *Br. J. Pharmacol.* **2007**, *151*, 580–590. [CrossRef]
16. Zoellner, H.; Hofler, M.; Beckmann, R.; Hufnagl, P.; Vanyek, E.; Bielek, E.; Wojta, J.; Fabry, A.; Lockie, S.; Binder, B.R. Serum albumin is a specific inhibitor of apoptosis in human endothelial cells. *J. Cell Sci.* **1996**, *109*, 2571–2580. [CrossRef]
17. Iwao, Y.; Ishima, Y.; Yamada, J.; Noguchi, T.; Kragh-Hansen, U.; Mera, K.; Honda, D.; Suenaga, A.; Maruyama, T.; Otagiri, M. Quantitative evaluation of the role of cysteine and methionine residues in the antioxidant activity of human serum albumin using recombinant mutants. *IUBMB Life* **2012**, *64*, 450–454. [CrossRef]

18. Quinlan, G.J.; Martin, G.S.; Evans, T.W. Albumin: Biochemical properties and therapeutic potential. *Hepatology* **2005**, *41*, 1211–1219. [CrossRef]
19. Setoyama, H.; Tanaka, M.; Nagumo, K.; Naoe, H.; Watanabe, T.; Yoshimaru, Y.; Tateyama, M.; Sasaki, M.; Watanabe, H.; Otagiri, M.; et al. Oral branched-chain amino acid granules improve structure and function of human serum albumin in cirrhotic patients. *J. Gastroenterol.* **2017**, *52*, 754–765. [CrossRef]
20. Soejima, A.; Kaneda, F.; Manno, S.; Matsuzawa, N.; Kouji, H.; Nagasawa, T.; Era, S.; Takakuwa, Y. Useful markers for detecting decreased serum antioxidant activity in hemodialysis patients. *Am. J. Kidney Dis.* **2002**, *39*, 1040–1046. [CrossRef]
21. Fujii, R.; Ueyama, J.; Aoi, A.; Ichino, N.; Osakabe, K.; Sugimoto, K.; Suzuki, K.; Hamajima, N.; Wakai, K.; Kondo, T. Oxidized human serum albumin as a possible correlation factor for atherosclerosis in a rural Japanese population: The results of the Yakumo Study. *Environ. Health Prev. Med.* **2018**, *23*, 1. [CrossRef]
22. Vaziri, N.D. Roles of oxidative stress and antioxidant therapy in chronic kidney disease and hypertension. *Curr. Opin. Nephrol. Hypertens.* **2004**, *13*, 93–99. [CrossRef] [PubMed]
23. Sato, K.; Dohi, Y.; Kojima, M.; Miyagawa, K.; Takase, H.; Katada, E.; Suzuki, S. Effects of ascorbic acid on ambulatory blood pressure in elderly patients with refractory hypertension. *Arzneimittelforschung* **2006**, *56*, 535–540. [CrossRef]
24. Keaney, J.F., Jr.; Larson, M.G.; Vasan, R.S.; Wilson, P.W.; Lipinska, I.; Corey, D.; Massaro, J.M.; Sutherland, P.; Vita, J.A.; Benjamin, E.J. Obesity and systemic oxidative stress: Clinical correlates of oxidative stress in the Framingham Study. *Arterioscler. Thromb. Vasc. Biol.* **2003**, *23*, 434–439. [CrossRef] [PubMed]
25. Oettl, K.; Birner-Gruenberger, R.; Spindelboeck, W.; Stueger, H.P.; Dorn, L.; Stadlbauer, V.; Putz-Bankuti, C.; Krisper, P.; Graziadei, I.; Vogel, W.; et al. Oxidative albumin damage in chronic liver failure: Relation to albumin binding capacity, liver dysfunction and survival. *J. Hepatol.* **2013**, *59*, 978–983. [CrossRef] [PubMed]
26. Terawaki, H.; Yoshimura, K.; Hasegawa, T.; Matsuyama, Y.; Negawa, T.; Yamada, K.; Matsushima, M.; Nakayama, M.; Hosoya, T.; Era, S. Oxidative stress is enhanced in correlation with renal dysfunction: Examination with the redox state of albumin. *Kidney Int.* **2004**, *66*, 1988–1993. [CrossRef] [PubMed]
27. Suzuki, Y.; Suda, K.; Matsuyama, Y.; Era, S.; Soejima, A. Close relationship between redox state of human serum albumin and serum cysteine levels in non-diabetic CKD patients with various degrees of renal function. *Clin. Nephrol.* **2014**, *82*, 320–325. [CrossRef]
28. Bissinger, R.; Bhuyan, A.A.M.; Qadri, S.M.; Lang, F. Oxidative stress, eryptosis and anemia: A pivotal mechanistic nexus in systemic diseases. *FEBS J.* **2019**, *286*, 826–854. [CrossRef]
29. Weiss, S.J. Tissue destruction by neutrophils. *N. Engl. J. Med.* **1989**, *320*, 365–376. [CrossRef]
30. Masudo, R.; Yasukawa, K.; Nojiri, T.; Yoshikawa, N.; Shimosaka, H.; Sone, S.; Oike, Y.; Ugawa, A.; Yamazaki, T.; Shimokado, K.; et al. Evaluation of human nonmercaptalbumin as a marker for oxidative stress and its association with various parameters in blood. *J. Clin. Biochem. Nutr.* **2017**. [CrossRef]
31. Yasunari, K.; Maeda, K.; Nakamura, M.; Yoshikawa, J. Oxidative stress in leukocytes is a possible link between blood pressure, blood glucose and C-reacting protein. *Hypertension* **2002**, *39*, 777–780. [CrossRef]
32. Chen, Z.; Zhong, C. Oxidative stress in Alzheimer's disease. *Neurosci. Bull.* **2014**, *30*, 271–281. [CrossRef]
33. Ashikawa, H.; Adachi, T.; Ueyama, J.; Yamada, S. Association between redox state of human serum albumin and exercise capacity in older women: A cross-sectional study. *Geriatr. Gerontol. Int.* **2020**, *20*, 256–260. [CrossRef]
34. Imagama, S.; Hasegawa, Y.; Matsuyama, Y.; Sakai, Y.; Ito, Z.; Hamajima, N.; Ishiguro, N. Influence of sagittal balance and physical ability associated with exercise on quality of life in middle-aged and elderly people. *Arch. Osteoporos.* **2011**, *6*, 13–20. [CrossRef]
35. Tanaka, S.; Ando, K.; Kobayashi, K.; Hida, T.; Ito, K.; Tsushima, M.; Morozumi, M.; Machino, M.; Ota, K.; Suzuki, K.; et al. Utility of the Serum Cystatin C Level for Diagnosis of Osteoporosis among Middle-Aged and Elderly People. *Biomed. Res. Int.* **2019**, *2019*, 5046852. [CrossRef]
36. Muramoto, A.; Imagama, S.; Ito, Z.; Hirano, K.; Tauchi, R.; Ishiguro, N.; Hasegawa, Y. Threshold values of physical performance tests for locomotive syndrome. *J. Orthop. Sci.* **2013**, *18*, 618–626. [CrossRef]
37. Imagama, S.; Hasegawa, Y.; Ando, K.; Kobayashi, K.; Hida, T.; Ito, K.; Tsushima, M.; Nishida, Y.; Ishiguro, N. Staged decrease of physical ability on the locomotive syndrome risk test is related to neuropathic pain, nociceptive pain, shoulder complaints, and quality of life in middle-aged and elderly people—The utility of the locomotive syndrome risk test. *Mod. Rheumatol.* **2017**, *27*, 1051–1056. [CrossRef]
38. Seichi, A.; Hoshino, Y.; Doi, T.; Akai, M.; Tobimatsu, Y.; Iwaya, T. Development of a screening tool for risk of locomotive syndrome in the elderly: The 25-question Geriatric Locomotive Function Scale. *J. Orthop. Sci.* **2012**, *17*, 163–172. [CrossRef]
39. Sogami, M.; Era, S.; Nagaoka, S.; Kuwata, K.; Kida, K.; Miura, K.; Inouye, H.; Suzuki, E.; Hayano, S.; Sawada, S. HPLC-studies on nonmercapt-mercapt conversion of human serum albumin. *Int. J. Pept. Protein Res.* **1985**, *25*, 398–402. [CrossRef]
40. Ueyama, J.; Ishikawa, Y.; Kondo, T.; Motoyama, M.; Matsumoto, H.; Matsushita, T. A revised method for determination of serum mercaptalbumin and non-mercaptalbumin by high-performance liquid chromatography coupled with postcolumn bromocresol green reaction. *Ann. Clin. Biochem.* **2015**, *52*, 144–150. [CrossRef]
41. Maeda, K.; Yoshizaki, S.; Iida, T.; Terada, T.; Era, S.; Sakashita, K.; Arikawa, H. Improvement of the fraction of human mercaptalbumin on hemodialysis treatment using hydrogen-dissolved hemodialysis fluid: A prospective observational study. *Ren. Replace. Ther.* **2016**, *2*, 42. [CrossRef]

42. Oettl, K.; Marsche, G. Redox state of human serum albumin in terms of cysteine-34 in health and disease. *Methods Enzymol.* **2010**, *474*, 181–195. [CrossRef] [PubMed]
43. Anraku, M.; Chuang, V.T.; Maruyama, T.; Otagiri, M. Redox properties of serum albumin. *Biochim. Biophys. Acta* **2013**, *1830*, 5465–5472. [CrossRef] [PubMed]
44. Ishibashi, H. Locomotive syndrome in Japan. *Osteoporos Sarcopenia* **2018**, *4*, 86–94. [CrossRef]
45. Michaud, M.; Balardy, L.; Moulis, G.; Gaudin, C.; Peyrot, C.; Vellas, B.; Cesari, M.; Nourhashemi, F. Proinflammatory cytokines, aging, and age-related diseases. *J. Am. Med. Dir. Assoc.* **2013**, *14*, 877–882. [CrossRef]
46. Arena, S.K.; Doherty, D.J.; Bellford, A.; Hayman, G. Effects of Aerobic Exercise on Oxidative Stress in Patients Diagnosed with Cancer: A Narrative Review. *Cureus* **2019**, *11*, e5382. [CrossRef]

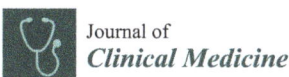 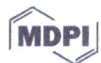

Article

Prevalence and Characteristics of Spinal Sagittal Malalignment in Patients with Osteoporosis

Takayuki Matsunaga [1], Masayuki Miyagi [1,*], Toshiyuki Nakazawa [1], Kosuke Murata [1], Ayumu Kawakubo [1], Hisako Fujimaki [1], Tomohisa Koyama [1], Akiyoshi Kuroda [1], Yuji Yokozeki [1], Yusuke Mimura [1], Eiki Shirasawa [1], Wataru Saito [1], Takayuki Imura [1], Kentaro Uchida [1], Yuta Nanri [2], Kazuhide Inage [3], Tsutomu Akazawa [4], Seiji Ohtori [4], Masashi Takaso [1] and Gen Inoue [1]

[1] Department of Orthopaedic Surgery, School of Medicine, Kitasato University, Kanagawa 252-0374, Japan; auaa.0718.aaui@gmail.com (T.M.); nakazawa@kitasato-u.ac.jp (T.N.); nineball5121@yahoo.co.jp (K.M.); ayumukawakubo0827@gmail.com (A.K.); hisako19830608@yahoo.co.jp (H.F.); tomohisakoyama1989@gmail.com (T.K.); akiyoshikvroda@yahoo.co.jp (A.K.); yuji0328yoko@yahoo.co.jp (Y.Y.); msm.men.36@gmail.com (Y.M.); eeiikkii922@yahoo.co.jp (E.S.); boatwataru0712@gmail.com (W.S.); tk2003@kitasato-u.ac.jp (T.I.); kuchida@med.kitasato-u.ac.jp (K.U.); mtakaso@kitasato-u.ac.jp (M.T.); ginoue@kitasato-u.ac.jp (G.I.)

[2] Department of Rehabilitation, Kitasato University Hospital, Sagamihara 252-0374, Japan; nanriyuta.rpt-103@hotmail.co.jp

[3] Department of Orthopedic Surgery, Graduate School of Medicine, Chiba University, Chiba 260-8670, Japan; kazuhideinage@chiba-u.jp

[4] Department of Orthopaedic Surgery, School of Medicine, St. Marianna University, Kawasaki 216-8511, Japan; cds00350@par.odn.ne.jp (T.A.); sohtori@faculty.chiba-u.jp (S.O.)

* Correspondence: masayuki008@aol.com; Tel.: +81-42-778-8111

Citation: Matsunaga, T.; Miyagi, M.; Nakazawa, T.; Murata, K.; Kawakubo, A.; Fujimaki, H.; Koyama, T.; Kuroda, A.; Yokozeki, Y.; Mimura, Y.; et al. Prevalence and Characteristics of Spinal Sagittal Malalignment in Patients with Osteoporosis. J. Clin. Med. 2021, 10, 2827. https://doi.org/10.3390/jcm10132827

Academic Editor: Alexandra Lucas

Received: 27 April 2021
Accepted: 24 June 2021
Published: 26 June 2021

Publisher's Note: MDPI stays neutral with regard to jurisdictional claims in published maps and institutional affiliations.

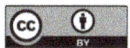

Copyright: © 2021 by the authors. Licensee MDPI, Basel, Switzerland. This article is an open access article distributed under the terms and conditions of the Creative Commons Attribution (CC BY) license (https://creativecommons.org/licenses/by/4.0/).

Abstract: Spinal sagittal malalignment due to vertebral fractures (VFs) induces low back pain (LBP) in patients with osteoporosis. This study aimed to elucidate spinal sagittal malalignment prevalence based on VF number and patient characteristics in individuals with osteoporosis and spinal sagittal malalignment. Spinal sagittal alignment, and VF number were measured in 259 patients with osteoporosis. Spinal sagittal malalignment was defined according to the SRS-Schwab classification of adult spinal deformity. Spinal sagittal malalignment prevalence was evaluated based on VF number. In patients without VFs, bone mineral density, bone turnover markers, LBP scores and health-related quality of life (HRQoL) scores of normal and sagittal malalignment groups were compared. In 205 of the 259 (79.2%) patients, spinal sagittal malalignment was detected. Sagittal malalignment prevalence in patients with 0, 1, or ≥2 VFs was 72.1%, 86.0%, and 86.3%, respectively. All LBP scores and some subscale of HRQoL scores in patients without VFs were significantly worse for the sagittal malalignment group than the normal alignment group ($p < 0.05$). The majority of patients with osteoporosis had spinal sagittal malalignment, including ≥70% of patients without VFs. Patients with spinal sagittal malalignment reported worse LBP and HRQoL. These findings suggest that spinal sagittal malalignment is a risk factor for LBP and poor HRQoL in patients with osteoporosis.

Keywords: spinal sagittal alignment; osteoporosis; low back pain; health-related quality of life

1. Introduction

Patients with osteoporosis often report low back pain (LBP), particularly intermittent LBP such as vague LBP due to standing or walking for a long stretch of time. In clinical settings, the types of LBP reported tend be difficult to treat. Whether osteoporosis causes LBP is controversial because its pathological mechanism has not been fully elucidated. Several factors, including high bone turnover [1], low muscle mass [2], and vertebral fractures (VFs) [3], have been reported to be associated with increased risk of LBP and osteoporosis. In addition, it is well known that VFs induce spinal sagittal malalignment in osteoporosis patients [4].

Patients with spinal sagittal malalignment presenting as adult spinal deformity often complained of severe LBP that induced the deterioration of health-related quality of life (HRQoL), requiring treatment [5]. Patients with spinal deformity tend to be elderly individuals who also have osteoporosis. Therefore, osteoporosis might be associated with adult spinal deformity. Furthermore, it has been reported that osteoporotic patients with VFs showed worse spinal sagittal alignment and LBP and HRQoL scores [6]. However, the prevalence of spinal sagittal malalignment in osteoporosis patients remains unclear. Improving our understanding of the characteristics of patients with spinal sagittal malalignment may lead to the improvement of spinal sagittal malalignment treatment. The aim of this study was to elucidate the prevalence of spinal sagittal malalignment based on VF number and the characteristics of patients with osteoporosis and spinal sagittal malalignment.

2. Materials and Methods

2.1. Patient Population

The records of patients with osteoporosis who first visited these facilities from June 2015 to March 2017 were reviewed in this cross-sectional study. We excluded patients who developed new vertebral fractures within three months. The remaining 259 patients (48 men, 211 women; mean age: 71.5 years) were included.

2.2. Measurements

In all patients, we evaluated bone mineral density (BMD) of the lumbar spine (LS: L2–L4), femoral neck (FN), and total hip (TH), using dual-energy X-ray absorptiometry (DXA: Horizon DXA System; Hologic Inc., Santa Clara, CA, USA), and serum levels of bone turnover markers including bone-specific alkaline phosphatase (BAP; Beckman Coulter Inc. Brea, CA, USA) and tartrate-resistant acid phosphatase 5b (TRACP5b; DS Pharma Biomedical Inc., Osaka, Japan).

2.2.1. Radiographical Evaluation

X-ray images taken in frontal and lateral views of the whole spine, including the hip joints, in the standing position were reviewed to evaluate spinal sagittal alignment and VFs. For the evaluation of spinal sagittal alignment, three spinal sagittal alignment parameters were measured. To assess pelvic tilt (PT), the angle between the line joining the midpoint of the bilateral center of the femoral head to the center of the S1 endplate and a vertical reference line was measured. Pelvic incidence (PI) was determined by measuring the angle between a line joining the midpoint of the bilateral center of the femoral head to the center of the S1 endplate, and a line orthogonal to the S1 endplate, as previously reported [7]. To measure lumbar lordosis (LL), we assessed the angles between the first line parallel to the upper endplate of L1 and the second line parallel to the superior endplate of the sacral base on lateral views of the whole-spine radiograph. Then, PI-LL was used to evaluate spinal sagittal alignment. For measuring the sagittal vertical axis (SVA), the horizontal distance between the posterior-superior corner of the sacrum and a vertical line from the center of C7 was measured, as previously reported [8]. In accordance with the SRS-Schwab classification scheme [9], patients were categorized using three sagittal spinopelvic modifiers, including PT, PI-LL, and SVA. SVA > 40 mm, PT > 20°, or PI-LL > 10° was defined as spinal sagittal malalignment. Based on these data, subjects were divided into a normal alignment group and a sagittal malalignment group.

2.2.2. Clinical Outcome Evaluation

LBP was evaluated using the Japanese Orthopedic Association Back Pain Evaluation Questionnaire (JOABPEQ), the Oswestry Disability Index (ODI), and the visual analogue scale (VAS). JOABPEQ consists of five functional scores: pain-related disorders, lumbar spine dysfunction, gait disturbance, social life dysfunction, and psychological disorders. Each domain score ranges from 0 to 100, and higher scores corresponded to an improved patient condition.

In addition, HRQoL was evaluated using the MOS 36-Item Short-Form Health Survey (SF-36). SF-36 consists of 8 subscales, as follows: physical function, PF; role physical, RP; body pain, BP; general health, GH; vitality, VT; social functioning, SF; role emotional, RE; and mental health, MH. The score for each domain ranged from 0 to 100, and higher scores indicated a better condition.

2.3. Statistical Analysis

First, the prevalence of a spinal sagittal malalignment was evaluated based on the number of VFs identified. Factors including age, BMD, serum levels of bone turnover markers, and parameters of spinal sagittal alignment of the three groups of patients with 0, 1, and ≥2 VFs were compared using the Bonferroni test for multiple comparisons. Sex and the spinal sagittal alignment differences were compared using the chi-squared test.

Characteristics of spinal sagittal malalignment evaluated in sagittal malalignment and normal alignment groups in patients without VFs were compared. Leven's test was used to assess variance for variables of interest. To assess data with unequal variance, the Mann–Whitney U test was applied. An unpaired t-test was used to assess data with equal variance. All data were analyzed using IBM SPSS Statistics version 26 (IBM, Atmonk, NY, USA), and $p < 0.05$ were considered significant.

2.4. Ethics

Ethical approval from Institutional Review Board in Kitasato University was obtained for this study (Approval code, #B17–197), which was conducted in accordance with the ethical principles specified in the 1964 Declaration of Helsinki and its later amendments.

3. Results

Characteristics of the patient population and BMD, serum levels of bone turnover markers, and parameters of spinal sagittal alignment, are listed in Table 1. Spinal malalignment was observed in 205 of 259 (79.2%) patients. BMDs of the FN and TH in the group with ≥2 VF were significantly lower than those of the 0 group. The BMD of the TH in the group with 1 VF was significantly lower than that of the 0 VF group ($p < 0.05$).

Table 1. The patient population of this study.

			Total		VF: 0		VF: 1		VF: ≥2		Comparison
	N		259		129		50		80		-
	Sex (M:W)		48:211		18:111		9:41		21:59		N.S.
			mean	SD	mean	SD	mean	SD	mean	SD	
	Age		71.5	10.3	69.6	9.5	72.4	10.8	73.8	10.8	N.S.
		LS	0.783	0.169	0.776	0.166	0.786	0.153	0.791	0.185	N.S.
BMD		FN	0.558	0.118	0.586	0.122	0.543	0.099	0.522	0.113	VF: 0 vs. ≥2 $p < 0.05$
		TH	0.623	0.132	0.652	0.136	0.591	0.126	0.596	0.121	VF: 0 vs. 1, 0 vs. ≥2 $p < 0.05$
Bone turnover marker		BAP	14.8	12.5	14.2	14.6	15.3	10.0	15.5	9.9	N.S.
		TRACP5b	407	244	390	198	406	231	436	309	N.S.
Spinal sagittal alignment		PT	24.8	11.9	22.4	11.2	26.2	10.4	27.6	13.3	VF: 0 vs. ≥2 $p < 0.05$
		PI-LL	15.1	21.3	13.1	20.3	16.5	18.4	17.6	24.4	N.S.
		SVA	60.4	68.4	48.6	64.8	69.1	62.8	74.0	74.5	VF: 0 vs. ≥2 $p < 0.05$
JOABPEQ	pain-related disorders		77.3	31.6	77.3	31.6	62.2	32.4	66.1	32.2	VF: 0 vs. 1, 0 vs. ≥2 $p < 0.05$
	lumbar spine dysfunction		69.9	29.1	78.1	26.3	64.1	26.8	60.4	31.1	VF: 0 vs. 1, 0 vs. ≥2 $p < 0.05$
	gait disturbance		61.5	34.7	72.6	31.5	54.1	34.0	48.1	34.3	VF: 0 vs. 1, 0 vs. ≥2 $p < 0.05$
	social life dysfunction		58.2	27.5	68.2	25.8	52.4	26.7	45.5	24.5	VF: 0 vs. 1, 0 vs. ≥2 $p < 0.05$
	psychological disorders		49.6	17.3	54.7	17.3	44.2	15.9	44.9	15.8	VF: 0 vs. 1, 0 vs. ≥2 $p < 0.05$
	ODI		26.7	20.7	20.3	18.5	29.3	19.6	35.5	21.3	VF: 0 vs. 1, 0 vs. ≥2 $p < 0.05$
	VAS		3.3	3.8	2.6	2.4	3.7	3.0	4.2	5.5	VF: 0 vs. ≥2 $p < 0.05$

Table 1. Cont.

		Total		VF: 0		VF: 1		VF: ≥2		Comparison
SF-36	PF	63.7	43.3	74.7	52.4	57.8	27.4	49.9	28.1	VF: 0 vs. ≥2 $p < 0.05$
	RP	60.3	31.7	71.5	26.8	54.0	32.1	46.3	32.2	VF: 0 vs. 1, 0 vs. ≥2 $p < 0.05$
	BP	53.4	25.4	59.3	24.1	46.8	25.1	47.9	25.6	VF: 0 vs. 1, 0 vs. ≥2 $p < 0.05$
	GH	44.9	16.8	48.2	15.8	42.4	18.0	41.2	16.9	VF: 0 vs. ≥2 $p < 0.05$
	VT	51.7	21.6	55.8	21.5	49.5	22.4	46.5	20.0	VF: 0 vs. ≥2 $p < 0.05$
	SF	69.7	28.7	76.4	27.3	64.0	26.3	62.4	29.9	VF: 0 vs. 1, 0 vs. ≥2 $p < 0.05$
	RE	63.8	33.4	74.1	28.8	56.1	32.0	51.9	36.2	VF: 0 vs. 1, 0 vs. ≥2 $p < 0.05$
	MH	63.7	20.8	68.3	20.0	59.7	21.7	58.8	20.1	VF: 0 vs. 1, 0 vs. ≥2 $p < 0.05$
		N	%	N	%	N	%	N	%	
	normal alignment	54	20.8	36	27.9	7	14.0	11	13.8	$p < 0.05$
	malalignment	205	79.2	93	72.1	43	86.0	69	86.3	

BMD: body mass index, LS: lumbar spine, FN: femoral neck, TH: total hip, BAP: bone-specific alkaline phosphatase, TRACP5b: tartrate-resistant acid phosphatase 5b, PT: pelvic tilt, PI-LL: pelvic incidence minus lumbar lordosis, SVA: sagittal vertical axis, VF: vertebral fracture, JOABPEQ: Japanese Orthopedic Association Back Pain Evaluation Questionnaire, ODI: Oswestry Disability Index, VAS: visual analogue scale of low back pain, SF-36: MOS 36-Item Short-Form Health Survey, PF: physical function, RP: role physical, BP: body pain, GH: general health, VT: vitality, SF: social functioning, RE: role emotional, MH: mental health.

With regard to spinal sagittal alignment parameters, PT and SVA values of the ≥2 VF group was significantly higher than that of the 0 VF group ($p < 0.05$). No significant differences between 0, 1, ≥2 VF groups were observed with regard to BMD, bone turnover markers, and PI-LL ($p > 0.05$). The prevalence of a spinal sagittal malalignment in patients with 0, 1, or ≥2 VFs was 72.1%, 86.0%, and 86.3%, respectively, and differences among the three groups were determined as significant ($p < 0.05$) (Table 1).

With regard to LBP and the HRQoL score, all five domains of JOABPEQ, ODI, and VAS, as well as all eight subscales of the SF-36 of the ≥2 VF group, were significantly worse than those of the 0 VF group ($p < 0.05$). In addition, the values of all five domains of JOABPEQ, ODI, RP, BP, SF, RE, and MH of SF-36 in the 1 VF group were significantly worse than those in the 0 VF group ($p < 0.05$) (Table 1).

In a sub-analysis of patients without VFs, no significant differences were observed between the sagittal malalignment group and the normal alignment group with regard to age; LS, FN, and TH of BMD; or bone turnover markers, including BAP and TRACP5b ($p > 0.05$) (Figure 1). In contrast, all five JOABPEQ functional scores (including pain-related disorders, lumbar spine dysfunction, gait disturbance, social life dysfunction, and psychological disorders) of the sagittal malalignment group were significantly lower than those of the normal alignment group ($p < 0.05$) (Figure 2A). Furthermore, ODI and the VAS values determined for LBP in patients without VFs were significantly higher in the sagittal malalignment group than in the normal alignment group ($p < 0.05$) (Figure 2B,C). Additionally, PF, RP, VT, RE, and MH of SF-36 values of the sagittal malalignment group were significantly lower than those of the normal alignment group ($p < 0.05$) (Figure 3).

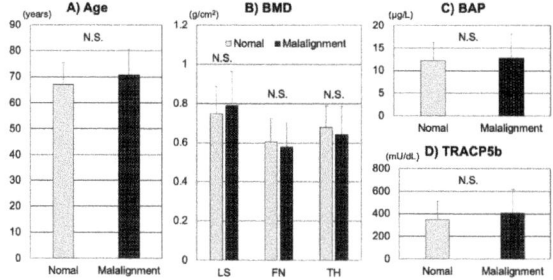

Figure 1. In patients without VFs, comparisons of (**A**) age, (**B**) BMD, (**C**) BAP, and (**D**) TRACP5b values determined in patients of the normal alignment and sagittal malalignment groups are shown. VF, vertebral fracture; N.S.: not significant; BMD, bone mineral density; BAP, bone-specific alkaline phosphatase; TRACP5b, tartrate-resistant acid phosphatase 5b.

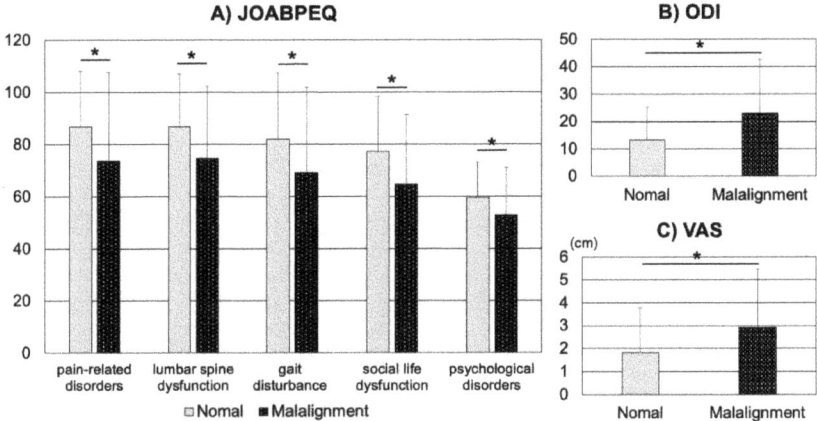

Figure 2. In patients without VFs, comparisons of (**A**) JOABPEQ, (**B**) ODI, and (**C**) VAS of LBP for patients of the normal alignment and sagittal malalignment groups are shown. VF, vertebral fracture; LBP, low back pain; ODI, Oswestry Disability Index; JOABPEQ, Japanese Orthopedic Association Back Pain Evaluation Questionnaire; VAS, Visual Analogue Scale, * $p < 0.05$.

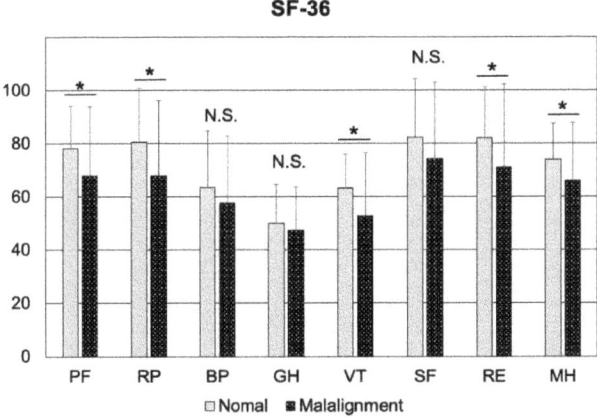

Figure 3. A comparison of MOS 36-Item Short-Form Health Survey scores of normal alignment and sagittal malalignment groups in patients without VFs is shown. VF, vertebral fracture; PF: Physical function, RP: Role physical, BP: Body pain, GH: General health, VT: Vitality, SF: Social functioning, RE: Role emotional, MH: Mental health, N.S.: not significant, * $p < 0.05$.

4. Discussion

In the current study, the prevalence of spinal sagittal malalignment in osteoporosis patients was determined to be 79.2%. Furthermore, as the number of VFs increased, the prevalence of spinal sagittal malalignment also increased and LBP and HRQoL scores worsened. Interestingly, more than 70% of osteoporosis patients without VFs had spinal sagittal malalignment. Additionally, in patients without VFs, patients with spinal sagittal malalignment had worse LBP and HRQoL scores than patients with normal alignment.

Regarding the relationship between VFs and spinal sagittal alignment, as the number of VFs increased, the prevalence of spinal sagittal malalignment also increased, and LBP and HRQoL scores worsened in this study. Mochizuki et al. previously reported that spinal sagittal alignment is associated with age and VF in patients with rheumatoid arthritis [10]. In addition, osteoporosis patients with VFs have worse global sagittal alignment and a worsened quality of life [6]. Scaturro et al. reported that the severity of LBP is correlated with the number of vertebral fractures [11]. These findings indicate that VFs are closely correlated with sagittal spinal malalignment and affect LBP as well as HRQoL.

With regard to cause-and-effect relationships between VFs and spinal sagittal malalignment, Zhang et al. reported that multiple VFs lead to spinal sagittal malalignment in patients with osteoporosis [12]. In contrast, several authors reported that spinal sagittal malalignment was a potential risk factor for increased VF incidence in patients with osteoporosis [4,13,14]. These findings indicate that VFs induce spinal sagittal malalignment; spinal sagittal malalignment also leads to VFs in patients with osteoporosis.

In the current study, more than 70% of patients with osteoporosis without VFs had spinal sagittal malalignment. In a longitudinal study with a minimum of 10 years of follow-up, Takeda et al. reported that spinal sagittal malalignment, decreased lumbar lordosis, and increased SVA were correlated with age in patients without VFs [15]. Regarding the underlying mechanism of spinal sagittal malalignment in patients without VFs, several authors reported a relationship between spinal sagittal malalignment and decreased muscle mass in patients with spinal diseases [16,17]. Additionally, Scaturro et al. reported that combination treatments with medication and postural training/resistance exercises showed improvements in the pain and QoL for patients with osteoporosis undergoing rehabilitation [18]. These findings indicate that decreasing muscle mass may induce spinal sagittal malalignment.

In the current study, the majority of osteoporosis patients had spinal sagittal malalignment. In recent years, several authors reported that long spinal fusion and corrective surgery for spinal sagittal malalignment could be used to achieve good spinal alignment. Improvements were due to recent, remarkable developments in surgical techniques and spinal instruments and contributed to improvements in ADL and LBP outcomes [19,20]. However, high perioperative complication rates for long spinal fusion and corrective surgery have been reported [21]. Therefore, performing the highly invasive and costly surgery in all osteoporosis patients is not advisable. Alternatively, we should consider early intervention for spinal sagittal malalignment in osteoporosis patients, which may prevent the need for surgery to correct adult spinal deformity.

When investigating relationships between spinal sagittal alignment and LBP or HRQoL, Schwab et al. reported that high SVA, PI-LL, and PT values induced the deterioration of HRQoL in elderly adult patients with spinal deformity and a defined SRS-Schwab classification [9]. Similarly, the current study reported that osteoporosis patients with spinal sagittal malalignment and a defined SRS-Schwab Classification had some reduced HRQoL subscale values, including PF, RP, VT, RE, and MH. On the other hand, results of a meta-analysis by Chun et al. indicated that LBP was strongly correlated with decreased LL, especially when affected patients were compared with age-matched healthy controls [22]. Additionally, Miyakoshi et al. reported that decreased LL and the limitation of total spinal extension are important risk factors for gait disturbance in patients with chronic LBP [23]. These findings indicate that osteoporosis patients with spinal sagittal malalignment, even those without VFs, had worse HRQoL and LBP compared with patients with normal spinal sagittal alignment. Further, spinal sagittal malalignment is a potential risk factor for LBP and HRQoL in patients with osteoporosis.

The current study had some limitations. First, we did not evaluate medication status, such as use of painkillers and osteoporosis medications. In addition, we included patients with osteoporosis who first visited our department, although many patients had already undergone an intervention during their consultation. Painkillers and osteoporosis medication use might affect HRQoL as well as LBP. Second, this was a cross-sectional study; therefore, we could not evaluate cause-and-effect relationships among spinal sagittal malalignment, VFs, LBP, and HRQoL. Additionally, the patho-mechanism of spinal sagittal malalignment in patients without VFs remains unclear. To further understand these mechanisms, additional studies with larger sample sizes and a longitudinal design are needed.

5. Conclusions

The majority of patients with osteoporosis had spinal sagittal malalignment, and more than 70% of patients without VFs, had spinal sagittal malalignment. Furthermore, patients with spinal sagittal malalignment had worse LBP and HRQoL compared with patients with normal spinal sagittal alignment. These findings suggest that spinal sagittal malalignment is a potential risk factor for LBP and HRQoL in patients with osteoporosis.

Author Contributions: T.M. and M.M. revised the manuscript and participated in the formulation of the study design. T.N. drafted the manuscript and collected clinical data. K.M., A.K. (Ayumu Kawakubo), H.F., T.K., A.K. (Akiyoshi Kuroda), Y.Y., Y.M. and Y.N. collected clinical data, and E.S., W.S., T.I., K.I., T.A. and S.O. helped to revise the manuscript. K.U. carried out statistical analyses, and M.T. and G.I. conceived the study, participated in the formulation of its design and coordinated the work. T.M. and M.M. equally contributed in this study. All authors have read and agreed to the published version of the manuscript.

Funding: This investigation was supported in part by JOA-Subsidized Science Project Research 2018-2.

Institutional Review Board Statement: The study was conducted according to the guidelines of the Declaration of Helsinki, and approved by Institutional Review Board in Kitasato University (Approval code, #B17–197).

Informed Consent Statement: Informed consent was obtained from all subjects involved in the study.

Data Availability Statement: The data presented in this study are available on request from the corresponding author.

Acknowledgments: We thank Motoki Makabe, Yukie Arai, Kazue Takakura and Ikumi Sekihara for their assistance with this study. M.M., Y.A., K.T. and I.S. have agreed to the published version of the manuscript.

Conflicts of Interest: The authors declare that there is no conflict of interest.

References

1. Ohtori, S.; Akazawa, T.; Murata, Y.; Kinoshita, T.; Yamashita, M.; Nakagawa, K.; Inoue, G.; Nakamura, J.; Orita, S.; Ochiai, N.; et al. Risedronate decreases bone resorption and improves low back pain in postmenopausal osteoporosis patients without vertebral fractures. *J. Clin. Neurosci.* **2010**, *17*, 209–213. [CrossRef]
2. Hori, Y.; Hoshino, M.; Inage, K.; Miyagi, M.; Takahashi, S.; Ohyama, S.; Suzuki, A.; Tsujio, T.; Terai, H.; Dohzono, S.; et al. ISSLS PRIZE IN CLINICAL SCIENCE 2019: Clinical importance of trunk muscle mass for low back pain, spinal balance, and quality of life-a multicenter cross-sectional study. *Eur. Spine J.* **2019**, *28*, 914–921. [CrossRef]
3. Ahmadi, S.A.; Takahashi, S.; Hoshino, M.; Takayama, K.; Sasaoka, R.; Tsujio, T.; Yasuda, H.; Kanematsu, F.; Kono, H.; Toyoda, H.; et al. Association between MRI findings and back pain after osteoporotic vertebral fractures: A multicenter prospective cohort study. *Spine J.* **2019**, *19*, 1186–1193. [CrossRef] [PubMed]
4. Dai, J.; Yu, X.; Huang, S.; Fan, L.; Zhu, G.; Sun, H.; Tang, X. Relationship between sagittal spinal alignment and the incidence of vertebral fracture in menopausal women with osteoporosis: A multicenter longitudinal follow-up study. *Eur. Spine J.* **2015**, *24*, 737–743. [CrossRef]
5. Matsuyama, Y. Surgical treatment for adult spinal deformity: Conceptual approach and surgical strategy. *Spine Surg. Relat. Res.* **2017**, *1*, 56–60. [CrossRef]
6. Hu, Z.; Man, G.C.W.; Kwok, A.K.L.; Law, S.W.; Chu, W.W.C.; Cheung, W.H.; Qiu, Y.; Cheng, J.C.Y. Global sagittal alignment in elderly patients with osteoporosis and its relationship with severity of vertebral fracture and quality of life. *Arch. Osteoporos.* **2018**, *13*, 95. [CrossRef] [PubMed]
7. Duval-Beaupère, G.; Schmidt, C.; Cosson, P. A Barycentremetric study of the sagittal shape of spine and pelvis: The conditions required for an economic standing position. *Ann. Biomed. Eng.* **1992**, *20*, 451–462. [CrossRef]
8. Van Royen, B.J.; Toussaint, H.M.; Kingma, I.; Bot, S.D.; Caspers, M.; Harlaar, J.; Wuisman, P.I. Accuracy of the sagittal vertical axis in a standing lateral radiograph as a measurement of balance in spinal deformities. *Eur. Spine J.* **1998**, *7*, 408–412. [CrossRef] [PubMed]
9. Schwab, F.; Ungar, B.; Blondel, B.; Buchowski, J.; Coe, J.; Deinlein, D.; DeWald, C.; Mehdian, H.; Shaffrey, C.; Tribus, C.; et al. Scoliosis research society-schwab adult spinal deformity classification: A validation study. *Spine* **2012**, *37*, 1077–1082. [CrossRef]
10. Mochizuki, T.; Yano, K.; Shirahata, T.; Ikari, K.; Hiroshima, R.; Nasu, Y.; Okazaki, K. Spinal sagittal balance associated with age, vertebral fracture, and functional disability in patients with rheumatoid arthritis: A cross-sectional study. *Mod. Rheumatol.* **2020**, *30*, 1002–1008. [CrossRef]

11. Scaturro, D.; Lauricella, L.; Tumminelli, L.G.; Tomasello, S.; Mauro, G.L. Is there a relationship between mild-moderate back pain and fragility fractures? Original investigation. *Acta Med. Mediterr.* **2020**, *36*, 2149–2153. [CrossRef]
12. Zhang, Y.L.; Shi, L.T.; Tang, P.F.; Sun, Z.J.; Wang, Y.H. Correlation analysis of osteoporotic vertebral compression fractures and spinal sagittal imbalance. *Orthopade* **2017**, *46*, 249–255. [CrossRef]
13. Kobayashi, T.; Takeda, N.; Atsuta, Y.; Matsuno, T. Flattening of sagittal spinal curvature as a predictor of vertebral fracture. *Osteoporos. Int.* **2008**, *19*, 65–69. [CrossRef] [PubMed]
14. Ohnishi, T.; Iwata, A.; Kanayama, M.; Oha, F.; Hashimoto, T.; Iwasaki, N. Impact of spino-pelvic and global spinal alignment on the risk of osteoporotic vertebral collapse. *Spine Surg. Relat. Res.* **2018**, *2*, 72–76. [CrossRef]
15. Takeda, N.; Kobayashi, T.; Atsuta, Y.; Matsuno, T.; Shirado, O.; Minami, A. Changes in the sagittal spinal alignment of the elderly without vertebral fractures: A minimum 10-year longitudinal study. *J. Orthop. Sci.* **2009**, *14*, 748–753. [CrossRef]
16. Eguchi, Y.; Suzuki, M.; Yamanaka, H.; Tamai, H.; Kobayashi, T.; Orita, S.; Yamauchi, K.; Suzuki, M.; Inage, K.; Fujimoto, K.; et al. Influence of skeletal muscle mass and spinal alignment on surgical outcomes for lumbar spinal stenosis. *Asian Spine J.* **2018**, *12*, 556–562. [CrossRef] [PubMed]
17. Hiyama, A.; Katoh, H.; Sakai, D.; Sato, M.; Tanaka, M.; Nukaga, T.; Watanabe, M. Correlation analysis of sagittal alignment and skeletal muscle mass in patients with spinal degenerative disease. *Sci. Rep.* **2018**, *8*, 15492. [CrossRef] [PubMed]
18. Scaturro, D.; Rizzo, S.; Sanfilippo, V.; Giustino, V.; Messina, G.; Martines, F.; Falco, V.; Cuntrera, D.; Moretti, A.; Iolascon, G.; et al. Effectiveness of rehabilitative intervention on pain, postural balance, and quality of life in women with multiple vertebral fragility fractures: A prospective cohort study. *J. Funct. Morphol. Kinesiol.* **2021**, *6*, 24. [CrossRef]
19. Kondo, R.; Yamato, Y.; Nagafusa, T.; Mizushima, T.; Hasegawa, T.; Kobayashi, S.; Togawa, D.; Oe, S.; Kurosu, K.; Matsuyama, Y. Effect of corrective long spinal fusion to the ilium on physical function in patients with adult spinal deformity. *Eur. Spine J.* **2017**, *26*, 2138–2145. [CrossRef]
20. Hayashi, K.; Boissière, L.; Guevara-Villazón, F.; Larrieu, D.; Núñez-Pereira, S.; Bourghli, A.; Gille, O.; Vital, J.M.; Pellisé, F.; Sánchez Pérez-Grueso, F.J.; et al. Factors influencing patient satisfaction after adult scoliosis and spinal deformity surgery. *J. Neurosurg. Spine* **2019**, *31*, 408–417. [CrossRef]
21. Yoshida, G.; Hasegawa, T.; Yamato, Y.; Kobayashi, S.; Oe, S.; Banno, T.; Mihara, Y.; Arima, H.; Ushirozako, H.; Yasuda, T.; et al. Predicting perioperative complications in adult spinal deformity surgery using a simple sliding scale. *Spine* **2018**, *43*, 562–570. [CrossRef] [PubMed]
22. Chun, S.W.; Lim, C.Y.; Kim, K.; Hwang, J.; Chung, S.G. The relationships between low back pain and lumbar lordosis: A systematic review and meta-analysis. *Spine J.* **2017**, *17*, 1180–1191. [CrossRef] [PubMed]
23. Miyakoshi, N.; Kasukawa, Y.; Ishikawa, Y.; Nozaka, K.; Shimada, Y. Spinal alignment and mobility in subjects with chronic low back pain with walking disturbance: A community-dwelling study. *Tohoku J. Exp. Med.* **2010**, *221*, 53–59. [CrossRef] [PubMed]

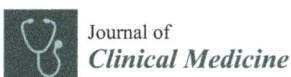 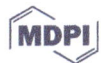

Article

The Level of Conus Medullaris in 629 Healthy Japanese Individuals

Hiroaki Nakashima [1,*], Keigo Ito [2], Yoshito Katayama [2], Mikito Tsushima [2], Kei Ando [1], Kazuyoshi Kobayashi [1], Masaaki Machino [1], Sadayuki Ito [1], Hiroyuki Koshimizu [1], Naoki Segi [1], Hiroyuki Tomita [1] and Shiro Imagama [1]

[1] Department of Orthopaedic Surgery, Nagoya University Graduate School of Medicine, Nagoya 466-8560, Japan; andokei@med.nagoya-u.ac.jp (K.A.); k_koba1@f2.dion.ne.jp (K.K.); masaaki_machino_5445_2@yahoo.co.jp (M.M.); sadaito@med.nagoya-u.ac.jp (S.I.); love_derika@yahoo.co.jp (H.K.); naoki.s.n@gmail.com (N.S.); hiro_tomi_1031@yahoo.co.jp (H.T.); imagama@med.nagoya-u.ac.jp (S.I.)

[2] Department of Orthopedic Surgery, Chubu Rosai Hospital, 1-10-6 Komei, Minato-ku, Nagoya 455-8530, Japan; spine.ort@chubuh.johas.go.jp (K.I.); yokatayama@hotmail.com (Y.K.); meikeihan@hotmail.com (M.T.)

* Correspondence: hirospine@med.nagoya-u.ac.jp

Abstract: The conus medullaris typically terminates at the L1 level; however, variations in its level and the factors associated with the conus medullaris level are unclear. We investigated the level of conus medullaris on magnetic resonance imaging in healthy volunteers. In total, 629 healthy adult volunteers (≥50 individuals of each sex and in each decade of age from 20 to 70) were enrolled. The level of the conus medullaris was assessed based on the T2-weighted sagittal magnetic resonance images, and factors affecting its level were investigated employing multivariate regression analysis including the participants' background and radiographical parameters. L1 was the most common conus medullaris level. Participant height was significantly shorter in the caudally placed conus medullaris ($p = 0.013$). With respect to the radiographical parameters, pelvic incidence ($p = 0.003$), and pelvic tilt ($p = 0.03$) were significantly smaller in participants with a caudally placed conus medullaris. Multiple regression analysis showed that the pelvic incidence ($p < 0.0001$) and height ($p < 0.0001$) were significant factors affecting the conus medullaris level. These results indicated that the length of the spinal cord varies little among individuals and that skeletal differences affect the level of the conus medullaris.

Keywords: conus medullaris; height; pelvic incidence; magnetic resonance imaging; healthy volunteers

1. Introduction

The conus medullaris is located at the terminal end of the spinal cord. The lowermost tapering extremity of the spinal cord is called the conus medullaris [1–6]. The thoracolumbar junction includes the conus medullaris and cauda equina. Injury to these neurological structures is associated with functional consequences. The conus medullaris and cauda equina are a transition point from the central to the peripheral nervous system, and injury to this point can result in a series of upper and lower motor neuron symptoms, depending on the location of the injury.

Although its level varies between T12 and lower L2, it typically lies at the inferior aspect of the L1 vertebra in adults [1–6]. The level of the conus medullaris is important in spinal anesthesia and spinal surgeries. However, few studies have investigated the factors affecting the conus medullaris level; sex, and age have been reported as potential factors [5–8]. With respect to children, the conus medullaris is placed caudally to L2 vertebrae in children younger than 1 year of age; however, it is found in the lower third of L1 after 1 year of age [6,8]. There remains controversy as to whether age affects the conus medullaris level in adults [9], and the influence of sex is also controversial.

The problems with previous studies are that (1) few large-scale studies involving older adults have been performed employing magnetic resonance imaging (MRI); (2) few studies have investigated the physical aspect of the participants, such as height and weight; and (3) there are no reports on the relationship between spinal alignment on X-ray photographs (Xp) and conus medullaris on MRI. Also, the significant factors affecting the level of the conus medullaris in adults are unclear. The aim of the current study was to investigate the levels of conus medullaris on MRI in healthy individuals and identify the factors that determine the conus medullaris location, including body size and radiographical spinal alignment.

2. Materials and Methods

2.1. Study Participants

Japanese volunteers were prospectively recruited after the purpose of this study was officially announced and after obtaining institutional review board approval from the Chubu Rosai Hospital (IRB approval no., 2009-2). Written informed consent was obtained from all participants. As part of a comprehensive medical examination, the study was conducted after consent was obtained from subjects who wanted spinal examinations. Participants were offered free feedback on findings from spine radiographs and MRIs, rather than monetary rewards. All of the included volunteers understood the negative effects of radiation exposure and agreed to undergo an X-ray examination. We prospectively recruited the subjects using newspaper advertisements and posters in facilities having some sort of relationship with our hospital. The majority of the subjects were not patients at our hospital but relatively healthy residents of the area. This study was registered in the research database at the Rosai Hospital in Japan.

The exclusion criteria included a history of brain or spinal surgery; comorbid neurological disease, such as cerebral infarction or neuropathy; symptoms related to sensory or motor disorders (numbness, clumsiness, motor weakness, or gait disturbances); intermittent claudication; and severe low back pain. Visual analogue scale (VAS) measurements of the lower back, buttock, and leg pain were taken before deciding on the inclusion of patients in this study and excluded cases with severe pain anywhere above 80 mm as cases with severe pain. Pregnant women and individuals who received worker's compensation or who presented with symptoms after a motor vehicle accident were also excluded. If radiographic measurements of the sagittal parameters were difficult to assess due to lumbosacral transitional anomalies, the participants were also excluded. We also excluded cases with a previous medical history of vertebral fracture, spinal infection, rheumatoid arthritis, autoimmune diseases, or chronic renal failure. In contrast, we included cases with diabetes mellitus or smoking history. Finally, 629 individuals with appropriate images were enrolled: the study population included at least 50 participants of each sex and each decade of age from 20 to 70. The study included 308 men (50 in their 20s, 51 in their 30s, 50 in their 40s, 56 in their 50s, 51 in their 60s, and 50 in their 70s) and 321 women (53 in their 20s, 50 in their 30s, 57 in their 40s, 51 in their 50s, 60 in their 60s, and 50 in their 70s).

2.2. Radiographical Examinations

We performed MRI scans on a 1.5-Tesla superconducting magnet (Signa Horizon Excite HD version 12; GE Healthcare, UK). Scans were taken at slice thicknesses of 3 mm in the respective sagittal planes. We obtained T1-weighted images (fast spin-echo repetition time (TR), 450 ms; echo time (TE), 13 ms), and T2-weighted images (fast spin-echo TR, 4000 ms; TE, 85 ms). All images were transferred to the computer as Digital Imaging and Communications in Medicine (DICOM) data. The tip of the conus medullaris can be identified on midline sagittal T1- and T2-weighted MRI.

Furthermore, full-length, free-standing spinal radiographs with fists on the clavicles were obtained from all the participants. All the images were transferred to a computer as DICOM data. The sagittal vertical axis (SVA), cervical lordosis, thoracic kyphosis, lumbar lordosis (LL), pelvic incidence (PI), and pelvic tilt (PT) were measured. Each parameter was manually measured by experienced radiation technologists (single measurements by random raters) under the supervision of a certified spine surgeon, using imaging software (Osiris version4; Icestar Media Ltd., Essex, UK).

2.3. Statistical Analysis

Each variable was reported as the mean ± standard deviation. At first, we assessed the standard distribution of each parameter (age, height, weight, BMI, and radiographical parameters using the Kolmogorov-Smirnov test. After confirmation of the normal distribution, we employed the one-way ANOVA (post hoc Tukey) to investigate the differences for each parameter at the different conus medullaris levels. The Chi-square test was used for testing relationships between categorical variables. In addition, a multivariate regression analysis was performed to determine the significant contributory factors at each level of the conus medullaris. We employed the step-wise method for the multivariate regression analysis and included factors with a p-value of <0.05. p-values of <0.05 were considered to be indicative of statistical significance. All analyses were performed with the IBM SPSS Statistics for Windows, Version 27.0 (IBM Corp., Armonk, NY, USA).

3. Results

The conus medullaris level was Th11-12, T12, T12-L1, L1, L1-2, and L2 in 3 (0.5%), 46 (7.3%), 204 (32.4%), 288 (45.8%), 79 (12.6%), and 9 (1.4%) participants, respectively, and L1 was the most common level.

Next, we investigated the effect of the physique on the level of the conus medullaris. The participants' heights were significantly shorter in the caudally placed conus medullaris cases (163.7, 163.9, 163.2, 162.7, 159.5, and 157.4 cm in the Th11-12, T12, T12-L1, L1, L1-2, and L2 conus medullaris levels, respectively; $p = 0.013$). On the other hand, there were no significant differences related to gender ($p = 0.48$), body weight ($p = 0.14$) or body mass index (BMI) ($p = 0.96$) (Table 1). Age was also not significantly different among the conus medullaris levels ($p = 0.86$ in Table 1).

With respect to the relationship between the radiographical parameters and the conus medullaris levels, PI (62.0°, 58.0°, 55.0°, 52.7°, 50.9°, and 49.6° in the Th11-12, T12, T12-L1, L1, L1-2, and L2 conus medullaris level, respectively; $p = 0.003$) and PT (18.4°, 18.2°, 15.7°, 13.9°, 14.6°, and 12.4° in the Th11-12, T12, T12-L1, L1, L1-2, and L2 conus medullaris level, respectively; $p = 0.03$) were significantly smaller in the participants with caudal cauda equina (Table 2). The LL was smaller in the caudal levels of conus medullaris (56.7°, 52.1°, 50.5°, 49.1°, 46.9°, and 46.0° in the Th11-12, T12, T12-L1, L1, L1-2, and L2 conus medullaris level, respectively; $p = 0.10$), although the difference did not reach statistical significance. However, there were no significant differences in cervical lordosis, thoracic kyphosis, or SVA (Table 2).

In order to analyze the data in further detail, height, PI, and PT were divided into categories and examined again (Table 3). With respect to the PI, there was a significant difference ($p = 0.045$) when the conus medullaris was located in the cranial side in the case of high PI, but there was no significant difference in the cases of other heights ($p = 0.67$) and PT ($p = 0.12$).

Multiple regression analysis showed that PI (standardized β coefficient: −0.18, $p < 0.0001$) and height (standardized β coefficient: −0.16, $p < 0.0001$) were significant factors affecting the level of the conus medullaris, although age, sex, weight, BMI, and other radiographical parameters were not significant.

Table 1. The association between the conus medullaris level and patients' backgrounds.

	T11-12	T12	T12-L1	L1	L1-2	L2	p
age (yr)	39.7 ± 15.0	49.2 ± 15.5	49.0 ± 15.9	50.3 ± 17.0	49.6 ± 16.2	48.2 ± 23.4	0.86
gender (male/female)	0/3	20/26	96/108	146/142	41/38	5/4	0.48
height (cm)	163.7 ± 6.8	163.9 ± 9.8	163.2 ± 8.9	162.7 ± 8.7	159.5 ± 8.9	157.4 ± 10.8	0.013
body weight (kg)	60.7 ± 8.1	60.3 ± 12.1	60.6 ± 12.4	59.9 ± 10.6	56.8 ± 12.1	54.3 ± 6.7	0.14
BMI	22.7 ± 2.7	22.3 ± 3.5	22.6 ± 3.4	22.6 ± 3.1	22.2 ± 3.7	22.0 ± 2.4	0.97

yr: years of age, BMI: body mass index.

Table 2. The association between the conus medullaris level and radiographical parameters.

	T11-12	T12	T12-L1	L1	L1-2	L2	p
CL (°)	8.7 ± 8.5	4.0 ± 15.0	3.3 ± 10.8	4.5 ± 12.5	3.9 ± 11.7	12.6 ± 9.1	0.29
TK (°)	43.7 ± 8.3	32.8 ± 14.9	32.5 ± 19.7	34.9 ± 14.6	30.0 ± 18.6	36.2 ± 6.0	0.19
LL (°)	56.7 ± 11.4	52.1 ± 11.5	50.5 ± 11.9	49.1 ± 11.9	46.9 ± 14.3	46.0 ± 8.1	0.10
PI (°)	62.0 ± 12.2	58.0 ± 13.5	55.0 ± 12.0	52.7 ± 11.0	50.9 ± 11.5	49.6 ± 9.6	0.003
PT (°)	18.4 ± 7.8	18.2 ± 9.5	15.7 ± 9.0	13.9 ± 8.2	14.6 ± 10.6	12.4 ± 7.8	0.03
SVA (cm)	2.1 ± 4.9	3.0 ± 5.0	1.2 ± 5.4	1.8 ± 5.5	1.9 ± 6.5	1.7 ± 5.1	0.55

CL: cervical lordosis, TK: thoracic kyphosis, LL: lumbar lordosis, PI: pelvic incidence, PT: pelvic tilt, SVA: sagittal vertical axis.

Table 3. The distribution of each factor at the different levels of conus medullaris.

	Total Number of Cases	T11-12	T12	T12-L1	L1	L1-2	L2	p
Height								
≤150 cm	51	1	4	22	19	5	0	
150 to 175 cm	530	2	37	167	248	68	8	0.67
>175 cm	48	0	5	15	21	6	1	
PI								
<30°	4	0	0	2	1	1	0	
30–45°	139	0	7	41	69	19	3	0.045
45–60°	330	1	22	96	154	50	6	
>60°	156	2	17	64	64	9	0	
PT								
<20°	472	1	29	149	226	61	6	
20–30°	127	2	14	40	54	14	3	0.12
>30°	30	0	3	15	8	4	0	

Each number shows the number of cases. Statistical analysis was performed by using a Chi-square test.

4. Discussion

This study investigated the anatomical level of the conus medullaris and analyzed factors associated with the conus medullaris levels in 629 healthy volunteers. In the present study, the majority (92.2%) of the participants had the conus medullaris at the caudal level of the T12-L1 disk, and the conus medullaris was located cranially to the T12 vertebral level in only 7.8% of the participants. Among them, the T12-L1 disk and L1 vertebral body were the most common conus medullaris levels, which were 32.4% and 45.8%, respectively.

Our study demonstrated that shorter height and smaller PI were significantly associated with a caudally placed conus medullaris. This result might indicate that the length of the spinal cord varies little among individuals and that the skeletal difference affects the conus medullaris level. In addition to height, PI was a key driver of the conus medullaris level. Individuals with a larger PI typically have greater LL and thoracic kyphosis, and the end of the spinal cord might be located more cranially in the twisted spinal canal. However, as far as we know, there is no paper showing the relationship between the PI and the conus level due to the lack of studies investigating the conus level by using both lumbar MRI and X-rays. For this reason, the current results will need to be verified in future studies.

The location of the conus medullaris varies by developmental stage [6,8]. At birth, the cord fills the vertebral canal and terminates at the lumbosacral junction [8]. The distal end of the spinal cord then moves toward the cranial direction with infant development [6,8], probably because of the differential growth between the spinal column and spinal cord. In adults, the tip usually terminates at the mid aspect of the L1 vertebra. However, its position varies between the lower 11th thoracic and upper third lumbar vertebrae [5]. In a cadaveric study, the spinal cord measured roughly 45 cm in the adult male and 42 cm in the adult female [10]. The current results might indicate that the variation in spinal cord length is limited, and the skeletal anatomy of height and spino-pelvic sagittal alignment varies among individuals.

PI is one of the most important radiographical parameters in the case of spinal sagittal alignment [11]. The PI increases during childhood as the spine adapts to bipedal walking and stabilizes after adulthood [12]. PI strongly correlates with LL through the sacral slope (SS), and the larger PI is associated with a larger LL. Despite its great importance, PI varies from 33° to 85° among adults [13] and largely affects spinal sagittal alignment. Recent retrospective studies suggested that distal LL (L4-S1) is comparable between low to moderate and high PI groups. Proximal LL (L1-L4), however, is significantly influenced by the PI value (greater PI, and greater proximal lumbar lordosis) [14,15]. Furthermore, not only does the LL magnitude increase in cases of a larger PI but also the LL apex and inflection point are located more toward the cranial side [14]. Thus, in cases with a large PI the local lordosis around L1, where the conus medullaris is often located [1–6], might be greater, and the conus medullaris might be located more toward the cranial side in the twisted spinal canal. The present study did not measure local sagittal alignment around L1, and so this discussion is only speculative. The relationship between PI and conus medullaris needs to be further investigated.

Strengths and Limitations

A strength of this study was that it was a relatively large-scale study including ≥50 individuals of each sex and decade of age (20s–70s). Furthermore, both MRI and Xp were obtained in all subjects. As a limitation of the current study, the participants were a single race of Japanese. This limitation might affect the size and place of the spinal column and spinal cord. An international large-scale multicenter study is warranted to validate our results. As a second limitation, cases with lumbosacral transitional anomalies were excluded in the current study, however, it is necessary to examine the level of conus in these cases of transitional vertebra in the future. Lastly, we could not compare spinal alignment and the level of conus medullaris by degrees of pain, although the degrees of pain might affect the results. Future detailed studies assessing the pain are needed.

5. Conclusions

The majority of participants had the conus medullaris at the caudal level of the T12-L1 disk (92.2%), and the conus medullaris was located cranially to the T12 vertebral level in only 7.8% of the 629 healthy volunteers. Lower height and smaller PI were associated with the caudally placed conus medullaris; thus, skeletal differences were significantly associated with the conus medullaris level.

Author Contributions: H.N. designed the study and wrote the manuscript; K.I., Y.K. and M.T. performed the data collection; K.A., K.K., M.M., S.I. (Sadayuki Ito), H.K., N.S. and H.T. provided clinical experience; S.I. (Shiro Imagama) supervised the entire study. All authors have read and agreed to the published version of the manuscript.

Funding: This study was supported by institutional funds and by grant research funds, which are intended for promoting hospital functions, of the Japan Labor Health and Welfare Organization (Kawasaki, Japan).

Institutional Review Board Statement: The Japanese volunteers were recruited after the purpose of this study was officially announced and after obtaining institutional review board approval from the

Chubu Rosai Hospital (IRB approval no., 2009-2). All participants provided written informed consent prior to participation. The research procedure was carried out in accordance with the principles of the Declaration of Helsinki.

Informed Consent Statement: All participants gave written informed consent prior to participation.

Data Availability Statement: The data of this study are available from the corresponding authors upon request.

Acknowledgments: We are grateful to Fumihiko Kato and Yasutsugu Yukawa at Chubu Rosai Hospital for their assistance throughout this study.

Conflicts of Interest: The authors declare that there is no conflict of interest regarding the publication of this paper.

References

1. Bauer, D.F.; Shoja, M.M.; Loukas, M.; Oakes, W.J.; Tubbs, R.S. Study of the effects of flexion on the position of the conus medullaris. *Child's Nerv. Syst.* **2008**, *24*, 1043–1045. [CrossRef]
2. Gatonga, P.; Ogeng'o, J.A.; Awori, K.O. Spinal cord termination in adult Africans: Relationship with intercristal line and the transumbilical plane. *Clin. Anat.* **2010**, *23*, 563–565. [CrossRef] [PubMed]
3. Hedaoo, K.; Kumar, A.; Singh, B.K.; Sharma, R.K.; Sinha, M.; Yadav, Y. Morphometric analysis of thoracolumbar junction (T11-L2) in central Indian population: A computerized tomography based study of 800 vertebrae. *J. Clin. Orthop. Trauma* **2021**, *15*, 139–144. [CrossRef] [PubMed]
4. Nasr, A.Y.; Hussein, A.M.; Zaghloul, S.A. Morphometric parameters and histological Study of the Filum Terminale of Adult human cadavers and MR images. *Folia Morphol.* **2018**, *77*, 609–619. [CrossRef] [PubMed]
5. Soleiman, J.; Demaerel, P.; Rocher, S.; Maes, F.; Marchal, G. Magnetic Resonance Imaging Study of the Level of Termination of the Conus Medullaris and the Thecal Sac: Influence of Age and Gender. *Spine* **2005**, *30*, 1875–1880. [CrossRef] [PubMed]
6. Van Schoor, A.N.; Bosman, M.C.; Bosenberg, A.T. Descriptive study of the differences in the level of the conus medullaris in four different age groups. *Clin. Anat.* **2015**, *28*, 638–644. [CrossRef] [PubMed]
7. Macdonald, A.; Chatrath, P.; Spector, T.; Ellis, H. Level of termination of the spinal cord and the dural sac: A magnetic resonance study. *Clin. Anat.* **1999**, *12*, 149–152. [CrossRef]
8. Malas, M.A.; Salbacak, A.; Büyükmumcu, M.; Seker, M.; Köylüoğlu, B.; Karabulut, A.K. An investigation of the conus medullaris termination level during the period of fetal development to adulthood. *Kaibogaku Zasshi* **2001**, *76*, 453–459. [PubMed]
9. Demiryürek, D.; Aydingöz, Ü.; Akşit, M.D.; Yener, N.; Geyik, P.Ö. MR imaging determination of the normal level of conus medullaris. *Clin. Imaging* **2002**, *26*, 375–377. [CrossRef]
10. Cho, T.A. Spinal cord functional anatomy. *Continuum (Minneap Minn)* **2015**, *21*, 13–35. [CrossRef] [PubMed]
11. Legaye, J.; Duval-Beaupere, G.; Hecquet, J.; Marty, C. Pelvic incidence: A fundamental pelvic parameter for three-dimensional regulation of spinal sagittal curves. *Eur. Spine J.* **1998**, *7*, 99–103. [CrossRef] [PubMed]
12. Mac-Thiong, J.M.; Roussouly, P.; Berthonnaud, E.; Guigui, P. Age- and sex-related variations in sagittal sacropelvic morphology and balance in asymptomatic adults. *Eur. Spine J.* **2011**, *20*, 572–577. [CrossRef] [PubMed]
13. Mac-Thiong, J.M.; Roussouly, P.; Berthonnaud, É.; Guigui, P. Sagittal parameters of global spinal balance: Normative values from a prospective cohort of seven hundred nine Caucasian asymptomatic adults. *Spine* **2010**, *35*, E1193–E1198. [CrossRef] [PubMed]
14. Li, Y.; Sun, J.; Wang, G. Lumbar lordosis morphology correlates to pelvic incidence and erector spinae muscularity. *Sci. Rep.* **2021**, *11*, 802. [CrossRef] [PubMed]
15. Pesenti, S.; Lafage, R.; Stein, D.; Elysee, J.C.; Lenke, L.G.; Schwab, F.J.; Kim, H.J.; Lafage, V. The Amount of Proximal Lumbar Lordosis Is Related to Pelvic Incidence. *Clin. Orthop. Relat. Res.* **2018**, *476*, 1603–1611. [CrossRef] [PubMed]

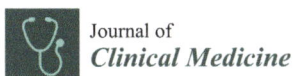

Article

Early Gender Differences in Pain and Functional Recovery Following Thoracolumbar Spinal Arthrodesis

Matthew T. Gulbrandsen [1,*], Nina Lara [2], James A. Beauchamp [3], Andrew Chung [4], Michael Chang [2,4] and Dennis Crandall [2,4]

1. Department of Orthopedic Surgery, Loma Linda University, Loma Linda, CA 92354, USA
2. Department of Orthopedic Surgery, Mayo Clinic, Phoenix, AZ 85054, USA; Nina.J.Lara@gmail.com (N.L.); msc@sonoranspine.com (M.C.); dennis@sonoranspine.com (D.C.)
3. Department of Biomedical Engineering, Northwestern University, Evanston, IL 60208, USA; james.beauchamp@northwestern.edu
4. Sonoran Spine Center, Tempe, AZ 85281, USA; andrewchung84@gmail.com
* Correspondence: mgulbrandsen@llu.edu

Abstract: Background: To analyze gender differences regarding the recovery experience (pain, function, complications) after spinal arthrodesis surgery. Methods: Pre-operative and post-operative gender-based differences in patient-reported outcomes for open posterior spinal arthrodesis at 6 weeks, 3 months, 6 months, and 1 year were studied, including age, comorbidities, body mass index (BMI), diagnosis, number of vertebrae fused, type of surgery, primary vs. revision surgery, and complications. Statistical analysis included the use of Student's t-test, Chi square, linear regression, Mann–Whitney U test, and Spearman's rho. Results: Primary or revision posterior arthrodesis was performed on 1931 consecutive adults (1219 females, 712 males) for deformity and degenerative pathologies. At surgery, females were older than males (61.7 years vs. 59.7 years, $p < 0.01$), had slightly more comorbidities (1.75 vs. 1.5, $p < 0.01$), and were more likely to undergo deformity correction (38% vs. 22%, $p < 0.01$). Females described more pre-op pain (female VAS = 6.54 vs. male VAS = 6.41, $p < 0.01$) and lower pre-op function (female ODI = 49.73 vs. male ODI = 46.52, $p < 0.01$). By 3 months post-op, there was no significant gender difference in VAS or ODI scores. Similar pain and function scores between males and females continued through 6 months and 12 months. Conclusion: Although females have more pain and dysfunction before undergoing spinal surgery, the differences in these values do not reach the Minimum Clinically Important Difference (MCID). Post-operatively, there is no difference in pain and function scores among males and females at 3, 6, and 12 months.

Keywords: gender differences; spine arthrodesis; spinal fusion; spine; deformity

1. Introduction

Historically, common stereotypes exist regarding the differences in how males and females perceive pain. Females have been reported to describe higher levels of pain when presented with equal amounts of thermal stimuli compared to males [1]. Females have also shown a lower threshold for thermal pain and lower pain tolerance than males [2]. Tonelli et al. reported female joint arthroplasty patients experienced more pain and dysfunction than males, even in the setting of less severe osteoarthritis [3].

However, in the setting of low back pain, much is unknown regarding gender perceived differences in pain and functional outcomes. Chenot et al. found that females had a lower pain threshold and lower functional capacity than males with chronic low back pain [4]. On the other hand, females with chronic low back pain treated with spinal fusion have been shown to experience similar pain and functional outcomes when compared to males [5]. For patients undergoing laminectomy alone or with fusion, similar ultimate clinical outcomes have been reported without gender differences [6].

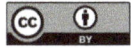

Specifically, gender differences in pain perception and function after spinal fusion surgery have not been studied in the setting of lumbar degenerative disease or thoracolumbar deformity. Consequently, gender-based outcome differences remain unclear in patients undergoing spinal surgery for these conditions. The purpose of this study is therefore to analyze how a patient's gender impacts self-reported pain and functional recovery after spinal arthrodesis surgery for thoracolumbar deformity and lumbar degenerative disease.

2. Materials and Methods

2.1. Patient Sample

This was a retrospective cohort study utilizing patient data from a single center's prospectively collected surgical database that received IRB exemption. Only adult patients (>18 years old) undergoing open posterior instrumented arthrodesis were included in this study. Included were both primary and revision surgeries of any length, with or without interbody fusions, for lumbar degenerative conditions and thoracolumbar deformity. Patients without a minimum 1 year of clinical and radiographic follow-up data were excluded. Trauma, tumor, and infection cases were additional grounds for exclusion. All surgeries were performed by 5 fellowship trained spine surgeons.

A similar strategy for post-operative pain management and limited narcotic use was used throughout this study, with an effort to have all patients off opiate analgesics by 3 months post-op. Post-operative bracing was optional and provided at the request of individual patients. Post-operative physical therapy was typically instituted at 8–12 weeks post-op, and continued for 4 weeks. All patients were placed on a home exercise program after formal physical therapy was completed.

All patient demographic information and baseline characteristics including comorbidities, smoking status, body mass index (BMI), and indication for surgery were noted. Surgical factors were additionally collected.

2.2. Outcome Measures

Clinical outcome measurements included the Visual Analogue Scale (VAS) and the Oswestry Disability Index (ODI). These scores were collected pre-operatively, at 6 weeks, 3 months, 6 months, and 1 year after surgery. Radiographic data were additionally collected at similar time points. Radiographic evidence of fusion included no implant–bone interface lucency, apparent bridging bone either posterolaterally or through the interspace, and no motion on flexion-extension radiographs at the 1 year post-operative follow-up. All peri-operative complications were noted.

2.3. Statistical Analysis

Mann–Whitney U test, was employed to determine potential gender differences in ODI and VAS scores. Student's t-test was used to compare gender differences in age at the time of surgery. Spearman's rho analysis was used to determine the strength of association between either VAS or ODI scores and a patient's gender, BMI, and age. A Chi-Square test was used to determine potential gender differences in the presence of complications, type of diagnosis (degenerative vs. deformity), and number of comorbidities. Linear regression models were used to estimate and compare the differential effects of a patient's gender, diagnosis (degenerative vs. deformity), age, number of comorbidities, BMI, levels of fusion, revision status, and presence of complications on ODI and VAS scores over time. Statistical significance was set at $p < 0.01$. All statistical analyses were conducted with IBM SPSS Statistics for Windows (IBM Corp., Armonk, NY, USA).

3. Results

3.1. Patient Characteristics

A total of 1931 consecutive patients (female: 1219, male: 712) met inclusion criteria. Mean follow-up was 84 months; range, 12–192 months) (Table 1). Males had a slightly higher BMI than females (29.7 vs. 28.7; $p < 0.01$) and were more likely to require surgery for degenerative disease compared to other diagnoses (78% vs. 62%; $p < 0.01$) (Table 2). Females tended to be older than males at the time of surgery (61.7 years ± 12.8 vs. 59.7 years ± 14.1; $p < 0.01$). In general, females had a greater number of comorbidities compared to males (1.75 vs. 1.5; $p < 0.01$, Table 3). Comorbidities included in this study were autoimmune disorders, gastrointestinal disorders, depression, fibromyalgia, and thyroid disease. There was no difference in smoking status between groups ($p > 0.01$).

Table 1. Patient characteristics separated by gender.

Characteristics	Male n = 712	Female n = 1219	p Value
Age (years)	59 ± 14.07	61 ± 12.83	<0.01
Pre-op BMI (kg/m^2)	29.7	28.7	<0.01
Degenerative [#]	562 (78.9%)	765 (62.8%)	<0.01
Deformity	150 (21.1%)	454 (37.2%)	<0.01
Smoker	146 (20.5%)	154 (12.6%)	NS
Revision Surgery	334 (46.9%)	552 (45.3%)	NS
Prior Laminectomy	128 (18.0%)	167 (13.6%)	NS
Prior Fusion	206 (28.9%)	385 (31.6%)	NS
Deformity Average Levels Fused	8.20	8.64	NS
Degenerative Average Levels Fused	2.09	2.13	NS

[#] Degenerative pathology includes degenerative and spondylolisthesis diagnoses. NS = not statistically significant.

Table 2. Comparison of patient diagnosis by gender.

Diagnosis	Male n = 712	Female n = 1219	p Value
Degenerative	287 (40.3%)	324 (26.6%)	<0.01
Spondylolisthesis	275 (38.6%)	441 (36.2%)	NS
Adult Idiopathic Scoliosis	20 (2.80%)	135 (11.1%)	<0.01
Degenerative Scoliosis	48 (6.74%)	162 (13.3%)	<0.01
Scheuermann's Kyphosis	18 (2.52%)	5 (0.41%)	<0.01
Neuromuscular Scoliosis	2 (0.28%)	7 (0.57%)	NS
Other Kyphosis	41 (5.76%)	77 (6.32%)	NS
Kyphoscoliosis	21 (2.95%)	68 (5.58%)	<0.01

Table 3. Patient comorbidities separated by gender.

Comorbidities	Male n = 712	Female n = 1219	p Value
Number of Comorbidities	1.50 ± 1.33	1.75 ± 1.42	<0.01
Rheumatoid Arthritis, Systemic Lupus Erythematosus	34 (4.78%)	82 (6.73%)	NS
Bowel/Bladder Dysfunction	33 (4.63%)	93 (7.63%)	NS
Cancer	80 (11.2%)	127 (10.4%)	NS
Stroke, Transient Ischemic Attack	18 (2.53%)	37 (3.04%)	NS
Pulmonary	101 (14.2%)	223 (18.3%)	NS
Vascular Disease	63 (8.85%)	145 (11.9%)	NS

A total of 1045 patients (54.1%) underwent primary fusion (Table 1). There were no statistical differences in levels fused between the two groups. On average, males with deformity disease underwent 8.2 level fusions and females underwent 8.64 level fusions. For degenerative disease, males underwent 2.09 level fusions and females underwent 2.13 level fusions.

3.2. Pain and Function

Females reported slightly higher pain scores pre-operatively (6.54 vs. 6.14; $p < 0.01$). At 6 weeks post-op, females continued to describe marginally more pain than males (VAS 4.36 vs. 3.99; $p < 0.01$). By 3 months, there was no gender-based difference in pain scores (female VAS: 3.73 vs. male VAS: 3.76; $p > 0.01$). Furthermore, there was no significant gender difference in pain scores at 6 months ($p > 0.01$), or 1 year post-operatively ($p > 0.01$).

Both male and female patients demonstrated significant clinical improvement in pain scores by 1 year follow-up (Table 4).

Table 4. Visual Analog Scale (VAS) for pain pre-operatively and at 6 weeks, 3 months, 6 months, and 1 year post-operatively, separated by gender. Oswestry Disability Index (ODI) score pre-operatively and post-operatively at 1 year, separated by gender.

	Male $n = 712$	Female $n = 1219$	p Value
VAS pre-op (mean)	6.14 (std = 2.16)	6.54 (std = 2.12)	<0.01
VAS 6 weeks (mean)	3.99 (std = 2.32)	4.36 (std = 2.29)	<0.01
VAS 3 months (mean)	3.76 (std = 2.38)	3.73 (std = 2.32)	NS
VAS 6 months (mean)	3.58 (std = 2.57)	3.61 (std = 2.45)	NS
VAS 1 year (mean)	3.50 (std = 2.61)	3.47 (std = 2.61)	NS
Change in VAS from pre-op to 1 year	−2.65 (std = 2.78)	−3.06 (std = 2.82)	<0.01
Pre-operative ODI (mean)	46.52 (std = 16.19)	49.73 (std = 16.44)	<0.01
1 year post-operative ODI (mean)	29.9 (std = 21.6)	29.79 (std = 20.89)	NS
Change in ODI from pre-op to 1 year post-op	−16.63 (std = 18.48)	−20.01 (std = 19.29)	<0.01

Females reported lower pre-op dysfunction scores (ODI scores, Table 4) when compared to males (F = 49.73 vs. M = 46.52; $p < 0.01$). Functional improvements in both genders were significant at 1 year ($p < 0.01$). At one year, there was no gender difference in ODI scores noted ($p > 0.01$). Females experienced a slightly greater mean overall improvement in ODI by 1 year (20 points in females vs. 16.6 points for males; $p < 0.01$).

3.3. Gender-Based Complication Rates

Comparing post-operative complications in our study group, there were no gender differences in pseudarthrosis rates, re-operation rates, or other complications (Table 5). Death is listed as a complication for any patient who died within 2 years of surgery.

Table 5. Complications separated by gender.

Complications	Male ($n = 712$)	Female ($n = 1219$)	p Value
Nonunion	16 (2.25%)	53 (4.35%)	NS
Adjacent Level Fracture	9 (1.26%)	23 (1.89%)	NS
Implant Loosening	3 (0.42%)	10 (0.82%)	NS
Implant Failure	5 (0.70%)	9 (0.74%)	NS
Neuro Deficit	7 (0.98%)	10 (0.82%)	NS
Death	14 (1.97%)	21 (1.72%)	NS
Deep Venous Thrombosis	3 (0.42%)	3 (0.25%)	NS
Pulmonary Embolus	1 (0.14%)	4 (0.33%)	NS
Deep Infection	22 (3.09%)	27 (2.21%)	NS
Iliac Screw Removal	6 (0.84%)	28 (2.30%)	NS
Revision Laminectomy	25 (3.51%)	46 (3.77%)	NS
Revision Fusion	42 (5.90%)	97 (7.96%)	NS

3.4. Predictors of Pain and Function

Predictors of pain and function were estimated through a linear regression model of 1 year post-operative VAS scores (Table 7) and ODI scores (Table 6), respectively. Separate models were fit for each gender and prediction estimates were based on the parameter coefficients (β), with significant coefficients ($p < 0.05$) interpreted as the estimated change in VAS or ODI for a unit change in the respective factor. As can be seen in Table 6, number of comorbidities, type of diagnosis, presence of complications, and BMI were found to significantly contribute to female 1 year post-operative ODI scores, while number of comorbidities, level of fusion, type of diagnosis, presence of complications, and BMI were found to significantly contribute to male 1 year post-operative ODI scores. Likewise, as shown in Table 7, number of comorbidities, presence of complications, BMI, and age were found to significantly contribute to female 1 year post-operative VAS scores, while number of comorbidities, level of fusion, type of diagnosis, presence of complications, and age were found to significantly contribute to male 1 year post-operative VAS scores.

Table 6. Linear regression model of post-op ODI at 1 year for male and female.

	Male 1 Year Post-Operative ODI			Female 1 Year Post-Operative ODI		
	β	Standard Error	p-Value	β	Standard Error	p-Value
Constant	11.562	5.866	0.049	15.711	4.109	<0.0005
Comorbidities	1.283	0.650	0.049	2.056	0.441	<0.0005
Level of Fusion (Single: 0, Multi: 1)	6.453	1.886	0.001	0.709	1.583	0.654
Diagnosis (Degen.: 0, Deformity: 1)	−4.282	2.094	0.041	−2.876	1.367	0.036
Complication (None: 0, Complications: 1)	3.440	1.638	0.036	4.474	1.188	<0.0005
Body Mass Index	0.483	0.151	0.001	0.481	0.095	<0.0005
Age at Operation	−0.056	0.061	0.364	−0.082	0.048	0.088

Table 7. Linear regression model of post-op VAS at 1 year for male and female.

	Male 1 Year Post-Operative Visual Analog Score			Female 1 Year Post-Operative Visual Analog Score		
	β	Standard Error	p-Value	β	Standard Error	p-Value
Constant	3.057	0.720	<0.0005	2.992	0.526	<0.0005
Comorbidities	0.213	0.079	0.007	0.229	0.056	<0.0005
Level of Fusion (Single: 0, Multi: 1)	0.475	0.231	0.040	0.179	0.203	0.377
Diagnosis (Degen.: 0, Deformity: 1)	−0.732	0.255	0.004	−0.341	0.175	0.051
Complication (None: 0, Complications: 1)	0.535	0.200	0.008	0.359	0.152	0.018
Body Mass Index	0.020	0.019	0.270	0.032	0.012	0.009
Age at Operation	−0.016	0.007	0.035	−0.017	0.006	0.007

4. Discussion

Numerous studies suggest certain patient characteristics and comorbidities affect outcomes after spinal fusion [7–12]. The few risk factors that have been shown to consistently result in worse outcomes include BMI, age, cardiovascular disease, smoking, and receiving worker's compensation or disability benefits [7–10]. However, the effect of patient gender on outcome after spinal arthrodesis has not been solidified.

In 2002, Gehrchen et al. conducted a retrospective review including 112 patients with degenerative disc disease (DDD) and spondylolisthesis that showed female gender to be an independent risk factor for a nonoptimal outcome after lumbar fusion [12]. In 2009, Ekman conducted a randomized control trial that included 164 patients treated with spinal fusion for spondylolisthesis that suggested females had worse PROs post-operatively [10]. In 1984, when analyzing the outcomes after treatment for cervical disc disease, Eriksen et al. found that females have more pain and dysfunction post-operatively after fusion surgery [13].

However, the results of our study align more closely to those of Triebel et al. and Pochon et al. [5,6]. Triebel et al., in a study that included 4780 Swedish patients with lumbar degenerative disc disease and chronic low back pain, found that Swedish women reported similar pain and function outcomes to men after lumbar spinal fusion [5]. Additionally, a 2016 study by Pochon et al. that included 1518 patients found that females who underwent decompression alone or decompression with fusion ± instrumentation did not experience a difference in outcomes when compared to men [6].

Our study shows that while females reported slightly more pain and worse function than males at the time of surgery, by 3 months and beyond, no further gender differences in post-operative pain or function existed. Our findings support the ultimate conclusions of gender outcome equality by Triebel et al. and Pochon et al. However, our study further expands their findings to the realm of deformity surgery [5,6].

An important aspect to acknowledge when reviewing the results of our study is the MCID for VAS back pain and ODI score. Previous studies have suggested that the MCID for VAS and ODI are 2.1 and 14.9, respectively [14,15]. Both MCIDs are significantly higher than the difference found in at any time point in our study. Therefore, the slightly increased pain (F = 6.54 vs. M = 6.14; $p < 0.01$) and disability (F = 49.73 vs. M= 46.52; $p < 0.01$) that females present with prior to undergoing spinal arthrodesis is not clinically relevant.

Similar results have been echoed in the total joint arthroplasty literature. For instance, Holtzman and Katz showed that females have more pain and dysfunction prior to undergoing total joint arthroplasty. However, they found that females do not recover as well post-operatively compared to their male counterparts [16,17]. Another finding of our study was that females were slightly older than males when they underwent spinal arthrodesis (61.7 years ± 12.8 vs. 59.7 years ± 14.1; $p < 0.01$). As far as we are aware, why females wait longer and endure more pain before undergoing spine or total joint surgery has not been well studied. Possible explanations for this phenomenon include that (1) females are more reluctant to choose surgical intervention [18], (2) females spend more time gathering information about risks and benefits [19], and (3) females are more likely than males to be prescribed anti-depressants or referred to mental health before being offered surgical intervention [2,20]. Another possible explanation for delayed spinal arthrodesis in females is that many gender comparative studies performed prior to 2010 showed inferior outcomes in females after spine surgery which may differentially impact the decision making from the surgeon's standpoint [9,10,12,13].

Given the higher comorbidity burden of females, it is surprising that they ultimately achieved similar outcomes to males. There are several potential explanations. Physical therapy use has been associated with improved outcomes after lumbar fusion [21], and current literature shows that females are much more likely to utilize physical therapy [22,23]. Females are also more likely to follow-up with their physician after lumbar surgery [24]. Interestingly, a study analyzing patient compliance after total knee arthroplasty showed that females are more like to be compliant when compared to males [25]. Female patients' propensity to attend physical therapy and comply with a physician's recommendation may explain their increased margin of post-operative improvement compared to males. Once again, it is important to note that although this margin of improvement is statistically significant, it does not reach the MCID and, therefore, is unlikely to be clinically significant.

There are several limitations to this study. First, this study was retrospective in nature. All patients underwent open posterior spinal arthrodesis and results may differ for other approaches or decompression without fusion. Furthermore, patient-reported pain and functional scores are individually subjective. Additionally, although our analyses accounted for many variables, possible confounding variables that we were unable to account for include patient expectations, the operating surgeon, physical therapy effort by the patient, psychosocial factors, living environment, and psychological background. Additionally, this study focused on general VAS scores for pain and did not distinguish between back pain and leg pain. Additionally, the findings here are limited to a single center's experience and may not be broadly applicable.

5. Conclusions

Although females have more pain and dysfunction before undergoing spinal arthrodesis for thoracolumbar deformity and lumbar degenerative disease, the differences in these values do not reach the Minimum Clinically Important Difference (MCID). Post-operatively, there is no difference in pain and function scores among males and females at 3, 6, and 12 months.

Author Contributions: Conceptualization, D.C. and M.C.; methodology, M.T.G. and J.A.B.; software, J.A.B.; validation, M.T.G., J.A.B. and N.L.; formal analysis, J.A.B.; investigation, N.L., A.C. and M.T.G.; resources, M.C. and D.C.; data curation, D.C. and M.C.; writing—original draft preparation, M.T.G.; writing—review and editing, M.T.G., N.L., J.A.B., A.C., M.C. and D.C.; supervision, D.C. All authors have read and agreed to the published version of the manuscript.

Funding: This research received no external funding.

Institutional Review Board Statement: Ethical review and approval were waived for this study, due to the use of de-identified patient information.

Informed Consent Statement: Patient consent was waived due to the use of retrospective de-identified patient information.

Data Availability Statement: Raw data are from a private clinic database, not publicly available.

Conflicts of Interest: The authors declare no conflict of interest.

References

1. Paulson, P.E.; Minoshima, S.; Morrow, T.J.; Casey, K.L. Gender differences in pain perception and patterns of cerebral activation during noxious heat stimulation in humans. *Pain* **1998**, *76*, 223–229. [CrossRef]
2. Robinson, M.E.; Wise, E.A. Gender bias in the observation of experimental pain. *Pain* **2003**, *104*, 259–264. [CrossRef]
3. Tonelli, S.M.; Rakel, B.A.; Cooper, N.A.; Angstom, W.L.; Sluka, K.A. Women with knee osteoarthritis have more pain and poorer function than men, but similar physical activity prior to total knee replacement. *Biol. Sex Differ.* **2011**, *2*, 12. [CrossRef]
4. Chenot, J.-F.; Becker, A.; Leonhardt, C.; Keller, S.; Donner-Banzhoff, N.; Hildebrandt, J.; Basler, H.-D.; Baum, E.; Kochen, M.M.; Pfingsten, M. Sex Differences in Presentation, Course, and Management of Low Back Pain in Primary Care. *Clin. J. Pain* **2008**, *24*, 578–584. [CrossRef]
5. Triebel, J.; Snellman, G.; Sandén, B.; Strömqvist, F.; Robinson, Y. Women do not fare worse than men after lumbar fusion surgery: Two-year follow-up results from 4,780 prospectively collected patients in the Swedish National Spine Register with lumbar degenerative disc disease and chronic low back pain. *Spine J.* **2013**, *17*, 656–662. [CrossRef]
6. Pochon, L.; Kleinstück, F.S.; Porchet, F.; Mannion, A.F. Influence of gender on patient-oriented outcomes in spine surgery. *Eur. Spine J.* **2016**, *25*, 235–246. [CrossRef]
7. Mannion, A.F.; Elfering, A. Predictors of surgical outcome and their assessment. *Eur. Spine J.* **2005**, *15*, S93–S108. [CrossRef] [PubMed]
8. Mannion, A.F.; Elfering, A.; Staerkle, R.; Junge, A.; Grob, D.; Dvorak, J.; Jacobshagen, N.; Semmer, N.; Boos, N. Predictors of multidimensional outcome after spinal surgery. *Eur. Spine J.* **2006**, *16*, 777–786. [CrossRef] [PubMed]
9. Peolsson, A.; Hedlund, R.; Vavruch, L.; Öberg, B. Predictive factors for the outcome of anterior cervical decompression and fusion. *Eur. Spine J.* **2003**, *12*, 274–280. [CrossRef] [PubMed]
10. Ekman, P.; Möller, H.; Hedlund, R. Predictive Factors for the Outcome of Fusion in Adult Isthmic Spondylolisthesis. *Spine* **2009**, *34*, 1204–1210. [CrossRef]
11. Lehto, M.U.K.; Honkanen, P. Factors influencing the outcome of operative treatment for lumbar spinal stenosis. *Acta Neurochir.* **1995**, *137*, 25–28. [CrossRef] [PubMed]
12. Gehrchen, M.P.; Dahl, B.; Katonis, P.; Blyme, P.; Tøndevold, E.; Kiær, T. No difference in clinical outcome after posterolateral lumbar fusion between patients with isthmic spondylolisthesis and those with degenerative disc disease using pedicle screw instrumentation: A comparative study of 112 patients with 4 years of follow-up. *Eur. Spine J.* **2002**, *11*, 423–427. [CrossRef]
13. Eriksen, E.F.; Buhl, M.; Fode, K.; Klaerke, A.; Krøyer, L.; Lindeberg, H.; Madsen, C.B.; Strange, P.; Wohlert, L.; Espersen, J.O. Treatment of cervical disc disease using Cloward's technique the prognostic value of clinical preoperative data in 1,106 patients. *Acta Neurochir.* **1984**, *70*, 181–197. [CrossRef]
14. Copay, A.G.; Glassman, S.D.; Subach, B.R.; Berven, S.; Schuler, T.C.; Carreon, L.Y. Minimum clinically important difference in lumbar spine surgery patients: A choice of methods using the Oswestry Disability Index, Medical Outcomes Study questionnaire Short Form 36, and Pain Scales. *Spine J.* **2008**, *8*, 968–974. [CrossRef] [PubMed]
15. Parker, S.L.; Mendenhall, S.K.; Shau, D.N.; Adogwa, O.; Anderson, W.N.; Devin, C.J.; McGirt, M.J. Minimum clinically important difference in pain, disability, and quality of life after neural decompression and fusion for same-level recurrent lumbar stenosis: Understanding clinical versus statistical significance. *J. Neurosurg. Spine* **2012**, *16*, 471–478. [CrossRef] [PubMed]
16. Katz, J.N.; Wright, E.A.; Guadagnoli, E.; Liang, M.H.; Karlson, E.W.; Cleary, P.D. Differences between men and women undergoing major orthopedic surgery for degenerative arthritis. *Arthritis Rheum.* **1994**, *37*, 687–694. [CrossRef]
17. Holtzman, J.; Saleh, K.; Kane, R. Gender Differences in Functional Status and Pain in a Medicare Population Undergoing Elective Total Hip Arthroplasty. *Med. Care* **2002**, *40*, 461–470. [CrossRef]
18. Karlson, E.W.; Daltroy, L.H.; Liang, M.H.; Eaton, H.E.; Katz, J.N. Gender Differences in Patient Preferences May Underlie Differential Utilization of Elective Surgery. *Am. J. Med.* **1997**, *102*, 524–530. [CrossRef]

19. Hawker, G.A.; Wright, J.G.; Coyte, P.C.; Williams, J.I.; Harvey, B.; Glazier, R.; Badley, E.M. Differences between Men and Women in the Rate of Use of Hip and Knee Arthroplasty. *N. Engl. J. Med.* **2000**, *342*, 1016–1022. [CrossRef]
20. Hirsh, A.T.; Hollingshead, N.A.; Matthias, M.; Bair, M.J.; Kroenke, K. The Influence of Patient Sex, Provider Sex, and Sexist Attitudes on Pain Treatment Decisions. *J. Pain* **2014**, *15*, 551–559. [CrossRef]
21. Madera, M.; Brady, J.; Deily, S.; McGinty, T.; Moroz, L.; Singh, D.; Tipton, G.; Truumees, E. The role of physical therapy and rehabilitation after lumbar fusion surgery for degenerative disease: A systematic review. *J. Neurosurg. Spine* **2017**, *26*, 694–704. [CrossRef] [PubMed]
22. Swinkels, I.C.S.; Wimmers, R.H.; Groenewegen, P.P.; Bosch, W.J.H.V.D.; Dekker, J.; Ende, C.H.M.V.D. What factors explain the number of physical therapy treatment sessions in patients referred with low back pain: A multilevel analysis. *BMC Health Serv. Res.* **2005**, *5*, 74. [CrossRef] [PubMed]
23. Machlin, S.R.; Chevan, J.; Yu, W.W.; Zodet, M.W. Determinants of Utilization and Expenditures for Episodes of Ambulatory Physical Therapy among Adults. *Phys Ther.* **2011**, *91*, 1018–1029. [CrossRef] [PubMed]
24. Ha, K.-Y.; Kim, S.-I.; Kim, Y.-H.; Oh, I.-S. Predictive Factors for Postoperative Follow-up: Which Patients are Prone to Loss to Follow-up After Spinal Surgery? *Clin. Spine Surg.* **2018**, *31*, E25–E29. [CrossRef]
25. Choi, J.K.; Geller, J.A.; Patrick, D.A., Jr.; Wang, W.; Macaulay, W. How are those "lost to follow-up" patients really doing? A compliance comparison in arthroplasty patients. *World J. Orthop.* **2015**, *6*, 150–155. [CrossRef]

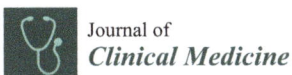

Article

Direct Lateral Corpectomy and Reconstruction Using an Expandable Cage Improves Local Kyphosis but Not Global Sagittal Alignment

Hidetomi Terai [1], Shinji Takahashi [1,*,†], Hiroyuki Yasuda [2], Sadahiko Konishi [2], Takafumi Maeno [3], Hiroshi Kono [3], Akira Matsumura [4], Takashi Namikawa [4], Minori Kato [4], Masatoshi Hoshino [1], Koji Tamai [1], Hiromitsu Toyoda [1], Akinobu Suzuki [1] and Hiroaki Nakamura [1]

1 Department of Orthopaedic Surgery, Osaka City University Graduate School of Medicine, Osaka 545-8585, Japan; hterai@med.osaka-cu.ac.jp (H.T.); hoshino717@gmail.com (M.H.); koji.tamai.707@gmail.com (K.T.); h-toyoda@msic.med.osaka-cu.ac.jp (H.T.); a-suzuki@msic.med.osaka-cu.ac.jp (A.S.); hnakamura@med.osaka-cu.ac.jp (H.N.)
2 Department of Orthopaedic Surgery, Osaka General Hospital of West Japan Railway Company, Osaka 545-0053, Japan; hiroyuki19780728@yahoo.co.jp (H.Y.); m1378921@med.osaka-cu.ac.jp (S.K.)
3 Department of Orthopaedic Surgery, Ishikiri Seiki Hospital, Osaka 579-8026, Japan; dzm02716@nifty.ne.jp (T.M.); hiroshikishikiri@gmail.com (H.K.)
4 Department of Orthopaedic Surgery, Osaka City General Hospital, Osaka 534-0021, Japan; amatsumura@med.osaka-cu.ac.jp (A.M.); namikawa@msic.med.osaka-cu.ac.jp (T.N.); minori202048@gmail.com (M.K.)
* Correspondence: shinji@med.osaka-cu.ac.jp; Tel.: +81-06-6645-3851
† Current Address: 1-4-3, Asahi-machi, Abeno-ku, Osaka 545-8585, Japan.

Citation: Terai, H.; Takahashi, S.; Yasuda, H.; Konishi, S.; Maeno, T.; Kono, H.; Matsumura, A.; Namikawa, T.; Kato, M.; Hoshino, M.; et al. Direct Lateral Corpectomy and Reconstruction Using an Expandable Cage Improves Local Kyphosis but Not Global Sagittal Alignment. J. Clin. Med. 2021, 10, 4012. https://doi.org/10.3390/jcm10174012

Academic Editor: Christian Carulli

Received: 5 July 2021
Accepted: 3 September 2021
Published: 5 September 2021

Publisher's Note: MDPI stays neutral with regard to jurisdictional claims in published maps and institutional affiliations.

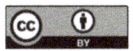

Copyright: © 2021 by the authors. Licensee MDPI, Basel, Switzerland. This article is an open access article distributed under the terms and conditions of the Creative Commons Attribution (CC BY) license (https://creativecommons.org/licenses/by/4.0/).

Abstract: Recently, an expandable cage equipped with rectangular footplates has been used for anterior vertebral replacement in osteoporotic vertebral fracture (OVF). However, the postoperative changes in global alignment have not been elucidated. The purpose of this study was to evaluate local and global spinal alignment after anterior and posterior spinal fixation (APSF) using an expandable cage in elderly OVF patients. This retrospective multicenter review assessed 54 consecutive patients who underwent APSF for OVF. Clinical outcomes were compared between postoperative sagittal vertical axis (SVA) > 95 mm and ≤95 mm groups to investigate the impact of malalignment. SVA improved by only 18.7 mm (from 111.8 mm to 93.1 mm). VAS score of back pain at final follow-up was significantly higher in patients with SVA > 95 mm than SVA ≤ 95 mm (42.4 vs. 22.6, $p = 0.007$). Adjacent vertebral fracture after surgery was significantly more frequent in the SVA > 95 mm (37% vs. 11%, $p = 0.038$). Multiple logistic regression showed significantly increased OR for developing adjacent vertebral fracture (OR = 4.76, 95% CI 1.10–20.58). APSF using the newly developed cage improves local kyphotic angle but not SVA. The main cause for the spinal malalignment after surgery was postoperative development of adjacent vertebral fractures.

Keywords: direct lateral corpectomy; expandable cage; global alignment; local kyphosis; osteoporosis vertebral fracture

1. Introduction

Maintenance of global sagittal balance in the standing position is important for minimizing energy expenditure and load on the musculoskeletal system [1]. Many mechanisms work together to maintain balance in the normal spine and extremities, including some compensatory mechanisms. However, once the compensatory mechanisms break down, there is severe deterioration in the patient's condition, pain, and reduction of quality of life (QOL) [2]. Other reports have shown that osteoporotic vertebral fracture (OVF) is strongly related to sagittal spinal imbalance in aged patients [3–5]. Several reports suggest that reduced muscle volume (i.e., sarcopenia) is one of the major causes of sagittal imbalance, causing reduction in the QOL of OVF patients [6–8]. Sarcopenia and osteoporosis show a high prevalence in old age and incur a high risk for falls, fractures, and further functional decline [9]. The term osteosarcopenia has been proposed to describe individuals suffering from both diseases [10]. With the aging of society and the associated increase in the amount of osteosarcopenia [11], the number of patients presenting with problems associated with an imbalanced sagittal spine is also likely to increase in the near future.

OVF mainly occurs at the thoracolumbar junction and negatively affects spinal alignment and QOL [5]. There are many surgical methods for the treatment of OVF, such as vertebroplasty (VP), balloon kyphoplasty (BKP), anterior vertebral replacement and posterior spinal fixation (APSF), and posterior osteotomy (PO) including posterior vertebral column resection (pVCR) [12,13]. The choice of surgical method is based on the goal of surgery, the patients' symptoms, the degree of deformity, the global spinal alignment, and the flexibility. However, few reports have described the correlation between local kyphotic changes and changes in global alignment after OVF surgery.

Recently, a newly developed expandable cage equipped with rectangular footplates has overcome the subsidence that is thought to be a disadvantage of anterior surgery for OVF. In addition, recent advances in the lateral approach enable minimally invasive anterior spinal reconstruction of thoracolumbar and lumbar lesions in elderly patients. Taiji et al. in a cohort of 16 OVF patients treated with the wide-foot-plate expandable cage reported a 30% correction loss (local kyphotic angle 22.6° before surgery, −1.5° immediately after surgery, and 7.0° at the final observation) [14]. However, there have been no reports about the changes in global alignment after anterior surgery for OVF. Our major clinical question in this study was whether sagittal imbalance following OVF could be improved by the anterior surgery or not. Therefore, the aim of this study was to report the correlation between local kyphotic changes and global spinal alignment after APSF in elderly OVF patients and to investigate the impact of global malalignment.

2. Materials and Methods

This multicenter retrospective cohort study was conducted at four institutions. Consecutive patients who underwent APSF for intra- or intervertebral instability after OVF were reviewed retrospectively.

The following were required of all patients eligible for participation in this retrospective study. (1) Osteoporotic vertebral fracture; (2) Intra- or intervertebral instability; (3) Neurologic deficit or severe back pain; and (4) Improvement of these symptoms in the supine position. Finally, the patients who were followed-up for at least 1 year were analyzed. Among them, patients with data of global spinal alignment before surgery and at final follow-up were included in the analysis. This study was approved by the institutional review board of our institution (approval no. 3170). The need to obtain informed consent was waived based on the retrospective design and anonymization of patient identifiers.

Patients' clinical records were reviewed for demographic data, instability type, operation time (min), estimated blood loss (mL), performance status (PS, Common Toxicity Criteria, version 2.0), comorbidities, and perioperative complications. Bone mineral density (BMD) at the femoral neck was determined using dual-energy x-ray absorptiometry. Information on previous surgeries at the corpectomy site was obtained and divided into lumbar decompression, VP/BKP, and posterior instrumentation. The severity of pain was subjectively assessed by the patients on a visual analogue scale (VAS), which was based on the average level of back pain that the patient felt over the previous week. The VAS was measured before surgery and at final follow-up. The rate of minimal clinically important differences (MCID) was evaluated. MCID score for lumbar fusion surgery [15] was used (≥21 mm) because there have been no reports about MCID for OVF treatment. The fracture level was divided into thoracolumbar (T11–L2) and lumbar (L3–L5) regions.

Radiographic evaluation was performed via whole spine x-ray on all patients before surgery and at final follow-up and included analysis of sagittal alignment (sagittal vertical axis: SVA; pelvic incidence: PI; lumbar lordosis: LL; sacral slope: SS; pelvic tilt: PT; thoracic kyphosis: TK; T1 pelvic angle: TPA) and incidence of cage subsidence. Local kyphotic angle was defined as the angle between the inferior endplate of the vertebra above and the superior endplate of the vertebra below the fractured vertebra and was given a negative value in patients with kyphotic deformity. Intravertebral instability was defined as angular motion of the fractured vertebral body with intravertebral cleft between flexed and extended positions. Intervertebral instability was defined as a change in disc height of >2 mm with deformation of the vertebral body between flexed and extended positions.

2.1. Surgical Indications and Techniques

The patient was placed in a lateral position and a true lateral film was obtained with fluoroscopy. The affected vertebral body and the upper and lower discs were exposed per transthoracic retropleural or retroperitoneal approaches. After removal of discs above and below the affected vertebral body and the ligation or coagulation of segmental vessels, corpectomy was performed using a large osteotome. The cartilaginous endplate was carefully removed by a disc knife and ring curettage to prevent inadvertent endplate violation. The vertebral segment was reconstructed with an expandable titanium cage comprising rectangular footplates (X-Core2®; NuVasive, San Diego, CA, USA). Bone grafting was performed inside and outside of the cage using artificial tricalcium phosphate particles, resected vertebral body, and resected rib fragments. After position change, posterior percutaneous pedicle screw fixation (PPS) fixation was performed without decompression. The range of posterior fixation was unregulated and depended on the surgeon's preference.

2.2. Statistical Analysis

Clinical outcomes were compared between postoperative SVA > 95 mm and ≤95 mm groups to investigate the impact of malalignment in patients who underwent this surgery [16]. In addition, baseline data, radiological parameters before surgery, and surgical complications were compared between SVA > 95 mm and ≤95 mm groups to investigate the factors related to SVA > 95 mm. Multiple logistic regression analysis was used to calculate odds ratios of variables for SVA > 95 mm. The model included age and variables with p-values < 0.10 in univariate analysis. The data on medication for osteoporosis including teriparatide, romosozumab, bisphosphonate, denosumab, and vitamin D within a month before index surgery were collected. We divided them into two groups in the analysis: bone-forming agents (teriparatide, romosozumab) and others.

Shapiro–Wilk tests were used to check normality assumptions for all parameters. The normality was confirmed in all continuous variables except for the VAS of back pain. The t-test (normality) or Mann–Whitney U test (non-normality) was used to compare continuous variables. The χ2 test or Fisher's exact test was used for categorical variables. To establish whether significant differences existed in postoperative clinical or radiologic outcomes between the two group, a restricted maximum likelihood, mixed-model regression was used. Statistical test results were considered significant for values of $p < 0.05$. All p-values were two-sided. All analyses were performed using SAS version 9.4 (SAS Institute, Cary, NC, USA).

3. Results

A total of 72 patients were enrolled in this study. Two patients were lost to follow-up and one patient died two months after surgery due to pneumonitis. Fifteen patients were excluded due to insufficient radiological data. Finally, 54 patients were included in the analysis. Patients with a mean age of 76.3 years ± standard deviation 6.1 were followed-up for 25.3 months ± 12.6. Twelve patients (22%) had a history of thoracic or lumbar surgery. Regarding medication for osteoporosis, 32 patients (59%) were treated by teriparatide, 3 patients (6%) by romosozumab, 8 patients (15%) by bisphosphonate, 4 patients (7%) by denosumab, and 7 patients (13%) by only vitamin D. Mean operative time and estimated blood loss was 269.8 ± 79.8 min and 289.5 ± 289.5 mL, respectively. Regarding fixation range, 32 patients (59%) were one above and one below fixation. Adjacent vertebral fractures were observed in 11 patients (20%) after surgery.

Table 1 shows the radiological parameters before and after surgery. Local kyphosis, thoracic kyphosis, lumbar lordosis, SVA, TPA and PI-LL significantly improved at final follow-up compared with before surgery, although there was no improvement in PT and SS. Local kyphosis improved from −17.5 degrees to 4.1 degrees immediately after surgery but was −0.6 degrees at final follow-up with 22.4% of correction loss. SVA was improved by only 18.7 mm (from 111.8 mm to 93.1 mm).

Table 1. Comparison of local and global alignment pre- and postoperatively.

	Mean (SD)		p-Value
Local kyphosis			
Preop	−17.5	(19.2)	
Immediate postop	4.1	(13.1)	
Final	−0.6	(14.8)	
Δ (preop-final)	21.7	(13.3)	<0.001
Correction loss (%)	22.4	(42.5)	<0.001
TK			
Preop	26.8	(17.1)	
Final	32.8	(12.3)	
Δ (preop-final)	6.1	(15.2)	<0.001
LL			
Preop	14.6	(16.9)	
Final	25.5	(13.8)	
Δ (preop-final)	10.9	(14.7)	<0.001
SVA			
Preop	111.8	(45.6)	
Final	93.1	(46.6)	
Δ (preop-final)	18.7	(56.7)	0.018
PT			
Preop	28.4	(7.9)	
Final	27	(8.2)	
Δ (preop-final)	1.4	(8)	0.209
SS			
Preop	21.5	9.8	
Final	22.8	10.0	
Δ (preop-final)	1.2	7.4	0.229
TPA			
Preop	33.2	(10.4)	
Final	30.1	(9.3)	
Δ (preop-final)	3.1	(9.5)	0.019
PI-LL			
Preop	35.1	(17.7)	
Final	24.2	(14.4)	
Δ (preop-final)	10.9	(14.7)	<0.001

SD, standard deviation; TK, Thoracic kyphosis; LL, Lumbar lordosis; SVA, Sagittal vertical axis; PT, Pelvic tilt; SS, sacral slope; TPA, T1 Pelvic Angle; PI-LL, Pelvic incidence- Lumbar lordosis.

Nineteen of the 54 patients (35%) showed global malalignment (SVA > 95 mm) postoperatively. Table 2 shows a comparison of baseline data, radiological parameters before surgery, and surgical complications between SVA > 95 mm and ≤95 mm groups. Adjacent vertebral fracture after surgery was significantly more frequent in the SVA > 95 mm group than in the SVA ≤ 95 mm group (37% vs. 11%, p = 0.038). TPA before surgery tended to be higher in the SVA > 95 mm group. Table 3 shows a comparison of clinical outcomes between SVA > 95 mm and ≤95 mm groups. VAS of back pain at final follow-up was significantly higher in patients with SVA > 95 mm than those in whom SVA was ≤95 mm (42.4 vs. 22.6, p = 0.015). Regarding the MCID, the better improvement was also observed in patients with SVA ≤ 95 mm (83% vs. 58%, p = 0.046). Multiple logistic regression showed a significantly increased odds ratio (OR) of adjacent vertebral fracture presence and TPA increase (OR = 4.76, 95% CI 1.10–20.58 and OR = 1.07, 1.00–1.14, respectively) (Table 4).

Table 2. Comparison between SVA > 95 mm and ≤95 mm groups by univariate analysis.

	SVA > 95 mm (n = 19)		SVA ≤ 95 mm (n = 35)		p-Value
	Mean or N	(SD or %)	Mean or N	(SD or %)	
Age	76.9	(5.8)	76	(6.2)	0.577
Gender	13	(68)	26	(74)	0.646
Follow-up period (months)	28.9	(13.4)	23.3	(11.8)	0.121
BMD (T-score)	−2.4	(0.5)	−2.1	(0.9)	0.251
Medication for osteoporosis					
Teriparatide/Romosozumab	13	(68)	22	(63)	0.683
Previous surgery					
Lumbar decompression	1	(5)	4	(11)	
Vertebral augmentation	1	(5)	1	(3)	
Posterior instrumentation	1	(5)	4	(11)	0.781
Level					
Thoracolumbar	10	(53)	17	(49)	
Lumbar	9	(47)	18	(51)	1.000
Proximal fixation range					
1	11	(58)	21	(60)	
>1	8	(42)	14	(40)	1.000
Distal fixation range					
1	13	(68)	24	(69)	
>1	6	(32)	11	(31)	1.000
Adjacent vertebral fracture	7	(37)	4	(11)	0.038
Infection	1	(5)	1	(3)	1.000
Reoperation	3	(16)	2	(6)	0.332
Cage subsidence	9	(47)	15	(43)	0.750
Local kyphosis preop	−21.7	(15.3)	−15.3	(20.8)	0.248
Local kyphosis at final FU	−2.2	(12)	0.3	(16.2)	0.549
LL preop	9.8	(17.8)	17.2	(16)	0.126
PT preop	30.6	(7.7)	27.1	(7.9)	0.127
PI preop	52.1	(10.7)	48.4	(9.5)	0.190
SVA preop	122.4	(45.4)	106.1	(45.4)	0.217
TK preop	21.5	(16.6)	29.6	(17)	0.100
TPA preop	36.9	(10.6)	31.2	(9.9)	0.052

SD, standard deviation; BMD, Bone marrow density; TK, Thoracic kyphosis; LL, Lumbar lordosis; SVA, Sagittal vertical axis; PT, Pelvic tilt; SS, sacral slope; TPA, T1 Pelvic Angle; PI-LL, Pelvic incidence- Lumbar lordosis.

Table 3. Comparison of clinical outcomes between SVA > 95 mm and ≤95 mm groups.

	SVA > 95 mm (n = 19)		SVA ≤ 95 mm (n = 35)		p-Value
	Mean or N	(SD or %)	Mean or N	(SD or %)	
PS improvement (N)	15	(79)	33	(94)	0.087
JOA score					
Preop	10.9	(5.1)	9.5	(4.8)	0.311
Final	19.2 *	(5.4)	20.5 *	(4.7)	0.361
Improvement ratio	46.1	(19.8)	54.8	(28.7)	0.248
VAS of back pain					
Preop	73.7	(17.8)	77.3	(23)	0.301
Final	42.4 *	(28.7)	22.6 *	(23)	0.015
Δ (preop-final)	31.4	(23.2)	54.7	(30.8)	0.008
MCID (≥21 mm)	11	(58)	29	(83)	0.046

SD, standard deviation; PS, Performance Status; JOA score, The Japanese Orthopaedic Association score; MCID, minimal clinically important difference. * There were significant differences between preop and final scores of JOA score and VAS of back pain.

Table 4. Adjusted odds ratio for SVA > 95 mm at final follow-up.

	Adjusted OR *	95% CI		p-Value
TPA preop (per 1 degree)	1.07	1.00	1.14	0.047
Adjacent vertebral fracture	4.76	1.10	20.58	0.037

TPA, T1 Pelvic Angle; OR, odds ratio. * The odds ratio was adjusted for age, preoperative TPA and adjacent vertebral fracture.

4. Discussion

This is the first study to reveal details about changes in sagittal balance following the minimally invasive procedure of corpectomy and reconstruction using an expandable cage with rectangular foot plates (APSF). Although there was 22.4% correction loss, local kyphotic changes using this system was 21.7°, which was better than the previous reports for APSF [17–19]. As well, Kanayama et al. reported that 80% of patients with OVF could be successfully treated using Kaneda instrumentation without the need for posterior reinforcement [20]. However, nearly 40% of correction loss was observed at the final follow-up. Suk et al. compared anterior-posterior surgery versus closing wedge osteotomy for kyphotic OVF and reported that the correction loss of anterior-posterior surgery was 27.3% with a mean blood loss of 2892 mL, whereas that of posterior closing wedge osteotomy was 10.8% with a mean blood loss of 1930 mL [21]. Posterior closing wedge osteotomy might offer better kyphosis correction. However, the procedure is technically demanding with more blood loss compared with the system in this study.

Although it is reported that anatomical and biomechanical restoration of vertebra is an advantage of anterior surgery resulting from the placement of anterior struts, our results indicated that restoration of sagittal alignment was not achieved by anterior surgery with 1–2 level posterior fixation in OVF patients. The parameters of SVA and TPA were used to evaluate sagittal spinal balance in this study. SVA increases with aging, and it is affected by movement of the hip and knee joint, such as "sway back" TPA, which combines information of SVA and PT and is a reliable indicator to address sagittal balance, including pelvic inclination [22]. TPA in this series was 33.2° preoperatively and 30.1° postoperatively. Thus, the improvement in TPA might not be significant. Ryan et al. demonstrated that TPA > 20° was the severe deformity threshold [23]. The main reason for this observation in our study was postoperative development of adjacent vertebral fracture. Low BMD, older age, an upper instrumented vertebra (UIV) level at the thoracolumbar spine, and a high preoperative SVA have been reported as risk factors for proximal junctional failure following surgical treatment for adult spinal deformity [24]. In the current series, BMD, medicine for osteoporosis, and level of surgery was not different between SVA > 95 mm and SVA ≤ 95 mm groups, probably because all the patients had comparatively severe osteoporosis. Posterior tethers and vertebral augmentation might be effective in preventing the failure of instrumentation, especially in patients with a high risk for proximal junctional kyphosis [25].

The relationship between PI and LL (PI-LL) is also considered an important parameter to evaluate sagittal spinal balance. Schwab et al. reported that SVA of 47 mm or more, PI-LL > 11° or more, and PT < 22° predicted severe disability (ODI > 40) [26]. Yamato et al. [31] described that the ideal LL angle can be determined using the equation 'LL = 0.45 × PI + 31.8'. Inami et al. [27] reported that the optimum value of PI-LL is inconsistent, in that it depends on the individual PI. [28]. In this study, although PI-LL improved significantly (from 35.1° to 24.2°), the final PI-LL did not reach the ideal value. In addition, the preoperative decrease in SS did not change postoperatively, indicating absence of improvement of pelvic retroversion. If lumbar lordosis is restored by surgery, the retroverted sacrum must be improved to maintain spino-pelvic harmony. Otherwise, reciprocal changes in the thoracic spine might develop to maintain sagittal balance [29,30]. Our results showed an increase in TK from 26.8° to 32.8°, which concurred with the theory mentioned above. This reciprocal change might be one of the reasons SVA did not change significantly in the OVF patients in our study. Improvement of the retroverted sacrum requires extension of the hip joint, with the erector spinae and gluteus muscles playing an important role in this action. In aged OVF patients, weakness of these muscles is responsible for the pelvic retroversion [8,31]. The average age of patients in this study was 76.3 years; hence, although we did not measure muscle volumes in these patients, they might have had age-related muscle wasting and weakness. A retroverted pelvis can be managed surgically by osteotomy of the lower lumbar vertebra or long fixation involving the pelvis. However, these are extremely invasive surgeries and it is not clear whether such invasive correction surgery is necessary for aged OVF patients.

SVA changed from 111.8 mm to 93.1 mm, which, although a statistically significant change, might be an insufficient improvement to correct malalignment. Based on the classification of Scoliosis Research Society [16], SVA (>95 mm) was reported as a risk factor with the deterioration of QOL measures [32]. In the current study, the number of patients who acquired one or more level improvement of PS was 15/19 (78.9%) in SVA > 95 mm and 33/35 (94.3%) in SVA $\leq$ 95 mm groups, which although better in the SVA $\leq$ 95 mm group, was not significantly different. Postoperative VAS was better in the SVA $\leq$ 95 mm than the SVA > 95 mm group. As also reported by Hu et al. [5]. SVA correlated with back pain in this study, which significantly improved after surgery. However, age and preoperative comorbidities influence the complication rate in deformity surgery [33]. Thus, we thought that the strategy for aged OVF patients should differ from those in ASD patients to relieve pain and improve mobility. Our results also showed the significant improvement of JOA score and VAS even in the SVA > 95 mm group compared with those before surgery. It is not always necessary to restore sagittal imbalance in aged OVF patients to the same level as in young people, although the clinical results are worse in patients with SVA > 95 mm.

There are some limitations to this study. First, the number of patients was small because some patients were excluded due to lack of data from standing whole spine X-ray films before surgery because of intractable back pain. Second, due to the lack of apparatus, we did not take whole spine X-rays including the lower extremity. Hence, we could not evaluate knee and hip joint flexion, which might have been used to compensate for sagittal imbalance [34]. Despite these limitations, this is the first report describing the correlation between anterior spinal surgery and changes in sagittal alignment, which might contribute to preoperative planning in OVF patients. For further study, the prediction methods for postoperative sagittal balance are necessary, since this might contribute to decision-making in the surgical planning for OVF patients.

5. Conclusions

This study demonstrated the clinical and radiological outcomes of combined anterior–posterior procedures via a lateral corpectomy, vertebral reconstruction using an expandable cage with rectangular footplates and posterior percutaneous pedicle screw fixation. The procedure, which includes short segment fixation, did not improve global spinal alignment and pelvic retroversion. However, the procedure achieved significant reduction of local kyphosis and VAS of back pain. This indicated that the procedure is effective in elderly patients with severe back pain due to spinal deformity and instability caused by OVF despite the global spinal malalignment.

Author Contributions: Conceptualization, H.T. (Hidetomi Terai) and H.N.; methodology, H.Y., S.K., T.M. and H.K.; formal analysis, S.T.; data curation, A.M., T.N., M.K., M.H., K.T., H.T. (Hiromitsu Toyoda), and A.S.; writing—original draft preparation, H.T. (Hidetomi Terai); writing—review and editing, H.T. (Hiromitsu Toyoda); supervision, H.N. All authors have read and agreed to the published version of the manuscript.

Funding: No funds were received in support of this work.

Institutional Review Board Statement: The study was conducted according to the guidelines of the Declaration of Helsinki and approved by the Institutional Review Board of Osaka city university (protocol code 3170 and date of approval 30 June 2015).

Informed Consent Statement: The need to obtain informed consent was waived based on the retrospective design and anonymization of patient identifiers.

Conflicts of Interest: A.S. received fee for Speakers Bureaus. The other authors declare that they have no conflicts of interest.

References

1. Dubousset, J. Three-dimensional analysis of the scoliotic deformity. In *The Pediatric Spine: Principles and Practice*; Weinstein, S.L., Ed.; Raven Press Ltd.: New York, NY, USA, 1994; pp. 479–496.
2. Miyakoshi, N.; Hongo, M.; Kobayashi, T.; Abe, T.; Abe, E.; Shimada, Y. Improvement of spinal alignment and quality of life after corrective surgery for spinal kyphosis in patients with osteoporosis: A comparative study with non-operated patients. *Osteoporos. Int.* **2015**, *26*, 2657–2664. [CrossRef] [PubMed]
3. Dai, J.; Yu, X.; Huang, S.; Fan, L.; Zhu, G.; Sun, H.; Tang, X. Relationship between sagittal spinal alignment and the incidence of vertebral fracture in menopausal women with osteoporosis: A multicenter longitudinal follow-up study. *Eur. Spine J.* **2015**, *24*, 737–743. [CrossRef] [PubMed]
4. Ohnishi, T.; Iwata, A.; Kanayama, M.; Oha, F.; Hashimoto, T.; Iwasaki, N. Impact of spino-pelvic and global spinal alignment on the risk of osteoporotic vertebral collapse. *Spine Surg. Relat. Res.* **2018**, *2*, 72–76. [CrossRef]
5. Hu, Z.; Man, G.C.W.; Kwok, A.K.L.; Law, S.W.; Chu, W.W.C.; Cheung, W.H.; Qiu, Y.; Cheng, J.C. Global sagittal alignment in elderly patients with osteoporosis and its relationship with severity of vertebral fracture and quality of life. *Arch. Osteoporos.* **2018**, *13*, 95. [CrossRef] [PubMed]
6. Menezes-Reis, R.; Bonugli, G.P.; Salmon, C.E.G.; Mazoroski, D.; Herrero, C.; Nogueira-Barbosa, M.H. Relationship of spinal alignment with muscular volume and fat infiltration of lumbar trunk muscles. *PLoS ONE* **2018**, *13*, e0200198. [CrossRef]
7. Yagi, M.; Hosogane, N.; Watanabe, K.; Asazuma, T.; Matsumoto, M. The paravertebral muscle and psoas for the maintenance of global spinal alignment in patient with degenerative lumbar scoliosis. *Spine J.* **2016**, *16*, 451–458. [CrossRef]
8. Takayama, K.; Kita, T.; Nakamura, H.; Kanematsu, F.; Yasunami, T.; Sakanaka, H.; Yamano, Y. New Predictive Index for Lumbar Paraspinal Muscle Degeneration Associated With Aging. *Spine* **2016**, *41*, E84–E90. [CrossRef]
9. Drey, M.; Sieber, C.C.; Bertsch, T.; Bauer, J.M.; Schmidmaier, R.; The FiAT Intervention Group. Osteosarcopenia is more than sarcopenia and osteopenia alone. *Aging Clin. Exp. Res.* **2016**, *28*, 895–899. [CrossRef]
10. Hirschfeld, H.P.; Kinsella, R.; Duque, G. Osteosarcopenia: Where bone, muscle, and fat collide. *Osteoporos. Int.* **2017**, *28*, 2781–2790. [CrossRef] [PubMed]
11. Cooper, C.; Cole, Z.A.; Holroyd, C.R.; Earl, S.C.; Harvey, N.C.; Dennison, E.M.; Melton, L.J.; Cummings, S.R.; Kanis, J.A. Secular trends in the incidence of hip and other osteoporotic fractures. *Osteoporos. Int.* **2011**, *22*, 1277–1288. [CrossRef]
12. Hosogane, N.; Nojiri, K.; Suzuki, S.; Funao, H.; Okada, E.; Isogai, N.; Ueda, S.; Hikata, T.; Shiono, Y.; Watanabe, K.; et al. Surgical Treatment of Osteoporotic Vertebral Fracture with Neurological Deficit-A Nationwide Multicenter Study in Japan. *Spine Surg. Relat. Res.* **2019**, *3*, 361–367. [CrossRef]
13. Watanabe, K.; Katsumi, K.; Ohashi, M.; Shibuya, Y.; Hirano, T.; Endo, N.; Kaito, T.; Yamashita, M.; Fujiwara, H.; Nagamoto, Y.; et al. Surgical outcomes of spinal fusion for osteoporotic vertebral fracture in the thoracolumbar spine: Comprehensive evaluations of 5 typical surgical fusion techniques. *J. Orthop. Sci.* **2019**, *24*, 1020–1026. [CrossRef]
14. Taiji, R.; Takami, M.; Yukawa, Y.; Hashizume, H.; Minamide, A.; Nakagawa, Y.; Nishi, H.; Iwasaki, H.; Tsutsui, S.; Okada, M.; et al. A short-segment fusion strategy using a wide-foot-plate expandable cage for vertebral pseudarthrosis after an osteoporotic vertebral fracture. *J. Neurosurg. Spine* **2020**, *33*, 862–869. [CrossRef]
15. Parker, S.L.; Adogwa, O.; Paul, A.R.; Anderson, W.N.; Aaronson, O.; Cheng, J.S.; McGirt, M.J. Utility of minimum clinically important difference in assessing pain, disability, and health state after transforaminal lumbar interbody fusion for degenerative lumbar spondylolisthesis. *J. Neurosurg. Spine* **2011**, *14*, 598–604. [CrossRef] [PubMed]
16. Schwab, F.; Ungar, B.; Blondel, B.; Buchowski, J.; Coe, J.; Deinlein, D.; DeWald, C.; Mehdian, H.; Shaffrey, C.; Tribus, C.; et al. Scoliosis Research Society-Schwab adult spinal deformity classification: A validation study. *Spine* **2012**, *37*, 1077–1082. [CrossRef]
17. Kashii, M.; Yamazaki, R.; Yamashita, T.; Okuda, S.; Fujimori, T.; Nagamoto, Y.; Tamura, Y.; Oda, T.; Ohwada, T.; Yoshikawa, H.; et al. Surgical treatment for osteoporotic vertebral collapse with neurological deficits: Retrospective comparative study of three procedures—Anterior surgery versus posterior spinal shortening osteotomy versus posterior spinal fusion using vertebroplasty. *Eur. Spine J.* **2013**, *22*, 1633–1642. [CrossRef] [PubMed]
18. Takenaka, S.; Mukai, Y.; Hosono, N.; Fuji, T. Major surgical treatment of osteoporotic vertebral fractures in the elderly: A comparison of anterior spinal fusion, anterior-posterior combined surgery and posterior closing wedge osteotomy. *Asian Spine J.* **2014**, *8*, 322–330. [CrossRef]
19. Uchida, K.; Kobayashi, S.; Nakajima, H.; Kokubo, Y.; Yayama, T.; Sato, R.; Timbihurira, G.; Baba, H. Anterior expandable strut cage replacement for osteoporotic thoracolumbar vertebral collapse. *J. Neurosurg. Spine* **2006**, *4*, 454–462. [CrossRef] [PubMed]
20. Kanayama, M.; Ishida, T.; Hashimoto, T.; Shigenobu, K.; Togawa, D.; Oha, F.; Kaneda, K. Role of major spine surgery using Kaneda anterior instrumentation for osteoporotic vertebral collapse. *J. Spinal Disord. Tech.* **2010**, *23*, 53–56. [CrossRef] [PubMed]
21. Suk, S.I.; Kim, J.H.; Lee, S.M.; Chung, E.R.; Lee, J.H. Anterior-posterior surgery versus posterior closing wedge osteotomy in posttraumatic kyphosis with neurologic compromised osteoporotic fracture. *Spine* **2003**, *28*, 2170–2175. [CrossRef]

22. Qiao, J.; Zhu, F.; Xu, L.; Liu, Z.; Zhu, Z.; Qian, B.; Sun, X.; Qiu, Y. T1 pelvic angle: A new predictor for postoperative sagittal balance and clinical outcomes in adult scoliosis. *Spine* **2014**, *39*, 2103–2107. [CrossRef]
23. Ryan, D.J.; Protopsaltis, T.S.; Ames, C.P.; Hostin, R.; Klineberg, E.; Mundis, G.M.; Obeid, I.; Kebaish, K.; Smith, J.S.; Boachie-Adjei, O.; et al. T1 pelvic angle (TPA) effectively evaluates sagittal deformity and assesses radiographical surgical outcomes longitudinally. *Spine* **2014**, *39*, 1203–1210. [CrossRef]
24. Yagi, M.; Fujita, N.; Okada, E.; Tsuji, O.; Nagoshi, N.; Asazuma, T.; Ishii, K.; Nakamura, M.; Matsumoto, M.; Watanabe, K. Fine-tuning the Predictive Model for Proximal Junctional Failure in Surgically Treated Patients With Adult Spinal Deformity. *Spine* **2018**, *43*, 767–773. [CrossRef] [PubMed]
25. Yagi, M.; Nakahira, Y.; Watanabe, K.; Nakamura, M.; Matsumoto, M.; Iwamoto, M. The effect of posterior tethers on the biomechanics of proximal junctional kyphosis: The whole human finite element model analysis. *Sci. Rep.* **2020**, *10*, 3433. [CrossRef] [PubMed]
26. Schwab, F.J.; Blondel, B.; Bess, S.; Hostin, R.; Shaffrey, C.I.; Smith, J.S.; Boachie-Adjei, O.; Burton, D.C.; Akbarnia, B.A.; Mundis, G.M.; et al. Radiographical spinopelvic parameters and disability in the setting of adult spinal deformity: A prospective multicenter analysis. *Spine* **2013**, *38*, E803–E812. [CrossRef]
27. Yamato, Y.; Hasegawa, T.; Kobayashi, S.; Yasuda, T.; Togawa, D.; Arima, H.; Oe, S.; Iida, T.; Matsumura, A.; Hosogane, N.; et al. Calculation of the Target Lumbar Lordosis Angle for Restoring an Optimal Pelvic Tilt in Elderly Patients With Adult Spinal Deformity. *Spine* **2016**, *41*, E211–E217. [CrossRef] [PubMed]
28. Inami, S.; Moridaira, H.; Takeuchi, D.; Shiba, Y.; Nohara, Y.; Taneichi, H. Optimum pelvic incidence minus lumbar lordosis value can be determined by individual pelvic incidence. *Eur. Spine J.* **2016**, *25*, 3638–3643. [CrossRef]
29. Klineberg, E.; Schwab, F.; Ames, C.; Hostin, R.; Bess, S.; Smith, J.S.; Gupta, M.C.; Boachie, O.; Hart, R.A.; Akbarnia, B.A.; et al. Acute reciprocal changes distant from the site of spinal osteotomies affect global postoperative alignment. *Adv. Orthop.* **2011**, *2011*, 415946. [CrossRef]
30. Ferrero, E.; Liabaud, B.; Challier, V.; Lafage, R.; Diebo, B.G.; Vira, S.; Liu, S.; Vital, J.M.; Ilharreborde, B.; Protopsaltis, T.S.; et al. Role of pelvic translation and lower-extremity compensation to maintain gravity line position in spinal deformity. *J. Neurosurg. Spine* **2016**, *24*, 436–446. [CrossRef]
31. Li, Q.; Sun, J.; Cui, X.; Jiang, Z.; Li, T. Analysis of correlation between degeneration of lower lumbar paraspinal muscles and spinopelvic alignment in patients with osteoporotic vertebral compression fracture. *J. Back Musculoskelet. Rehabil.* **2017**, *30*, 1209–1214. [CrossRef]
32. Banno, T.; Togawa, D.; Arima, H.; Hasegawa, T.; Yamato, Y.; Kobayashi, S.; Yasuda, T.; Oe, S.; Hoshino, H.; Matsuyama, Y. The cohort study for the determination of reference values for spinopelvic parameters (T1 pelvic angle and global tilt) in elderly volunteers. *Eur. Spine J.* **2016**, *25*, 3687–3693. [CrossRef]
33. Yoshida, G.; Hasegawa, T.; Yamato, Y.; Kobayashi, S.; Oe, S.; Banno, T.; Mihara, Y.; Arima, H.; Ushirozako, H.; Yasuda, T.; et al. Predicting Perioperative Complications in Adult Spinal Deformity Surgery Using a Simple Sliding Scale. *Spine* **2018**, *43*, 562–570. [CrossRef] [PubMed]
34. Bailey, J.F.; Matthew, R.P.; Seko, S.; Curran, P.; Chu, L.; Berven, S.H.; Deviren, V.; Burch, S.; Lotz, J.C. ISSLS PRIZE IN BIOENGINEERING SCIENCE 2019: Biomechanical changes in dynamic sagittal balance and lower limb compensatory strategies following realignment surgery in adult spinal deformity patients. *Eur. Spine J.* **2019**, *28*, 905–913. [CrossRef]

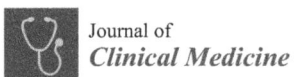

Article

Associations between Clinical Findings and Severity of Diffuse Idiopathic Skeletal Hyperostosis in Patients with Ossification of the Posterior Longitudinal Ligament

Takashi Hirai [1,*,†], Soraya Nishimura [2,†], Toshitaka Yoshii [1,†], Narihito Nagoshi [2,†], Jun Hashimoto [1,†], Kanji Mori [3,†], Satoshi Maki [4,†], Keiichi Katsumi [5,†], Kazuhiro Takeuchi [6,†], Shuta Ushio [1,†], Takeo Furuya [4,†], Kei Watanabe [5,†], Norihiro Nishida [7,†], Kota Watanabe [2,†], Takashi Kaito [8,†], Satoshi Kato [9,†], Katsuya Nagashima [10,†], Masao Koda [10,†], Hiroaki Nakashima [11,†], Shiro Imagama [11,†], Kazuma Murata [12,†], Yuji Matsuoka [12,†], Kanichiro Wada [13,†], Atsushi Kimura [14,†], Tetsuro Ohba [15,†], Hiroyuki Katoh [16,†], Masahiko Watanabe [16,†], Yukihiro Matsuyama [17,†], Hiroshi Ozawa [18,†], Hirotaka Haro [15,†], Katsushi Takeshita [14,†], Morio Matsumoto [2,†], Masaya Nakamura [2,†], Masashi Yamazaki [10,†], Yu Matsukura [1,†], Hiroyuki Inose [1,†], Atsushi Okawa [1,†] and Yoshiharu Kawaguchi [19,†]

1 Department of Orthopaedic Surgery, Tokyo Medical and Dental University, Bunkyo-ku, Tokyo 113-8510, Japan; yoshii.orth@tmd.ac.jp (T.Y.); 0123456789jun@gmail.com (J.H.); ushiorth20@gmail.com (S.U.); matsukura.orth@tmd.ac.jp (Y.M.); inose.orth@tmd.ac.jp (H.I.); okawa.orth@tmd.ac.jp (A.O.)
2 Department of Orthopedic Surgery, School of Medicine, Keio University, Shinjuku, Tokyo 160-8582, Japan; soraya.nishimura@gmail.com (S.N.); nagoshi@2002.jukuin.keio.ac.jp (N.N.); kw197251@keio.jp (K.W.); morio@a5.keio.jp (M.M.); masa@a8.keio.jp (M.N.)
3 Department of Orthopaedic Surgery, Shiga University of Medical Science, Ōtsu 520-2192, Japan; kanchi@belle.shiga-med.ac.jp
4 Department of Orthopaedic Surgery, School of Medicine, Chiba University Graduate, Chiba 260-0856, Japan; satoshi.maki@chiba-u.jp (S.M.); takeo251274@yahoo.co.jp (T.F.)
5 Department of Orthopedic Surgery, Niigata University Medical and Dental General Hospital, Niigata 951-8520, Japan; kkatsu_os@yahoo.co.jp (K.K.); keiwatanabe_39jp@live.jp (K.W.)
6 National Hospital Organization Okayama Medical Center, Department of Orthopedic Surgery, Okayama 701-1192, Japan; takeuchi@okayamamc.jp
7 Department of Orthopaedic Surgery, Graduate School of Medicine, Yamaguchi University, Yamaguchi 755-8505, Japan; nishida3@yamaguchi-u.ac.jp
8 Department of Orthopaedic Surgery, Graduate School of Medicine, Osaka University, Suita 565-0871, Osaka, Japan; takashikaito@gmail.com
9 Department of Orthopedic Surgery, Graduate School of Medical Sciences, Kanazawa University, Kanazawa 920-1192, Japan; skato323@gmail.com
10 Department of Orthopedic Surgery, Faculty of Medicine, University of Tsukuba, Tsukuba 305-8577, Japan; katsu_n103@yahoo.co.jp (K.N.); masaokod@gmail.com (M.K.); masashiy@md.tsukuba.ac.jp (M.Y.)
11 Department of Orthopedics, Graduate School of Medicine, Nagoya University, 65 Tsurumai, Shouwa-ku, Nagoya 466-8560, Japan; hirospine@med.nagoya-u.ac.jp (H.N.); imagama@med.nagoya-u.ac.jp (S.I.)
12 Department of Orthopedic Surgery, Tokyo Medical University, Shinjuku, Tokyo 160-8402, Japan; kaz.mur26@gmail.com (K.M.); yuji_kazu77@yahoo.co.jp (Y.M.)
13 Department of Orthopedic Surgery, Graduate School of Medicine, Hirosaki University, Hirosaki 036-8562, Japan; wadak39@hirosaki-u.ac.jp
14 Department of Orthopedics, Jichi Medical University, Shimotsuke 329-0498, Japan; akimura@jichi.ac.jp (A.K.); dtstake@gmail.com (K.T.)
15 Department of Orthopedic Surgery, University of Yamanashi, Chuo 409-3898, Japan; tooba@yamanashi.ac.jp (T.O.); haro@yamanashi.ac.jp (H.H.)
16 Department of Orthopedic Surgery, Surgical Science, School of Medicine, Tokai University, Isehara 259-1193, Japan; hero@tokai-u.jp (H.K.); masahiko@is.icc.u-tokai.ac.jp (M.W.)
17 Department of Orthopedic Surgery, School of Medicine, Hamamatsu University, Hamamatsu 431-3125, Japan; spine-yu@hama-med.ac.jp
18 Department of Orthopaedic Surgery, Tohoku Medical and Pharmaceutical University, Sendai 983-8536, Japan; hozawa@med.tohoku.ac.jp
19 Department of Orthopedic Surgery, Faculty of Medicine, University of Toyama, Toyama 930-0194, Japan; zenji@med.u-toyama.ac.jp
* Correspondence: hirai.orth@tmd.ac.jp; Tel.: +81-35-803-5279
† Japanese Organization of the Study for Ossification of Spinal Ligament (JOSL).

Abstract: Background: This study investigated how diffuse idiopathic skeletal hyperostosis (DISH) influences clinical characteristics in patients with cervical ossification of the posterior longitudinal ligament (OPLL). Although DISH is considered unlikely to promote neurologic dysfunction, this relationship remains unclear. Methods: Patient data were prospectively collected from 16 Japanese institutions. In total, 239 patients with cervical OPLL were enrolled who had whole-spine computed tomography images available. The primary outcomes were visual analog scale pain scores and the results of other self-reported clinical questionnaires. Correlations were sought between clinical symptoms and DISH using the following grading system: 1, DISH at T3-T10; 2, DISH at both T3–10 and C6–T2 and/or T11–L2; and 3, DISH beyond the C5 and/or L3 levels. Results: DISH was absent in 132 cases, grade 1 in 23, grade 2 in 65, and grade 3 in 19. There were no significant correlations between DISH grade and clinical scores. However, there was a significant difference in the prevalence of neck pain (but not in back pain or low back pain) among the three grades. Interestingly, DISH localized in the thoracic spine (grade 1) may create overload at the cervical spine and lead to neck pain in patients with cervical OPLL. Conclusion: This study is the first prospective multicenter cross-sectional comparison of subjective outcomes in patients with cervical OPLL according to the presence or absence of DISH. The severity of DISH was partially associated with the prevalence of neck pain.

Keywords: cervical spine; clinical findings; computed tomography; diffuse idiopathic skeletal hyperostosis; ossification of the posterior longitudinal ligament; pain; patient-reported outcomes; whole spine

1. Introduction

Ossification of the spinal ligaments impairs spinal mobility and occasionally leads to a spinal disorder [1,2]. Ossification of the posterior longitudinal ligament (OPLL) is common in Asian countries and can cause severe myelopathy [3]. Diffuse idiopathic skeletal hyperostosis (DISH), which is defined as ossification of the anterior longitudinal ligament bridging at least four vertebral segments of the thoracolumbar spine [4,5], has also been recognized as a pathological feature in patients predisposed to ossification and often coincides with the presence of OPLL [6–10]. Although DISH has been widely regarded as an asymptomatic disorder, it is unclear how it affects symptoms related to the whole spine. Few studies have compared patients with and without DISH in terms of clinical symptoms. Therefore, the Japanese Multicenter Research Organization for Ossification of the Spinal Ligament (JOSL), established a nationwide patient registry to prospectively collect the clinical and radiologic data, including whole-spine computed tomography (CT) scans, of OPLL patients. Using data from this registry, this paper focuses on differences in clinical and radiological findings between patients with and without DISH. We further sought to identify any significant associations between clinical symptoms and the severity of DISH in these patients based on patient-reported outcomes.

2. Materials and Methods

2.1. Patients and Methods

This multicenter prospective cross-sectional study used data from 16 member institutions of the JOSL established by the Japan Ministry of Health, Labour, and Welfare. The inclusion criteria were as follows: age ≥20 years; diagnosis of cervical OPLL based on radiographic findings; symptoms such as neck pain and upper and/or lower extremity numbness regardless of whether surgery was required, clumsiness, and gait disturbance; a visit made to a participating institution for symptoms between September 2015 and December 2017; and whole-spine CT scans available to determine the location of ossified lesions in the spine. The only exclusion criterion was a history of cervical spine surgery for OPLL. The study was approved by the institutional review board of each participating institution and conducted in accordance with the relevant guidelines and regulations.

2.2. Clinical Evaluation

Basic demographic and clinical data of patients were collected, including age, sex, diabetes mellitus (DM) status, body mass index (BMI), and presence of neck pain, back pain, and/or low back pain (LBP). Clinical status was evaluated using the following measures: cervical Japanese Orthopaedic Association (JOA) score [11], which is used for functional assessment of patients with cervical myelopathy, JOA Cervical Myelopathy Evaluation Questionnaire (JOA-CMEQ) [12], which assesses the function of the cervical spine, upper and lower extremities, and bladder as well as quality of life; and the JOA Back Pain Evaluation Questionnaire (JOA-BPEQ) [13], which assesses lumbar spine function, social dysfunction, mentality, locomotive function, and body pain. The degree of pain or stiffness in the neck or shoulders, pain or numbness in the arms or hands, and LBP was evaluated using a visual analog scale (VAS).

2.3. Radiologic Evaluations

CT images of the whole spine were collected for each patient. The images included the cervical, thoracic, and lumbosacral segments, spanning the occipital bone to the sacrum. The incidence of OPLL in the cervical spine from the clivus to C7 and in other spinal regions from T1 to S1 was evaluated on mid-sagittal CT images. Blinded to clinical outcomes, six senior spine surgeons (S.U., K.M., S.M., K.K., N.N., and K.T.) independently evaluated the images, as described previously [13]. OPLL was assessed as DISH if it completely bridged at least four contiguous adjacent vertebral bodies anywhere in the spine based on the criteria established by Resnick and Niwayama [5]. In accordance with a previous report [10], DISH was classified as follows: grade 1, DISH at T3–T10; grade 2, DISH at both T3–10 and C6–T2 and/or T11–L2; and grade 3, DISH extends beyond the C5 and/or L3 levels (Figure 1). To identify any significant differences in clinical findings, we compared patients with and without DISH and those with DISH according to grade. In addition, the ossification of the posterior longitudinal ligament index (OP-index), defined as the number of levels with OPLL in the whole spine [6], was also calculated for each patient.

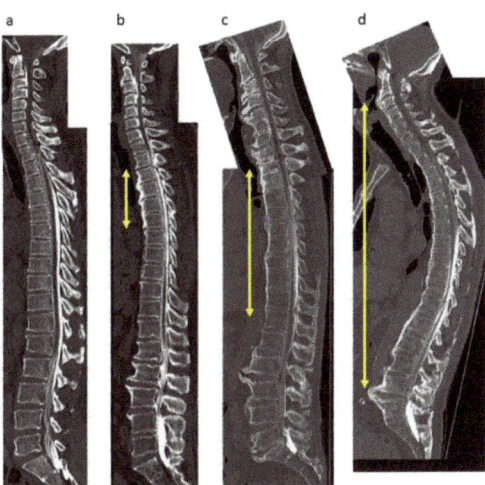

Figure 1. DISH grading system. (**a**) No DISH; (**b**) Grade 1 (bony bridge at T3–T6); (**c**) Grade 2 (T2–T12); (**d**) Grade 3 (C2–L5). DISH, diffuse idiopathic skeletal hyperostosis.

3. Results

3.1. Demographic and Clinical Data

The demographic and clinical characteristics of the patients are shown according to DISH status in Table 1. There was no significant difference in age, BMI, DM status, or cervical JOA score between the group with DISH (*n* = 107) and the group without DISH (*n* = 132). Table 1 shows the prevalence of pain and the JOA-CMEQ, JOA-BPEQ, and VAS scores for each domain. There was no significant between-group difference in these patient-reported outcomes except for lumbar spine function; however, there was a significant difference in the OP-index value.

Table 1. Demographic and clinical data for patients with OPLL according to presence or absence of DISH.

	No DISH (*n* = 132)	DISH (*n* = 107)	*p*-Value
Age (years)	60.9 ± 11.6	67.6 ± 12.1	<0.001 ***
Male (%)	61.4	76.6	0.01 *
Body mass index	26.1 ± 4.7	25.6 ± 4.2	0.38
Diabetes mellitus (%)	21.2	28.9	0.25
Cervical JOA score	12.5 (6–17)	11.9 (6–17)	0.22
OP-index	7.1 ± 0.5	10.5 ± 0.6	<0.001 ***
Prevalence of symptoms (%)			
Neck pain	59.8	58.9	0.94
Back pain	25.8	30.8	0.52
Low back pain	54.5	52.3	0.81
JOA-CMEQ score			
Cervical spine function	68.5 ± 28.2	62.5 ± 28.8	0.10
Upper extremity function	81.8 ± 20.6	78.0 ± 22.7	0.19
Lower extremity function	69.0 ± 29.5	62.3 ± 31.9	0.10
Bladder function	76.5 ± 19.8	72.0 ± 24.4	0.11
Quality of life	49.3 ± 20.0	50.7 ± 20.0	0.60
JOA-BPEQ score			
Lumbar spine function	72.3 ± 28.2	62.5 ± 35.0	0.02 *
Social dysfunction	57.7 ± 28.6	54.6 ± 30.4	0.47
Mentality	49.3 ± 19.5	49.0 ± 20.6	0.90
Locomotive function	67.1 ± 33.0	60.6 ± 37.7	0.19
Body pain	71.8 ± 32.7	69.6 ± 34.9	0.63
VAS score			
Neck pain	39.1 ± 30.2	38.4 ± 32.5	0.83
Upper extremity numbness	47.5 ± 32.8	42.1 ± 33.8	0.20
Chest constriction	11.1 ± 22.2	9.2 ± 21.3	0.48
Numbness below the chest	35.3 ± 32.7	39.0 ± 35.6	0.41
Low back pain	25.8 ± 26.6	30.0 ± 31.6	0.29
Lower extremity numbness	29.5 ± 32.7	32.8 ± 35.1	0.47
Lower extremity pain	24.0 ± 30.5	22.0 ± 29.9	0.57

Data are expressed as the mean ± standard deviation or as the percentage. BPEQ, Back Pain Evaluation Questionnaire; CMEQ, Cervical Myelopathy Evaluation Questionnaire; DISH, diffuse idiopathic skeletal hyperostosis; JOA, Japanese Orthopaedic Association; OP-index, ossification of the posterior longitudinal ligament index; OPLL, ossification of the posterior longitudinal ligament; VAS, visual analog scale.; * Significant at *p* < 0.05; *** significant at *p* < 0.001.

3.2. Demographic and Clinical Characteristics by DISH Grade

Patient demographics are shown according to DISH grade in Table 2 and Figure 2. There was a significant between-group difference in age (Figure 2a) but not in the sex distribution. No significant between-group difference was found in BMI (Figure 2b), DM status, or cervical JOA score among the three grades (Figure 2c). There was a significant correlation between the OP-index and DISH grade (Table 2).

Table 2. Demographics of patients with cervical OPLL according to DISH grade.

	Grade 1 (n = 23)	Grade 2 (n = 65)	Grade 3 (n = 19)	p-Value
Age (years)	65.4 ± 12.7	66.9 ± 12.3	72.8 ± 9.9	<0.001 ***
Male (%)	78.3	75.4	78.9	0.74
Body mass index	25.7 ± 5.0	25.9 ± 3.7	24.7 ± 4.9	0.55
Diabetes mellitus (%)	30.4	32.3	15.8	0.41
Cervical JOA score	12.4 (7.5–17)	11.8 (−2, 17)	11.9 (6–16)	0.36
OP-index	8.7 ± 1.1	10.4 ± 0.8	12.6 ± 1.0	<0.001 ***

Data are expressed as the mean ± standard deviation or as the percentage, DISH, diffuse idiopathic skeletal hyperostosis; JOA, Japanese Orthopaedic Association; OP-index, ossification of the posterior longitudinal ligament index; OPLL, ossification of the posterior longitudinal ligament; *** significant at $p < 0.001$.

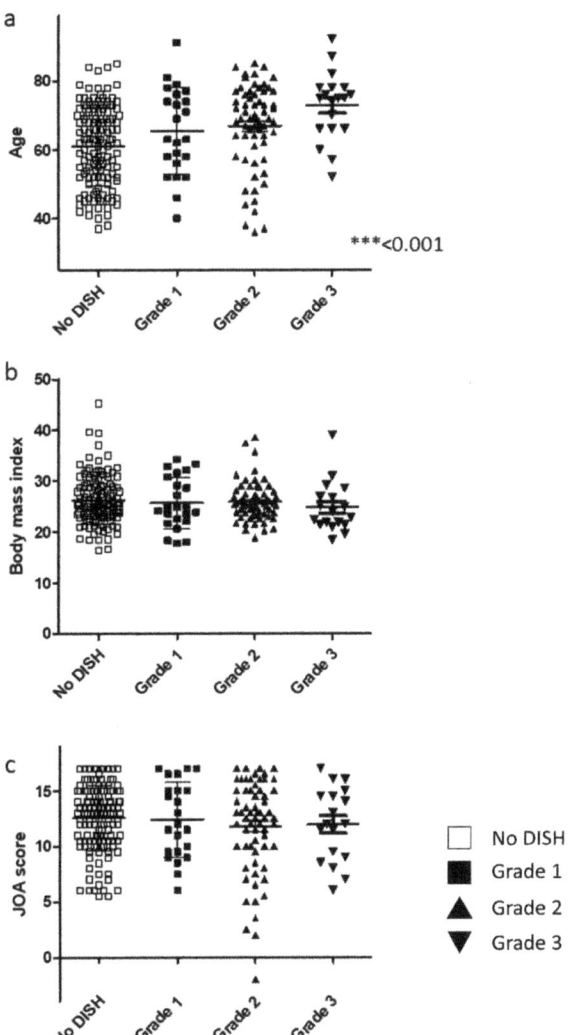

Figure 2. Relationship between basic demographic and clinical findings and DISH grade. (a) Patient age. (b) Body mass index. (c) JOA score. DISH, diffuse idiopathic skeletal hyperostosis; JOA, Japanese Orthopaedic Association.

3.3. Severity of DISH Was Not Associated with Myelopathic Symptoms or Lumbar Spine Function in Patients with Cervical OPLL

The score for each item in the JOA-CMEQ and JOA-BPEQ was evaluated to assess whether the severity of DISH in terms of cervical myelopathy and lumbar spine function affects the ability to perform activities of daily living. There were no significant correlations among the four groups for JOA-CMEQ scores (Figure 3a–e). Similarly, there were no significant differences among the three DISH grades in terms of lumbar spine function, social dysfunction, mentality, locomotive function, and body pain (Figure 4a–e).

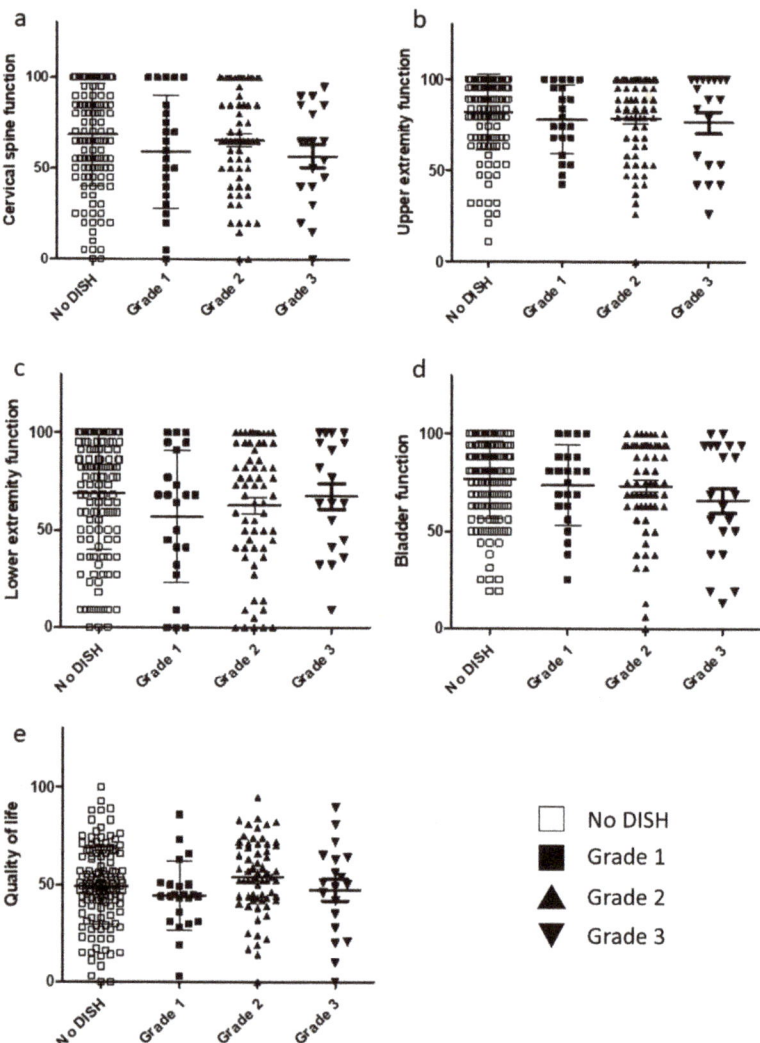

Figure 3. Relationship between JOA-CMEQ scores and DISH grade. (**a**) Cervical function. (**b**) Upper extremity function. (**c**) Lower extremity function. (**d**) Bladder function. (**e**) Quality of life. DISH, diffuse idiopathic skeletal hyperostosis; JOA-CMEQ, Japanese Orthopaedic Association Cervical Myelopathy Evaluation Questionnaire.

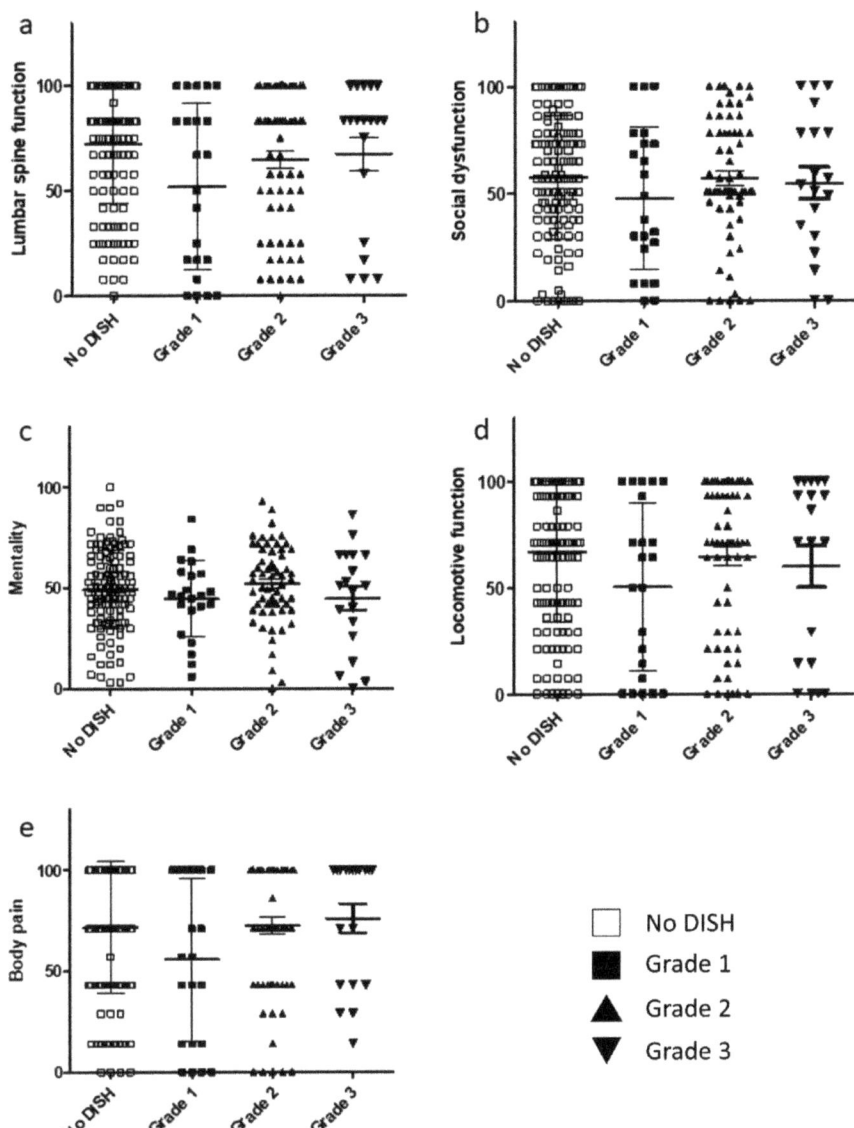

Figure 4. Relationship between JOA-BPEQ and DISH grade. (**a**) Lumbar function. (**b**) Social dysfunction. (**c**) Mentality. (**d**) Locomotive function. (**e**) Body pain. DISH, diffuse idiopathic skeletal hyperostosis; JOA-BPEQ, Japanese Orthopaedic Association Back Pain Evaluation Questionnaire.

3.4. Degree of DISH Correlated Negatively with Prevalence of Neck Pain but Not Back Pain or LBP in Patients with Cervical OPLL

The prevalence of neck pain was significantly correlated with degree of DISH, but back pain and LBP were not (Table 3). Furthermore, although there was no statistically significant difference in LBP among the three grades of DISH, LBP tended to decrease with increasing grade.

Table 3. Prevalence of symptoms in patients with cervical OPLL according to DISH grade.

	Grade 1 (n = 23)	Grade 2 (n = 65)	Grade 3 (n = 19)	p-Value
Prevalence of symptoms (%)				
Neck pain	78.3	56.9	36.8	<0.05 *
Back pain	30.4	32.3	26.3	0.65
Low back pain	60.9	53.8	36.8	0.14

Data are expressed as the mean ± standard deviation or as the percentage, DISH, diffuse idiopathic skeletal hyperostosis; OPLL, ossification of the posterior longitudinal ligament; * Significant at $p < 0.05$.

VAS scores from the JOA-CMEQ and JOA-BPEQ were investigated to clarify the relationship between degree of DISH and pain associated with cervical myelopathy. However, no significant difference was found in the VAS scores among the three DISH grades (Figures 5 and 6).

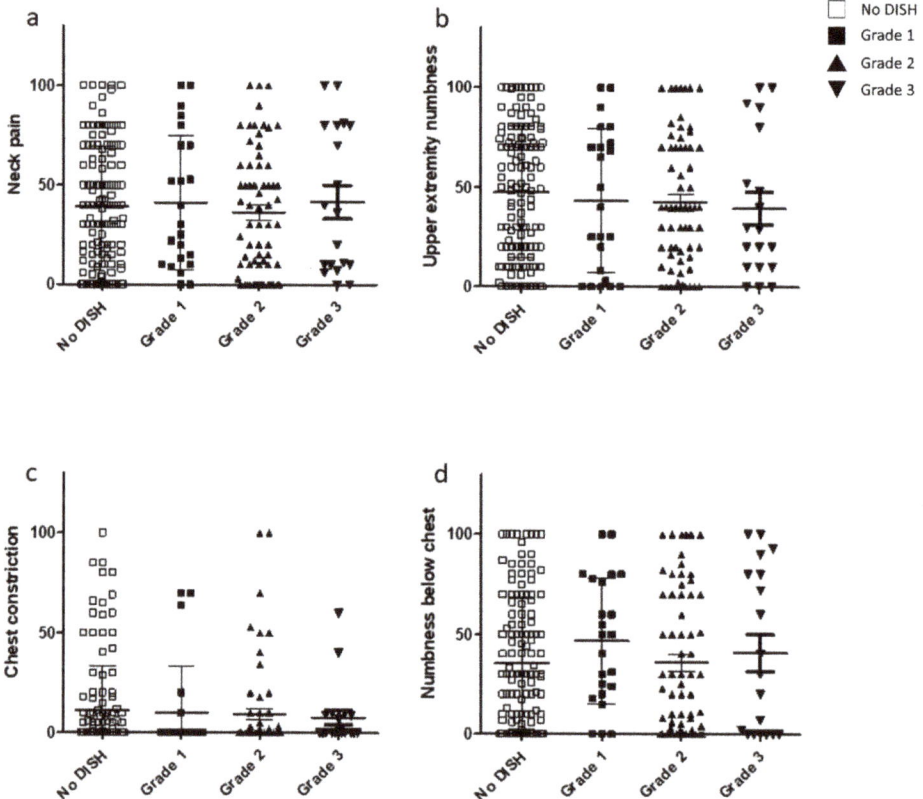

Figure 5. Relationship between the VAS scores included in the JOA-CMEQ and DISH grade. VAS scores for (**a**) neck pain, (**b**) upper extremity numbness, (**c**) chest constriction, and (**d**) numbness below the chest. DISH, diffuse idiopathic skeletal hyperostosis; JOA-CMEQ, Japanese Orthopaedic Association Cervical Myelopathy Evaluation Questionnaire; VAS, visual analog scale.

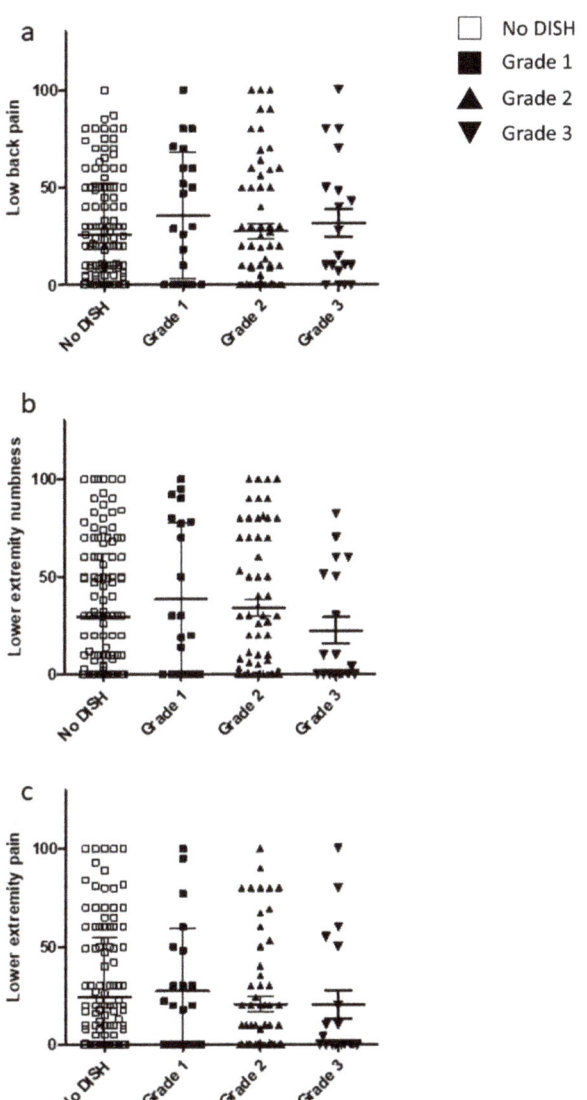

Figure 6. Relationship between the VAS scores included in the JOA-BPEQ and DISH grade. VAS scores for (**a**) low back pain, (**b**) lower extremity numbness, and (**c**) lower extremity pain. DISH, diffuse idiopathic skeletal hyperostosis; JOA-BPEQ, Japanese Orthopaedic Association Back Pain Evaluation Questionnaire; VAS, visual analog scale.

4. Discussion

DISH is a systemic condition characterized by ossification of ligaments and entheses throughout the body. Considered to be mostly an asymptomatic condition, DISH was largely ignored by clinicians and researchers until the 1990s. However, it is now known that DISH can sometimes result in specific symptoms, including back pain [14], stiffness [15], reduced range of articular motion [4] and dysphagia [16]. Notably, energy cannot be distributed over multiple segments in patients with DISH. Therefore, even minor trauma can lead to an unstable spinal fracture. A retrospective study [17,18] reviewed 289 patients with

DISH-related spinal fractures and demonstrated that these fractures frequently resulted in spinal cord injury and were sometimes associated with mortality. That study also found that the diagnosis was often delayed, leading to unexpected impairment of neurologic status, especially in patients with a thoracolumbar fracture. Therefore, it is important to recognize the presence of this pathology and the associated risks even after minor trauma, given that DISH creates longer bony lever arms, which increase spinal instability at the fracture site when a fracture occurs.

Patients with cervical OPLL often have ossification of other spinal ligaments, including the ligamentum flavum, anterior longitudinal ligament, and the interspinous and supraspinous ligaments. In earlier studies [4,19–22], 25–50% of patients with cervical OPLL had DISH. A previous retrospective study by our group [10] revealed that DISH was distributed primarily in the middle thoracic spine in younger patients but could extend to the cervical and/or lumbar spine in older patients. Toyoda et al. [23] reported that the prevalence of DISH increased with age in whole-spine radiographs of 345 patients in whom spinal surgery was required. Older patients in the present study also had a more severe DISH grade. Although a further longitudinal study is needed, the evidence to date suggests that ossification of the anterior longitudinal ligament might progress gradually from the thoracic spine to the cervical spine and lumbar spine with aging.

DISH has been recognized to be not only a structural abnormality in the human thoracic spine but also a result of metabolic syndrome. Okada et al. [24] compared subjects with and without DISH and demonstrated that the prevalence of metabolic syndrome was significantly higher in patients with DISH than in those without DISH (28.9% vs. 16.0%). Furthermore, using abdominal CT, Lantsman et al. [25] showed that areas of visceral fat were larger in patients with DISH than in healthy controls. Although there were no significant associations in terms of the prevalence of DM between patients with and without DISH or among the three grades in the present study, the onset and extent of DISH may be associated with a systemic metabolic disorder.

This prospective multicenter study is the first to investigate subjective outcomes in patients with cervical OPLL according to DISH status. Although we collected patient-reported outcomes for activities of daily living, we found no DISH-related differences in patients with cervical OPLL. These findings are consistent with the opinion of some clinicians that DISH should be considered a state rather than a disease [26]. DISH may be present not only by itself but can also accompany ossification of other spinal ligaments that often lead to spinal cord disorders [13,27]. Therefore, in the present study, to reduce selection bias in this regard, we enrolled only patients with cervical OPLL. Therefore, we believe that DISH does not directly impair neurologic status or quality of life.

Several studies have investigated the association between presence of DISH and physical pain. Mata et al. [28] compared clinical symptoms in 56 patients with DISH, 43 control patients with lumbar spondylosis, and healthy volunteers and demonstrated that patients with DISH were more likely to report a history of upper extremity pain, medial epicondylitis of the elbow, enthesitis of the patella or heel, and dysphagia than were patients with lumbar spondylosis. They also reported that neck rotation and thoracic movements were more limited in the patients with DISH than in the patients with spondylosis or the healthy controls, and lumbar movement was more restricted in the patients with DISH than in the healthy controls. However, the findings of a similar study were contradictory. Schlapbach et al. [29] demonstrated that the radiological findings for DISH were not associated with an increased frequency of back pain and had no clinical relevance. Moreover, Holton et al. [30] randomly collected data for 298 elderly men from a surveillance cohort of 5995 men and demonstrated that the frequency of LBP was reduced in 126 men with DISH compared with 172 men without DISH based on North American Spine Society questionnaires for back and neck pain. We have also shown that patients with continuous OPLL are less likely to have neck pain than those with other types of ossification in which the cervical spine has more mobility than in continuous OPLL [27]. Similarly, the present study revealed that the prevalence of neck pain decreased with increasing DISH grade. Given that patients with DISH are often found to have ossification of other spinal ligaments, the structural change caused by DISH alone cannot always explain their clinical status. Indeed, in this study, there was a significant increase in the OP-index value with increasing DISH grade, which may be a confounding factor. However, the present findings suggest that segmental motion at unstable intervertebral levels rather than bony bridging segments is likely to cause pain and that neck pain is likely to be less severe in patients with a more severely ankylosed spine (DISH grade 3) than in those with a less restricted spine. Therefore, DISH localized in the thoracic spine (grade 1) may create overload at the cervical and lumbar spine and lead to neck pain and LBP.

This study has several limitations. First, it was a cross-sectional cohort study of a specific disease and not population-based. Second, the study was not longitudinal and thus cannot reach conclusions on causality. Third, the presence of DISH was evaluated only on reconstructed sagittal CT images with no review of bony bridges at the lateral portion of the intervertebral segments. Fourth, we could not determine whether mobility of the segment adjacent to DISH affects neck pain or LBP. Fifth, the JOA-CMEQ could not evaluate pain states in detail. Further studies are required in the general population to clarify these clinical questions and eliminate confounding factors in terms of each spinal ligament. However, despite these limitations, we believe that our findings provide important information on the clinical features of DISH in patients with cervical OPLL.

5. Conclusions

This study is the first prospective multicenter cross-sectional comparison of subjective outcomes in patients with cervical OPLL according to the presence or absence of DISH. There were no significant correlations between DISH grade and clinical scores. However, there was a significant difference in the prevalence of neck pain among the three grades, albeit not in the prevalence of back pain or LBP. Interestingly, DISH localized in the thoracic spine (grade 1) could create overload at the cervical spine and lead to neck pain in patients with cervical OPLL.

Author Contributions: Conceptualization, T.H., S.N., T.Y., K.M. (Kanji Mori), S.U., S.M., K.K., N.N. (Narihito Nagoshi) and Y.K.; Methodology, T.H.; Software, T.H., S.U. and N.N. (Narihito Nagoshi); Validation, T.H., T.Y., K.M. (Kazuma Murata), S.U., S.M., K.K., N.N. (Narihito Nagoshi); Formal Analysis, T.H. and N.N. (Narihito Nagoshi); Investigation, K.M. (Kanji Mori), T.Y., T.H., N.N. (Narihito Nagoshi), S.N., K.T. (Kazuhiro Takeuchi), S.M. and K.K.; Resources, M.M., M.Y. (Masashi Yamazaki) and A.O.; Data Curation, T.H., T.Y., K.M. (Kanji Mori), S.U., S.M., K.K., N.N. (Narihito Nagoshi), M.M., M.N., K.W. (Kota Watanabe) and Y.K.; Conceptualization, T.H., T.Y., S.U., J.H., K.M. (Kanji Mori), S.M., K.K., N.N. (Narihito Nagoshi), K.T. (Katsushi Takeshita), T.F., K.W. (Kei Watanabe), N.N. (Norihiro Nishida), K.W. (Kota Watanabe), T.K., S.K., K.N., M.K., H.I., S.I., Y.M. (Yuji Matsuoka), K.W. (Kanichiro Wada), A.K., T.O., H.K., H.O., Y.M. (Yu Matsukura), H.I. and Y.K.; Writing—Original Draft Preparation, T.H., S.N., H.H., Y.M. (Yukihiro Matsuyama), K.T. (Katsushi Takeshita), H.O., A.O. and Y.K.; Writing—Review and Editing, T.H., S.N., T.Y., S.U., K.M. (Kanji Mori), S.M., K.K., N.N. (Norihiro Nishida), K.T. (Kazuhiro Takeuchi), T.F., K.W. (Kei Watanabe), N.N. (Norihiro Nishida), K.W. (Kota Watanabe), T.K., S.K., K.N., M.K., H.N., S.I., Y.M. (Yukihiro Matsuyama), K.W. (Kanichiro Wada), A.K., T.O., H.K., H.O. and Y.K.; Visualization, T.H., N.N. (Narihito Nagoshi), K.M.(Kazuma Murata) and S.U.; Supervision, M.M., M.W., M.N., M.Y., A.O. and Y.K.; Project Administration, T.H and Y.K.; Funding Acquisition, M.M., M.Y. and A.O. All authors have read and agreed to the published version of the manuscript.

Funding: This work was funded by a Health and Labour Science Research grant (number 201610008B) and a grant from the Japan Agency for Medical Research and Development (number 16ek0109136h0002).

Institutional Review Board Statement: The study was conducted according to the guidelines of the Declaration of Helsinki and approved by the institutional review board of each participating institution (protocol code 28-34; 14 March 2017).

Informed Consent Statement: Informed consent was obtained from all subjects involved in the study.

Data Availability Statement: The data generated and analyzed in this study are available from the corresponding author upon reasonable request.

Acknowledgments: We thank Nobuko Nakajima, Tomomi Kobayashi, Namiko Katayama, and Yukiko Oya for data collection.

Conflicts of Interest: The authors declare no conflict of interest. The funders had no role in the design of the study; in the collection, analyses, or interpretation of data; in the writing of the manuscript; or in the decision to publish the results.

References

1. Onishi, E.; Sakamoto, A.; Murata, S.; Matsushita, M. Risk factors for acute cervical spinal cord injury associated with ossification of the posterior longitudinal ligament. *Spine* **2012**, *37*, 660–666. [CrossRef] [PubMed]
2. Mochizuki, M.; Aiba, A.; Hashimoto, M.; Fujiyoshi, T.; Yamazaki, M. Cervical myelopathy in patients with ossification of the posterior longitudinal ligament. *J. Neurosurg. Spine* **2009**, *10*, 122–128. [CrossRef] [PubMed]
3. Matsunaga, S.; Sakou, T. Ossification of the posterior longitudinal ligament of the cervical spine: Etiology and natural history. *Spine* **2012**, *37*, E309–E314. [CrossRef] [PubMed]
4. Resnick, D.; Guerra, J.; Robinson, C.A.; Vint, V.C. Association of diffuse idiopathic skeletal hyperostosis (DISH) and calcification and ossification of the posterior longitudinal ligament. *AJR Am. J. Roentgenol.* **1978**, *131*, 1049–1053. [CrossRef] [PubMed]
5. Resnick, D.; Niwayama, G. Radiographic and pathologic features of spinal involvement in diffuse idiopathic skeletal hyperostosis (DISH). *Radiology* **1976**, *119*, 559–568. [CrossRef]
6. Hirai, T.; Yoshii, T.; Iwanami, A.; Takeuchi, K.; Mori, K.; Yamada, T.; Wada, K.; Koda, M.; Matsuyama, Y.; Takeshita, K.; et al. Prevalence and distribution of ossified lesions in the whole spine of patients with cervical ossification of the posterior longitudinal ligament a multicenter study (JOSL CT study). *PLoS ONE* **2016**, *11*, e0160117. [CrossRef]
7. Hirai, T.; Yoshii, T.; Nagoshi, N.; Takeuchi, K.; Mori, K.; Ushio, S.; Iwanami, A.; Yamada, T.; Seki, S.; Tsuji, T.; et al. Distribution of ossified spinal lesions in patients with severe ossification of the posterior longitudinal ligament and prediction of ossification at each segment based on the cervical OP index classification: A multicenter study (JOSL CT study). *BMC Musculoskelet. Disord.* **2018**, *19*, 107. [CrossRef]
8. Mori, K.; Yoshii, T.; Hirai, T.; Iwanami, A.; Takeuchi, K.; Yamada, T.; Seki, S.; Tsuji, T.; Fujiyoshi, K.; Furukawa, M.; et al. Prevalence and distribution of ossification of the supra/interspinous ligaments in symptomatic patients with cervical ossification of the posterior longitudinal ligament of the spine: A CT-based multicenter cross-sectional study. *BMC Musculoskelet. Disord.* **2016**, *17*, 492. [CrossRef]
9. Kawaguchi, Y.; Nakano, M.; Yasuda, T.; Seki, S.; Hori, T.; Kimura, T. Ossification of the posterior longitudinal ligament in not only the cervical spine, but also other spinal regions: Analysis using multidetector computed tomography of the whole spine. *Spine* **2013**, *38*, E1477–E1482. [CrossRef]
10. Nishimura, S.; Nagoshi, N.; Iwanami, A.; Takeuchi, A.; Hirai, T.; Yoshii, T.; Takeuchi, K.; Mori, K.; Yamada, T.; Seki, S.; et al. Prevalence and distribution of diffuse idiopathic skeletal hyperostosis on whole-spine computed tomography in patients with cervical ossification of the posterior longitudinal ligament: A multicenter study. *Clin. Spine Surg.* **2018**, *31*, E460–E465. [CrossRef]
11. Hirai, T.; Okawa, A.; Arai, Y.; Takahashi, M.; Kawabata, S.; Kato, T.; Enomoto, M.; Tomizawa, S.; Sakai, K.; Torigoe, I.; et al. Middle-term results of a prospective comparative study of anterior decompression with fusion and posterior decompression with laminoplasty for the treatment of cervical spondylotic myelopathy. *Spine* **2011**, *36*, 1940–1947. [CrossRef]
12. Fukui, M.; Chiba, K.; Kawakami, M.; Kikuchi, S.; Konno, S.; Miyamoto, M.; Seichi, A.; Shimamura, T.; Shirado, O.; Taguchi, T.; et al. JOA Back Pain Evaluation Questionnaire (JOABPEQ)/JOA Cervical Myelopathy Evaluation Questionnaire (JOACMEQ). The report on the development of revised versions. 16 April 2007. The Subcommittee of the Clinical Outcome Committee of the Japanese Orthopaedic Association on Low Back Pain and Cervical Myelopathy Evaluation. *J. Orthop. Sci.* **2009**, *14*, 348–365. [CrossRef]
13. Hirai, T.; Yoshii, T.; Ushio, S.; Hashimoto, J.; Mori, K.; Maki, S.; Katsumi, K.; Nagoshi, N.; Takeuchi, K.; Furuya, T.; et al. Associations between clinical symptoms and degree of ossification in patients with cervical ossification of the posterior longitudinal ligament: A prospective multi-institutional cross-sectional study. *J. Clin. Med.* **2020**, *9*, 4055. [CrossRef]
14. Beyeler, C.H.; Schlapbach, P.; Gerber, N.J.; Fahrer, H.; Hasler, F.; van der Linden, S.M.; Bürgi, U.; Fuchs, W.A.; Ehrengruber, H. Diffuse idiopathic skeletal hyperostosis (DISH) of the elbow: A cause of elbow pain? A controlled study. *Br. J. Rheumatol.* **1992**, *31*, 319–323. [CrossRef]
15. Utsinger, P.D. Diffuse idiopathic skeletal hyperostosis. *Clin. Rheum. Dis.* **1985**, *11*, 325–351. [CrossRef]
16. Verlaan, J.J.; Boswijk, P.F.E.; de Ru, J.A.; Dhert, W.J.A.; Oner, F.C. Diffuse idiopathic skeletal hyperostosis of the cervical spine: An underestimated cause of dysphagia and airway obstruction. *Spine J.* **2011**, *11*, 1058–1067. [CrossRef] [PubMed]
17. Okada, E.; Yoshii, T.; Yamada, T.; Watanabe, K.; Katsumi, K.; Hiyama, A.; Watanabe, M.; Nakagawa, Y.; Okada, M.; Endo, T.; et al. Spinal fractures in patients with Diffuse idiopathic skeletal hyperostosis: A nationwide multi-institution survey. *J. Orthop. Sci.* **2019**, *24*, 601–606. [CrossRef]

18. Katoh, H.; Okada, E.; Yoshii, T.; Yamada, T.; Watanabe, K.; Katsumi, K.; Hiyama, A.; Nakagawa, Y.; Okada, M.; Endo, T.; et al. A comparison of cervical and thoracolumbar fractures associated with diffuse idiopathic skeletal hyperostosis—A nationwide multicenter study. *J. Clin. Med.* **2020**, *9*, 208. [CrossRef] [PubMed]
19. Ehara, S.; Shimamura, T.; Nakamura, R.; Yamazaki, K. Paravertebral ligamentous ossification: DISH, OPLL and OLF. *Eur. J. Radiol.* **1998**, *27*, 196–205. [CrossRef]
20. Yoshimura, N.; Nagata, K.; Muraki, S.; Oka, H.; Yoshida, M.; Enyo, Y.; Kagotani, R.; Hashizume, H.; Yamada, H.; Ishimoto, Y.; et al. Prevalence and progression of radiographic ossification of the posterior longitudinal ligament and associated factors in the Japanese population: A 3-year follow-up of the ROAD study. *Osteoporos. Int.* **2014**, *25*, 1089–1098. [CrossRef] [PubMed]
21. Epstein, N.E. Simultaneous cervical diffuse idiopathic skeletal hyperostosis and ossification of the posterior longitudinal ligament resulting in dysphagia or myelopathy in two geriatric North Americans. *Surg. Neurol.* **2000**, *53*, 427–431, discussion 431. [CrossRef]
22. Fujimori, T.; Watabe, T.; Iwamoto, Y.; Hamada, S.; Iwasaki, M.; Oda, T. Prevalence, concomitance, and distribution of ossification of the spinal ligaments: Results of whole spine CT scans in 1500 Japanese patients. *Spine* **2016**, *41*, 1668–1676. [CrossRef]
23. Toyoda, H.; Terai, H.; Yamada, K.; Suzuki, A.; Dohzono, S.; Matsumoto, T.; Nakamura, H. Prevalence of diffuse idiopathic skeletal hyperostosis in patients with spinal disorders. *Asian Spine J.* **2017**, *11*, 63–70. [CrossRef]
24. Okada, E.; Ishihara, S.; Azuma, K.; Michikawa, T.; Suzuki, S.; Tsuji, O.; Nori, S.; Nagoshi, N.; Yagi, M.; Takayama, M.; et al. Metabolic syndrome is a predisposing factor for diffuse idiopathic skeletal hyperostosis. *Neurospine* **2021**, *18*, 109–116. [CrossRef]
25. Dan Lantsman, C.; Herman, A.; Verlaan, J.J.; Stern, M.; Mader, R.; Eshed, I. Abdominal fat distribution in diffuse idiopathic skeletal hyperostosis and ankylosing spondylitis patients compared to controls. *Clin. Radiol.* **2018**, *73*, 910.e915–910.e920. [CrossRef]
26. Hutton, C. DISH . . . a state not a disease? *Br. J. Rheumatol.* **1989**, *28*, 277–278. [CrossRef]
27. Hirai, T.; Yoshii, T.; Ushio, S.; Mori, K.; Maki, S.; Katsumi, K.; Nagoshi, N.; Takeuchi, K.; Furuya, T.; Watanabe, K.; et al. Clinical characteristics in patients with ossification of the posterior longitudinal ligament: A prospective multi-institutional cross-sectional study. *Sci. Rep.* **2020**, *10*, 5532. [CrossRef]
28. Mata, S.; Fortin, P.R.; Fitzcharles, M.A.; Starr, M.R.; Joseph, L.; Watts, C.S.; Gore, B.; Rosenberg, E.; Chhem, R.K.; Esdaile, J.M. A controlled study of diffuse idiopathic skeletal hyperostosis. Clinical features and functional status. *Medicine* **1997**, *76*, 104–117. [CrossRef] [PubMed]
29. Schlapbach, P.; Beyeler, C.; Gerber, N.J.; van der Linden, S.; Bürgi, U.; Fuchs, W.A.; Ehrengruber, H. Diffuse idiopathic skeletal hyperostosis (DISH) of the spine: A cause of back pain? A controlled study. *Br. J. Rheumatol.* **1989**, *28*, 299–303. [CrossRef] [PubMed]
30. Holton, K.F.; Denard, P.J.; Yoo, J.U.; Kado, D.M.; Barrett-Connor, E.; Marshall, L.M.; Osteoporotic Fractures in Men (MrOS) Study Group. Diffuse idiopathic skeletal hyperostosis and its relation to back pain among older men: The MrOS Study. *Semin. Arthritis Rheum.* **2011**, *41*, 131–138. [CrossRef] [PubMed]

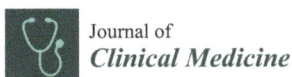

Article

Prevalence and Related Factors of Low Back Pain in the General Elderly Population: A Japanese Cross-Sectional Study Randomly Sampled from a Basic Resident Registry

Masashi Uehara [1,*], Shota Ikegami [1], Hiroshi Horiuchi [2], Jun Takahashi [1] and Hiroyuki Kato [1]

[1] Department of Orthopaedic Surgery, Shinshu University School of Medicine, Nagano 390-8621, Japan; sh.ikegami@gmail.com (S.I.); jtaka@shinshu-u.ac.jp (J.T.); hirokato@shinshu-u.ac.jp (H.K.)
[2] Rehabilitation Center, Shinshu University Hospital, Nagano 390-8621, Japan; horiuchih@aol.com
* Correspondence: masashi_u560613@yahoo.co.jp; Tel.: +81-263-37-2659

Abstract: Low back pain (LBP) is one of the main etiologies of disability in daily life. In the face of LBP increases in super-aged societies, there are serious concerns of escalating medical costs and deteriorations in the social economy. It is therefore important to identify the factors associated with LBP for prompt preventative and therapeutic measures. This study investigated the prevalence of LBP and the impact of subject-specific factors on LBP development in Japanese community-dwelling older adults. We established eight groups based on age (50's, 60's, 70's, and 80's) and gender after random sampling from a resident registry. A total of 411 participants (201 male and 210 female) were enrolled for a whole-spine lateral radiographic examination and dual-energy X-ray absorptiometry. All subjects were evaluated for the presence and degree of LBP. We analyzed the impact of clinical factors on LBP using multivariate analysis. Fifty-three (12.9%) participants (23 (11.4%) male and 30 (14.3%) female) were found to have LBP. The prevalence of LBP tended to increase with age, and similar results were found between genders. In univariate analysis, the subject-related factors of the sagittal vertebral axis, pelvic incidence minus lumbar lordosis (PI-LL) mismatch, and aging had significant associations with LBP. PI-LL mismatch was a significant independent factor in multivariate analysis. In conclusion, this study identified LBP prevalence and subject-specific factors on a general population basis. Multivariate analysis revealed PI-LL mismatch as an independent factor associated with LBP in the healthy community-dwelling elderly.

Keywords: low back pain; prevalence; influence factor; spinal alignment; aging

1. Introduction

As the elderly rate reached 28% of the Japanese population in 2019 (Ministry of Internal Affairs and Communications, Statistics Bureau, Population Census), it has become of social importance to clarify the impact of aging in order to extend healthy life expectancy. Low back pain (LBP) is one of the main etiologies of disability in daily life [1]. The lifetime prevalence of LBP is reportedly 80% [2] and has been found to increase with age [3]. Furthermore, LBP may cause depression in the elderly, which has a significant impact on quality of life [4]. LBP was shown to be associated with depression both in the elderly and in middle-aged individuals in the prime of their working life [5,6]. Not only does back pain lead to high medical costs, but the economic and social losses from LBP are considered enormous [7]; in the U.S., the financial loss to LBP has been calculated as up to 120 billion dollars yearly [7]. Several risk factors for LBP have been suggested, including old age, occupation, a sedentary lifestyle, obesity, spinal malalignment, pregnancy, and smoking [8,9]. However, those with the strongest influence on LBP onset remain unknown.

In the present population-based study of the elderly in Japan, we adopted random sampling from the basic resident registry of a suburban town to minimize selection bias and obtain cohort data that more closely resembled the general Japanese population. This epidemiological study was coined "the Obuse study", bearing the name of the cooperating local government. We have employed the Obuse study cohort for research on various musculoskeletal disorders [10–15].

Japan is currently facing a super-aged society unparalleled in the world, with serious concerns of escalating medical costs and significant losses in the social economy [16]. Therefore, it has become paramount to identify the factors associated with LBP development for appropriate early action. This investigation aimed to determine the prevalence of LBP in older Japanese adults using the Obuse study cohort and identify the impact of subject-specific factors, including age, sex, body mass index (BMI), lifestyle habits, comorbidities, and spinal alignment.

2. Methods

2.1. Study Design

Japanese resident cross-sectional study based on a municipal registry.

2.2. Settings

This study was conducted at a hospital in the town of Obuse from October 2014 to June 2017.

2.3. Bias

In order to minimize selection bias, we randomly selected candidates from the basic town resident registry.

2.4. Study Size

Assuming that the frequency of back pain in the comparison group was between 5% and 20%, sample size calculation estimated that 89 subjects per group would provide 80% statistical power (1 minus beta) with an alpha equal to 0.05. After estimating the possible cohort size in consideration of budget, time, and burden on subjects and research staff, we planned to establish eight groups by age (50's, 60's, 70's, and 80's) and gender (male and female) containing approximately 50 subjects each for a total of at least 400 subjects.

2.5. Data Source

The subject selection process in this study has been previously reported [10]. Briefly, we randomly sampled for candidates from the basic resident registry of the Obuse town (population: 11,326 in 2014). Sampling was conducted until the number of individuals providing consent for study participation reached the target number. A total of 1297 individuals were randomly selected from 5352 people aged between 50 and 89 years in the basic resident registry of the Obuse town in 2014 (Figure 1) [10]. Of them, 882 people were unwilling to participate for undisclosed reasons and excluded from this study.

2.6. Participation

After providing written consent, 415 subjects were enrolled in the Obuse study. The inclusion criteria were residents aged 50–90 years who were randomly selected by town administrative staff from the Obuse resident registry and who consented to participate in the study. The exclusion criteria were subjects with acute LBP, vertebral fracture, spinal infection, or spinal tumor within 3 months prior to the study, as well as those unable to undergo whole-spine radiographs in a standing position. Four people with missing radiographic data were excluded, leaving a total of 411 (201 male and 210 female) Japanese participants. All subjects were measured for physical characteristics and lifestyle habits. The baseline characteristics of the cohort are summarized in Table 1. The protocol of the investigation was approved by our Institutional Review Board (no. 2792). This study was reported in accordance with the STROBE guidelines.

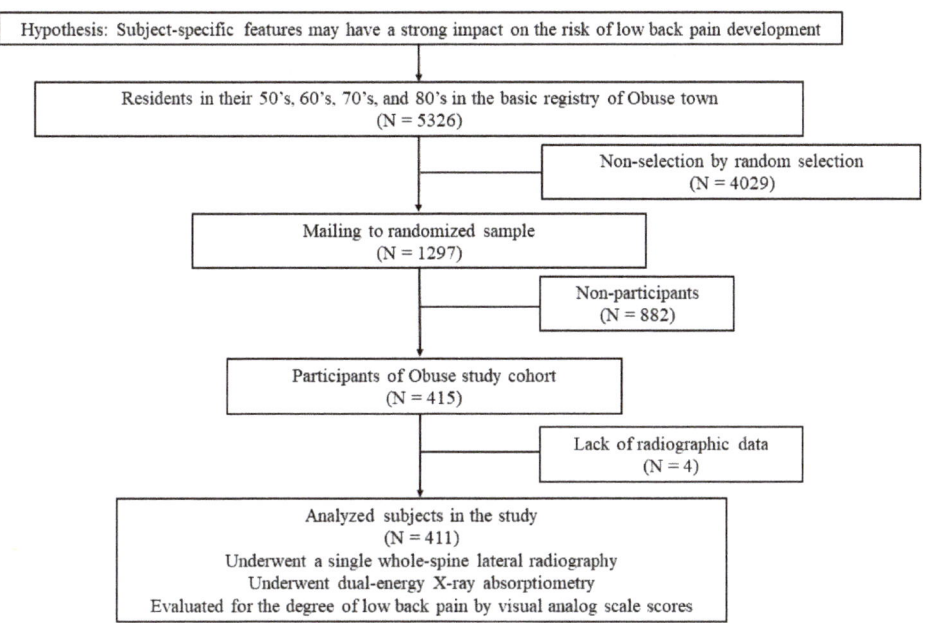

Figure 1. Obuse town resident participant flowchart.

Table 1. Baseline characteristics.

Gender	Age Group	N	Height, cm Mean (SD)	p-Value (vs. 50's)	Weight, kg Mean (SD)	p-Value (vs. 50's)	BMI Mean (SD)	p-Value (vs. 50's)
Male	50's	49	171.8 (6.0)		67.1 (9.1)		22.7 (2.9)	
	60's	53	166.7 (4.7)	<0.01	66.9 (7.7)	0.94	24.1 (2.7)	0.01
	70's	54	163.1 (5.0)	<0.01	59.9 (10.3)	<0.01	22.4 (3.5)	0.68
	80's	45	160.1 (5.7)	<0.01	57.5 (8.5)	<0.01	22.4 (2.8)	0.54
	Total	201	165.5 (6.8)		63 (9.8)		22.9 (3.1)	
Female	50's	47	158.1 (4.9)		55.4 (9.0)		22.2 (3.8)	
	60's	61	152.8 (5.4)	<0.01	52.2 (7.6)	0.06	22.3 (2.8)	0.86
	70's	54	149.7 (5.3)	<0.01	50.5 (7.9)	<0.01	22.5 (3.2)	0.68
	80's	48	144.6 (5.9)	<0.01	48.3 (7.9)	<0.01	23.1 (3.3)	0.21
	Total	210	151.3 (7.1)		51.6 (8.4)		22.5 (3.2)	

BMI: body mass index, SD: standard deviation.

2.7. Variables

Analyzed variables included age, gender, height, weight, BMI, smoking, visual analog scale (VAS) score for low back pain, spinal alignment parameters, bone mineral density (BMD), and skeletal muscle mass index (SMI).

2.8. Measurement

2.8.1. Measurements of Spinal Alignment

All subjects underwent a whole-spine lateral radiographic examination in a standing position with the hands on the clavicles [17] for the measurement of the sagittal vertical axis (SVA) as an indicator of total spinal alignment as well as pelvic incidence (PI) and lumbar lordosis (LL). A PI minus LL (PI-LL) mismatch was defined as PI-LL >10° [18].

The spinal alignment measurements were performed by 2 board-certified spine surgeons and a trained staff member. The calculated inter-rater reliability scores for each parameter were 0.95 for SVA, 0.80 for PI, and 0.65 for LL [10]. The calculated intra-rater reliability scores for each parameter were 0.91 for SVA, 0.97 for PI, and 0.96 for LL. For validity, our previous study demonstrated that our measurements were comparable to those of previous reports [10].

2.8.2. Evaluation of BMD and SMI

All subjects underwent dual-energy X-ray absorptiometry (GE Prodigy, GE healthcare, Chicago, IL, USA) of the lumbar spine. Osteoporosis was defined as a T-score ≤ -2.5 [19]. Skeletal muscle mass was calculated as the sum of the skeletal muscle mass of the arms and legs, assuming that the mass of lean soft tissue was representative of skeletal muscle mass. SMI was calculated as four-limb lean soft tissue mass in kilograms divided by height in meters squared.

2.8.3. Clinical Evaluation of Subjects

All subjects were evaluated for the degree of LBP by VAS scores (0–100 mm). In this study, subjects with moderate to severe LBP, defined as VAS > 50 mm, were considered as having LBP [20].

2.9. Statistical Methods

Welch's t-test was used to compare the mean values of continuous variables. Fisher's exact test was adopted to evaluate the differences between categorical variables. We employed a logistic regression model with the existence of moderate or severe LBP (i.e., VAS > 50 mm) as a response variable and subject-specific factor candidates as explanatory variables. Univariate and multivariate analyses using the forced entry method included the factors of sex, BMI, SMI, smoking, BMD, osteoporosis (i.e., T-score ≤ -2.5), SVA >50 mm, PI-LL mismatch, and aging as potential confounding factors of LBP according to previous reports [8,9]. Factors with $p < 0.2$ in the univariate analysis were included in the subsequent multivariate analysis with a stepwise algorithm. All statistical analyses were performed using EZR software (Saitama Medical Center, Jichi Medical University, Saitama, Japan), a modified graphical user interface of R commander (The Foundation for Statistical Computing, Vienna, Austria) designed to add statistical functions frequently used in biostatistics. The level of significance was set at $p < 0.05$.

3. Results

3.1. Descriptive Data

The prevalence of LBP in the cohort is summarized in Table 2.

Table 2. Prevalence of low back pain.

Age Group	Male	p-Value (vs. 50's)	Female	p-Value (vs. 50's)
50's	6.1% (3/49)		17.0% (8/47)	
60's	5.7% (3/53)	1	6.6% (4/61)	0.14
70's	14.5% (8/55)	0.34	14.8% (8/54)	1
80's	20.0% (9/45)	0.12	20.8% (10/48)	0.79
Total	11.4% (23/201)		14.3% (30/210)	

3.2. Outcome Data

A total of 53 (12.9%) participants (23 (11.4%) male and 30 (14.3%) female) were found to have LBP among subjects randomly selected from the basic resident registry of a suburb town. There were no cases of acute LBP at the time of data acquisition. The prevalence of

LBP for the 50's, 60's, 70's, and 80's age groups was 6.1%, 5.7%, 14.5%, and 20.0% in men and 17.0%, 6.6%, 14.8%, and 20.8% in women, respectively. The prevalence of LBP tended to increase with age, with the exception of 50's women. Similar results were observed between genders.

3.3. Main Result

In univariate analysis, the subject-specific factors of SVA, PI-LL mismatch, and aging had significant associations with LBP, while those of sex, BMI, BMD, SMI, and smoking did not. PI-LL mismatch was the only significant independent factor according to multivariate analysis, with an odds ratio of 1.91 (Table 3).

Table 3. Effects of subject-specific factors on low back pain.

Factor	Univariate Analysis		Multivariate Analysis	
	Odds Ratio (95% CI)	*p*-Value	Odds Ratio (95% CI)	*p*-Value
Sex (male)	1.29 (0.72–2.31)	0.39		
BMI	1.05 (0.96–1.15)	0.26		
SMI	1.04 (0.77–1.40)	0.81		
Smoking	0.77 (0.42–1.41)	0.40		
BMD	1.04 (0.33–3.26)	0.95		
Osteoporosis	0.61 (0.08–4.79)	0.64		
SVA >50 mm	2.3 (1.2–4.4)	0.011		
PI-LL mismatch	2.18 (1.22–3.91)	<0.01	1.91 (1.03–3.55)	0.041
Age (vs. 50's)				
60's	0.51 (0.19–1.36)	0.18	0.46 (0.17–1.25)	0.13
70's	1.33 (0.58–3.02)	0.50	1.24 (0.54–2.83)	0.62
80's	2.01 (0.90–4.50)	0.089	1.49 (0.64–3.48)	0.36

BMI: body mass index, SMI: skeletal muscle mass index, BMD: bone mineral density, SVA: sagittal vertical axis, PI: pelvic incidence, LL: lumbar lordosis.

4. Discussion

4.1. Key Result

This study evaluated the prevalence and related factors of LBP by random sampling from the basic resident registry of a suburb town for subject selection with age and gender clustering on a general population basis. LBP prevalence tended to increase comparably with age for both genders apart from 50's women, for which social activities and stress were possible reasons for the higher incidence. Multivariate analysis considering various confounders, such as age, gender, and BMI, revealed PI-LL mismatch as an independent factor associated with LBP. These findings may help in the early detection and treatment of LBP in subclinical or asymptomatic community-dwelling members.

Although numerous factors have been linked to LBP, their authenticity remains under debate [8,9]. Several reports have described an association between obesity and LBP [21,22]. In one population-based study, BMI was significantly associated with higher chronic LBP prevalence in women [22]. Hirano et al. also showed BMI to be strongly associated with lumbar spinal canal stenosis in community-living people [23]. On the other hand, Dario et al. witnessed that BMI did not increase the risk of chronic LBP in a population of Spanish adult twin [24]. In another study, although obesity was not associated with overall chronic LBP, its impact was more pronounced for severe chronic LBP [25]. In the present investigation, BMI did not significantly associate with LBP. Social factors and lifestyle have also been cited in relation to LBP, with reports implicating smoking with LBP [26,27]. In contrast, smoking and alcohol were not significantly linked to LBP in a cross-sectional prospective study of young twins [28], with conflicting associations for smoking [29,30]. We observed no remarkable associations for smoking with LBP.

Several reports have described a relationship between BMD and LBP [31–33]. A small-sample study argued that lower BMD of the lumbar spine was more frequent among LBP patients and that LBP could increase the risk of osteopenia [31]. On the other hand, another report found that participants with LBP had significantly higher lumbar BMD than did those without LBP, concluding that the presence of rotational asymmetry and associated motion restriction increased BMD in affected vertebrae [32]. A population-based cross-sectional study also showed an association for lumbar BMD with LBP [33]. In this investigation, however, BMD was not significantly related to LBP.

Regarding the influence of muscle mass, paraspinal muscle volume has been linked to sagittal spinal alignment [34–36]. Hori et al. described that trunk muscle mass was significantly associated with VAS scores in LBP patients visiting spinal outpatient clinics [37]. A systematic review showed that the cross-sectional area of the multifidus muscle was negatively related to LBP, with conflicting evidence for associations between the erector spinae, psoas, and quadratus lumborum cross-sectional area and LBP [38]. Our study found no significant impact for SMI on LBP.

In recent years, corrective surgeries for sagittal spinal deformity have been widely performed in older adults since such disorders were associated with impaired walking and mobility, respiratory and digestive symptoms, and LBP [39,40]. Multiple studies have stated that reduced lumbar lordosis is closely related to chronic LBP in adulthood [39,41]. Kitagawa et al. found that subjects with LBP showed significantly larger SVA and smaller LL as compared with the values of subjects without LBP in a study of total knee arthroplasty patients [42]. In our cohort, SVA > 50 mm, PI-LL mismatch, and aging were significantly associated with LBP in univariate analysis, although PI-LL mismatch alone remained associated with LBP in multivariate analysis (odds ratio: 1.91). A PI-LL mismatch is caused by a compensatory failure of the pelvis in spinal sagittal alignment. In a multicenter study of adult spinal deformity patients, a linear regression model demonstrated the threshold radiographical parameter for the Oswestry Disability Index of >40 to be PI-LL of 11° or more [43]. The results of our study suggest that individuals with LBP may more frequently suffer from pelvic compensatory insufficiency in postural abnormalities.

4.2. Limitation

The major limitation of this study was the small study group size due to the method of random sampling from a town population, with resource restrictions to 400 patients due to the inclusion of radiographical examination. Other limitations of the current investigation include a possibility of inter-observer bias and cross-sectional design; we are currently planning longitudinal studies to investigate the prevalence changes of LBP over time. Regional characteristics were also a shortcoming of this study as our subjects were sampled from a suburb area. Indeed, although epidemiological surveys are relatively easy in such regions due to less population displacement, there exists the possibility of differences with urban residents. Lastly, as this was a non-compulsory survey, the proportion of people randomly sampled who ultimately participated was less than one third. Since two thirds of candidates declined to enroll, incomplete selection bias could not be completely removed.

4.3. Generalizability

Nevertheless, the Obuse study cohort is presumed to resemble the average Japanese suburb population very closely due to its survey design.

4.4. Interpretation

Our findings showed spinal alignment to be significantly related to LBP onset and suggested that the early detection of lumbopelvic parameter mismatch by whole-spine radiographs might help prevent LBP occurrence, although further studies are warranted.

5. Conclusions

Based on data close to that of the general population, this cross-sectional study confirmed that LBP tended to increase with age in both men and women. Moreover, a high PI-LL mismatch was significantly associated with LBP development in the healthy community-dwelling elderly, which might serve as a simple indicator of health risk and aid in the prevention of back problems in this age group.

Author Contributions: Conceptualization, M.U. and S.I.; methodology, M.U., S.I. and J.T.; validation, M.U., and S.I.; formal analysis, M.U. and S.I.; investigation, M.U., S.I., H.H., J.T. and H.K.; data curation, M.U., S.I., H.H., J.T. and H.K.; writing—original draft preparation, M.U.; writing—review and editing, S.I., H.H., J.T. and H.K.; and supervision, H.K. All authors have read and agreed to the published version of the manuscript.

Funding: This work was supported by a grant from the Japan Orthopaedics and Traumatology Research Foundation, Inc. (no. 339), project research funds from the Japanese Orthopaedic Association, a research fund from the Japanese Society for Musculoskeletal Medicine, and a research fund from The Nakatomi Foundation.

Institutional Review Board Statement: The study was conducted according to the guidelines of the Declaration of Helsinki, and approved by the Institutional Review Board of Shinshu University Hospital (no. 2792).

Informed Consent Statement: Informed consent was obtained from all subjects involved in the study. Written informed consent has been obtained from the patients to publish this paper.

Data Availability Statement: The complete database of the cohort can be accessed at the Zenodo repository (doi.org/10.5281/zenodo.5512411).

Conflicts of Interest: The authors declare no conflict of interest.

References

1. GBD. 2015 Disease and Injury Incidence and Prevalence Collaborators. Global, regional, and national incidence, prevalence, and years lived with disability for 310 diseases and injuries, 1990–2015: A systematic analysis for the Global Burden of Disease Study 2015. *Lancet* **2016**, *388*, 1545–1602.
2. Fast, A. Low back disorders: Conservative management. *Arch. Phys. Med. Rehabil.* **1988**, *69*, 880–891. [PubMed]
3. Caron, T.; Bransford, R.; Nguyen, Q.; Agel, J.; Chapman, J.; Bellabarba, C. Spine fractures in patients with ankylosing spinal disorders. *Spine* **2010**, *35*, E458–E464. [CrossRef] [PubMed]
4. Calvo Lobo, C.; Vilar-Fernández, J.M.; Losa-Iglesias, M.E.; López-López, D.; Rodríguez-Sanz, D.; Palomo-López, P.; Becerro-de Bengoa-Vallejo, R. Depression Symptoms Among Older Adults with and Without Subacute Low Back Pain. *Rehabil. Nurs.* **2019**, *44*, 47–51. [CrossRef] [PubMed]
5. Calvo-Lobo, C.; Vilar Fernández, J.M.; Becerro-de-Bengoa-Vallejo, R.; Losa-Iglesias, M.E.; Rodríguez-Sanz, D.; Palomo López, P.; López, D. Relationship of depression in participants with nonspecific acute or subacute low back pain and no-pain by age distribution. *J. Pain Res.* **2017**, *10*, 129–135. [CrossRef] [PubMed]
6. Lopez-Lopez, D.; Vilar-Fernandez, J.M.; Calvo-Lobo, C.; Losa-Iglesias, M.E.; Rodriguez-Sanz, D.; Becerro-de-Bengoa-Vallejo, R. Evaluation of Depression in Subacute Low Back Pain: A Case Control Study. *Pain Physician* **2017**, *20*, E499–E505. [CrossRef]
7. Dagenais, S.; Caro, J.; Haldeman, S. A systematic review of low back pain cost of illness studies in the United States and internationally. *Spine J.* **2008**, *8*, 8–20. [CrossRef]
8. Hoy, D.; Bain, C.; Williams, G.; March, L.; Brooks, P.; Blyth, F.; Woolf, A.; Vos, T.; Buchbinder, R. A systematic review of the global prevalence of low back pain. *Arthritis Rheum.* **2012**, *64*, 2028–2037. [CrossRef]
9. Johansson, M.S.; Jensen Stochkendahl, M.; Hartvigsen, J.; Boyle, E.; Cassidy, J.D. Incidence and prognosis of mid-back pain in the general population: A systematic review. *Eur. J. Pain* **2017**, *21*, 20–28. [CrossRef]
10. Uehara, M.; Takahashi, J.; Ikegami, S.; Tokida, R.; Nishimura, H.; Sakai, N.; Kato, H. Sagittal spinal alignment deviation in the general elderly population: A Japanese cohort survey randomly sampled from a basic resident registry. *Spine J.* **2019**, *19*, 349–356. [CrossRef]
11. Uehara, M.; Takahashi, J.; Ikegami, S.; Tokida, R.; Nishimura, H.; Sakai, N.; Nakamura, Y.; Kato, H. Differences in bone mineral density and bone turnover markers between subjects with and without diffuse idiopathic skeletal hyperostosis. *Spine* **2020**, *45*, E1677–E1681. [CrossRef]
12. Ikegami, S.; Takahashi, J.; Uehara, M.; Tokida, R.; Nishimura, H.; Sakai, A.; Kato, H. Physical performance reflects cognitive function, fall risk, and quality of life in community-dwelling older people. *Sci. Rep.* **2019**, *9*, 12242. [CrossRef]

13. Uehara, M.; Takahashi, J.; Ikegami, S.; Tokida, R.; Nishimura, H.; Sakai, N.; Kato, H. Prevalence of diffuse idiopathic skeletal hyperostosis in the general elderly population: A Japanese cohort survey randomly sampled from a basic resident registry. *Clin. Spine Surg.* **2020**, *33*, 123–127. [CrossRef] [PubMed]
14. Tokida, R.; Uehara, M.; Ikegami, S.; Takahashi, J.; Nishimura, H.; Sakai, N.; Kato, H. Association between sagittal spinal alignment and physical function in the Japanese general elderly population: A Japanese cohort survey randomly sampled from a basic resident registry. *J. Bone Joint Surg. Am.* **2019**, *101*, 1698–1706. [CrossRef] [PubMed]
15. Uehara, M.; Takahashi, J.; Ikegami, S.; Tokida, R.; Nishimura, H.; Kuraishi, S.; Sakai, N.; Kato, H. Impact of diffuse idiopathic skeletal hyperostosis on sagittal spinal alignment in the general elderly population: A Japanese cohort survey randomly sampled from a basic resident registry. *JBJS Open Access* **2019**, *4*, e0062. [CrossRef]
16. Shinohara, S.; Okada, M.; Keira, T.; Ohwada, M.; Niitsuya, M.; Aizawa, Y. Prognosis of accidental low back pain at work. *Tohoku J. Exp. Med.* **1998**, *186*, 291–302. [CrossRef] [PubMed]
17. Liu, Y.; Liu, Z.; Zhu, F.; Qian, B.P.; Zhu, Z.; Xu, L.; Ding, Y.; Qiu, Y. Validation and reliability analysis of the new SRS-Schwab classification for adult spinal deformity. *Spine* **2013**, *38*, 902–908. [CrossRef]
18. Merrill, R.K.; Kim, J.S.; Leven, D.M.; Kim, J.H.; Cho, S.K. Beyond pelvic incidence-lumbar lordosis mismatch: The importance of assessing the entire spine to achieve global sagittal alignment. *Glob. Spine J.* **2017**, *7*, 536–542. [CrossRef]
19. Kanis, J.A. Assessment of fracture risk and its application to screening for postmenopausal osteoporosis: Synopsis of a WHO report. WHO Study Group. *Osteoporos Int.* **1994**, *4*, 368–381. [CrossRef] [PubMed]
20. Yamada, K.; Suzuki, A.; Takahashi, S.; Yasuda, H.; Koike, T.; Nakamura, H. Severe low back pain in patients with rheumatoid arthritis is associated with Disease Activity Score but not with radiological findings on plain X-rays. *Mod. Rheumatol.* **2015**, *25*, 56–61. [CrossRef]
21. Dario, A.B.; Ferreira, M.L.; Refshauge, K.M.; Lima, T.S.; Ordoñana, J.R.; Ferreira, P.H. The relationship between obesity, low back pain, and lumbar disc degeneration when genetics and the environment are considered: A systematic review of twin studies. *Spine J.* **2015**, *15*, 1106–1117. [CrossRef]
22. Dario, A.B.; Ferreira, M.L.; Refshauge, K.; Sánchez-Romera, J.F.; Luque-Suarez, A.; Hopper, J.L.; Ordoñana, J.R.; Ferreira, P.H. Are obesity and body fat distribution associated with low back pain in women? A population-based study of 1128 Spanish twins. *Eur. Spine J.* **2016**, *25*, 1188–1195. [CrossRef]
23. Hirano, K.; Imagama, S.; Hasegawa, Y.; Muramoto, A.; Ishiguro, N. Impact of spinal imbalance and BMI on lumbar spinal canal stenosis determined by a diagnostic support tool: Cohort study in community-living people. *Arch. Orthop. Trauma Surg.* **2013**, *133*, 1477–1482. [CrossRef] [PubMed]
24. Kakihana, H.; Jinnouchi, H.; Kitamura, A.; Matsudaira, K.; Kiyama, M.; Hayama-Terada, M.; Muraki, I.; Kubota, Y.; Yamagishi, K.; Okada, T.; et al. Overweight and hypertension in relation to chronic musculoskeletal pain among community-dwelling adults: The circulatory risk in communities study (CIRCS). *J. Epidemiol.* **2020**, in press. [CrossRef] [PubMed]
25. Dario, A.B.; Loureiro Ferreira, M.; Refshauge, K.; Refshauge, K.; Luque-Suarez, A.; Ordoñana, J.R.; Ferreira, P.H. Obesity does not increase the risk of chronic low back pain when genetics are considered. A prospective study of Spanish adult twins. *Spine J.* **2017**, *17*, 282–290. [CrossRef]
26. Schembri, E.; Massalha, V.; Spiteri, K.; Camilleri, L.; Lungaro-Mifsud, S. Nicotine dependence and the International Association for the Study of Pain neuropathic pain grade in patients with chronic low back pain and radicular pain: Is there an association? *Korean J. Pain* **2020**, *33*, 359–377. [CrossRef] [PubMed]
27. Shiri, R.; Karppinen, J.; Leino-Arjas, P.; Solovieva, S.; Viikari-Juntura, E. The association between smoking and low back pain: A meta-analysis. *Am. J. Med.* **2010**, *123*, e7–e35. [CrossRef]
28. Hestbaek, L.; Leboeuf-Yde, C.; Kyvik, K.O. Are lifestyle-factors in adolescence predictors for adult low back pain? A cross-sectional and prospective study of young twins. *BMC Musculoskelet. Disord.* **2006**, *7*, 27. [CrossRef]
29. Esquirol, Y.; Niezborala, M.; Visentin, M.; Leguevel, A.; Gonzalez, I.; Marquié, J.C. Contribution of occupational factors to the incidence and persistence of chronic low back pain among workers: Results from the longitudinal VISAT study. *Occup. Environ. Med.* **2017**, *74*, 243–251. [CrossRef]
30. Hashimoto, Y.; Matsudaira, K.; Sawada, S.S.; Gando, Y.; Kawakami, R.; Kinugawa, C.; Okamoto, T.; Tsukamoto, K.; Miyachi, M.; Naito, H. Obesity and low back pain: A retrospective cohort study of Japanese males. *J. Phys. Ther. Sci.* **2017**, *29*, 978–983. [CrossRef]
31. Gaber, T.A.; McGlashan, K.A.; Love, S.; Jenner, J.R.; Crisp, A.J. Bone density in chronic low back pain: A pilot study. *Clin. Rehabil.* **2002**, *16*, 867–870. [CrossRef] [PubMed]
32. Snider, K.T.; Johnson, J.C.; Degenhardt, B.F.; Snider, E.J. Low back pain, somatic dysfunction, and segmental bone mineral density T-score variation in the lumbar spine. *J. Am. Osteopath. Assoc.* **2011**, *111*, 89–96.
33. Lee, S.; Nam, C.M.; Yoon, D.H.; Kim, K.N.; Yi, S.; Shin, D.A.; Ha, Y. Association between low-back pain and lumbar spine bone density: A population-based cross-sectional study. *J. Neurosurg. Spine* **2013**, *19*, 307–313. [CrossRef]
34. Hiyama, A.; Katoh, H.; Sakai, D.; Tanaka, M.; Sato, M.; Watanabe, M. The correlation analysis between sagittal alignment and cross-sectional area of paraspinal muscle in patients with lumbar spinal stenosis and degenerative spondylolisthesis. *BMC Musculoskelet. Disord.* **2019**, *20*, 352. [CrossRef]

35. Yagi, M.; Hosogane, N.; Watanabe, K.; Asazuma, T.; Matsumoto, M.; Keio Spine Research Group. The paravertebral muscle and psoas for the maintenance of global spinal alignment in patient with degenerative lumbar scoliosis. *Spine J.* **2016**, *16*, 451–458. [CrossRef] [PubMed]
36. Ferrero, E.; Skalli, W.; Lafage, V.; Maillot, C.; Carlier, R.; Feydy, A.; Felter, A.; Khalifé, M.; Guigui, P. Relationships between radiographic parameters and spinopelvic muscles in adult spinal deformity patients. *Eur. Spine J.* **2020**, *29*, 1328–1339. [CrossRef]
37. Hori, Y.; Hoshino, M.; Inage, K.; Miyagi, M.; Takahashi, S.; Ohyama, S.; Suzuki, A.; Tsujio, T.; Terai, H.; Dohzono, S.; et al. ISSLS PRIZE IN CLINICAL SCIENCE 2019: Clinical importance of trunk muscle mass for low back pain, spinal balance, and quality of life—A multicenter cross-sectional study. *Eur. Spine J.* **2019**, *28*, 914–921. [CrossRef] [PubMed]
38. Ranger, T.A.; Cicuttini, F.M.; Jensen, T.S.; Peiris, W.L.; Hussain, S.M.; Fairley, J.; Urquhart, D.M. Are the size and composition of the paraspinal muscles associated with low back pain? A systematic review. *Spine J.* **2017**, *17*, 1729–1748. [CrossRef]
39. Glassman, S.D.; Bridwell, K.H.; Dimar, J.R.; Horton, W.; Berven, S.; Schwab, F. The impact of positive sagittal balance in adult spinal deformity. *Spine* **2005**, *30*, 2024–2029. [CrossRef] [PubMed]
40. Pellisé, F.; Vila-Casademunt, A.; Ferrer, M.; Domingo-Sàbat, M.; Bagó, J.; Pérez-Grueso, F.J.; Alanay, A.; Mannion, A.F.; Acaroglu, E.; European Spine Study Group (ESSG). Impact on health related quality of life of adult spinal deformity (ASD) compared with other chronic conditions. *Eur. Spine J.* **2015**, *24*, 3–11. [CrossRef]
41. Djurasovic, M.; Glassman, S.D. Correlation of radiographic and clinical findings in spinal deformities. *Neurosurg. Clin. N. Am.* **2007**, *18*, 223–227. [CrossRef] [PubMed]
42. Kitagawa, A.; Yamamoto, J.; Toda, M.; Hashimoto, Y. Spinopelvic Alignment and low back pain before and after total knee arthroplasty. *Asian Spine J.* **2021**, *15*, 9–16. [CrossRef] [PubMed]
43. Schwab, F.J.; Blondel, B.; Bess, S.; Hostin, R.; Shaffrey, C.I.; Smith, J.S.; Boachie-Adjei, O.; Burton, D.C.; Akbarnia, B.A.; Mundis, G.M.; et al. International Spine Study Group (ISSG). Radiographical spinopelvic parameters and disability in the setting of adult spinal deformity: A prospective multicenter analysis. *Spine* **2013**, *38*, E803–E812. [CrossRef] [PubMed]

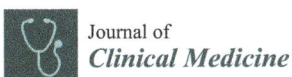 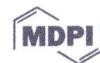

Article

Impact of Preoperative Total Knee Arthroplasty on Radiological and Clinical Outcomes of Spinal Fusion for Concurrent Knee Osteoarthritis and Degenerative Lumbar Spinal Diseases

Hong Jin Kim [1,†], Jae Hyuk Yang [2,†], Dong-Gune Chang [1,*], Seung Woo Suh [2], Hoon Jo [1], Sang-Il Kim [3], Kwang-Sup Song [4] and Woojin Cho [5]

[1] Department of Orthopedic Surgery, Inje University Sanggye Paik Hospital, College of Medicine, Inje University, Seoul 01757, Korea; hongjin0925@naver.com (H.J.K.); hunis121@gmail.com (H.J.)
[2] Department of Orthopedic Surgery, Korea University Guro Hospital, College of Medicine, Korea University, Seoul 08308, Korea; kuspine@naver.com (J.H.Y.); spine@korea.ac.kr (S.W.S.)
[3] Department of Orthopedic Surgery, College of Medicine, The Catholic University of Korea, Seoul 06591, Korea; sang1kim81@gmail.com
[4] Department of Orthopedic Surgery, Chung-Ang University Hospital, College of Medicine, Chung-Ang University, Seoul 06973, Korea; ksong70@cau.ac.kr
[5] Department of Orthopedic Surgery, Albert Einstein College of Medicine, Montefiore Medical Center, Bronx, NY 10467, USA; woojinchomd@aol.com
* Correspondence: dgchangmd@gmail.com; Tel.: +82-2-950-1284
† Hong Jin Kim and Jae Hyuk Yang equally contributed to this work, and should be considered co-first author.

Abstract: Concurrent knee osteoarthritis (KOA) and degenerative lumbar spinal disease (LSD) has increased, but the total knee arthroplasty (TKA) effect on degenerative LSD remains unclear. The aim of this study was to retrospectively analyze to compare radiological and clinical outcomes between spinal fusion only and preoperative TKA with spinal fusion for the patients with concurrent KOA and degenerative LSD. A total of 72 patients with concurrent KOA and degenerative LSDs who underwent spinal fusion at less than three levels were divided in two groups: non-TKA group (n = 50) and preoperative TKA group (n = 22). Preoperative lumbar lordosis (LL) was significantly lower in the preoperative TKA group than the non-TKA group ($p < 0.05$). Significantly higher preoperative pelvic incidence (PI), PI/LL mismatch, and pelvic tilt (PT) occurred in preoperative TKA group than non-TKA group (all $p < 0.05$). There was significant improvement of postoperative Oswestry Disability Index and leg Visual Analog Scale in the preoperative TKA group (all $p < 0.01$). Preoperative TKA could be a benefit for in proper correction of sagittal spinopelvic alignment by spinal fusion. Therefore, preoperative TKA could be considered a preceding surgical option for patients with severe sagittal spinopelvic parameters in concurrent KOA and degenerative LSD.

Keywords: spinal fusion; total knee arthroplasty; lumbar lordosis; sagittal spinopelvic parameters; clinical outcome

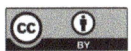

1. Introduction

With aging populations, the prevalence of concurrent degenerative musculoskeletal condition has increased, which has impacted global disease burden [1]. Degenerative lumbar spinal diseases (LSDs) are one of the most common musculoskeletal conditions caused by degenerative change in spinal joints, intervertebral disks, and ligament flavum, which can lead to load-bearing abnormalities including spinal stenosis, spondylolisthesis, herniated intervertebral disk, and degenerative lumbar scoliosis that are associated with adult spinal deformity [1–3]. Knee osteoarthritis (KOA) shares similar clinical presentations with degenerative LSD and is treated by total knee arthroplasty (TKA) in severe cases [4]. Patients frequently have concurrent KOA and degenerative LSD, and it is not uncommon that both disorders are severe enough to require surgical treatment [1,4].

Both degenerative diseases located in spine and knee have an effect on spinal alignment, which necessary for harmonious balances from upright posture to ambulation [3]. In particular, sagittal spinopelvic imbalances occurred in degenerative diseases in spine, as a result of the compensatory mechanism from loss of lordosis, pelvic retroversion, and knee flexion [2–5]. Furthermore, the stiffness of degenerative knee was reported to affect spinal malalignment because postural equilibrium was harmonized with coordinated movement of spine, hip, and knee [6]. Although knee stiffness significantly impacts on the biomechanical effect of spinal balances, few studies reported on the relationship between TKA and such malalignments to date [6–8]. In addition, there is lack of information on how resolution of knee stiffness by TKA affects spinal alignment. Furthermore, there are few studies on the effect of spinal balances between spine fusion and resolution of knee stiffness.

TKA is a well-established surgical treatment, as well as an efficacious way to decrease pain and improve functions for patients with KOA [9]. Surgical treatment of degenerative LSDs and KOA demonstrate uniformly favorable clinical outcomes, according to mid-term to long-term follow-up studies [10–12]. However, the effect of certain comorbidities on degenerative LSDs remains unclear. To date, decision-making for fusion surgery or TKA combines the patient's preferences and surgeons' assessment of the severity of both diseases [4]. When concurrent KOA and degenerative LSDs are of equally severe grade, there is insufficient evidence for the optimal order of surgical treatment [4]. To the best of our knowledge, there have been very few reports that performed a comparative analysis of spinal fusion in patients with and without TKA. Therefore, this study aimed to analyze the impact of TKA by comparing the clinical and radiological outcomes of spinal fusion for patients with concurrent severe KOA and degenerative LSDs.

2. Materials and Methods

This study was performed through retrospective comparative analysis at a single institute where spinal fusion and TKA were routinely performed. The concept and procedures of the study were approved by our institutional review board. All spinal fusion surgery procedures (posterior decompression with posterior lumbar interbody fusion and/or posterior lateral fusion with resected local bone graft and cages) and TKA were performed by senior surgeons (a spine surgeon and a knee surgeon) with vast experience in performing standard surgeries. The patients with hip and/or ankle osteoarthritis above moderate grade or patients who underwent hip arthroplasty, ankle fusion, ankle arthroplasty, and revision TKA were excluded from this study. The medical records data of 122 patients who underwent TKA before spinal fusion or underwent spinal fusion at less than three levels due to degenerative LSDs concurrent with KOA (more than Kellgren-Lawrence grade III) were collected from 2013 to 2018. A total of 72 patients were included, excluding loss to follow-up ($n = 17$) and those who underwent TKA during the postoperative follow-up period of spinal fusion ($n = 21$). The minimum interval between TKA and spinal fusion was set to one-year in consideration of TKA-related pain for at least 6 months. The patients were divided into two groups as follows: the non-TKA group ($n = 50$, patients who underwent spinal fusion only) and the preoperative TKA group ($n = 22$, patients who underwent spinal fusion after TKA)

All patient data were collected from the hospital database and retrospectively analyzed in 2021. Demographic and operative variables included age, height, weight, body mass index (BMI), bone mineral density (BMD), symptom duration, main diagnosis of LSD, spinal stenosis grade on magnetic resonance imaging (MRI), fusion levels, and Kellgren-Lawrence grade. Spinal stenosis grade on MRI was measured by qualitative grading system according to axial MRI on T2-weighted images [13]. Kellgren-Lawrence grade on plain radiograph of knee was evaluated as follows: grade I (doubtful joint space narrowing and possible osteolytic lipping), grade II (definite osteophytes and possible joint space narrowing), grade III (multiple osteophytes, definite joint space narrowing, sclerosis, possible bony deformity), and grade IV (large osteophytes, marked narrowing of joint space, severe sclerosis, and definite deformity of bone contour) [9].

Radiological variables included regional, global, coronal, and sagittal spinopelvic parameters preoperatively, immediate postoperatively (within 2 weeks), and at postoperative 2-year follow-up after spinal fusion. Lumbar lordosis (LL), thoracic kyphosis (TK), and cervical lordosis (CL) were collected as regional parameters. Sagittal vertical axis (SVA) and T1 pelvic angle (TPA) were collected as global parameters. Coronal parameters were measured by Cobb's angle reflecting local alignment and coronal balance reflecting global alignment. Sagittal spinopelvic parameters included pelvic incidence (PI), PI/LL mismatch, pelvic tilt (PT), and sacral slope. Regarding clinical outcomes, Oswestry Disability Index (ODI) and Visual Analog Scale (VAS) of the leg and back were used for clinical evaluation preoperatively, immediate postoperatively (discharge from hospital) and at postoperative 6-month follow-up after spinal fusion.

Statistical analysis was performed using SPSS Statistics for Windows, version 21.0 (IBM Corp., Armonk, NY, USA). A normal distribution was confirmed by Kolmogorov–Smirnov test. Regarding continuous variables, student-t-test and Mann–Whitney test were used for parametric data and non-parametric data, as appropriate. Regarding categorical variables, chi-square test and Fisher-exact test were used for parametric and non-parametric data, as appropriate. In the case of variables with negative or positive values based on the measured reference point, such as coronal balance and SVA, statistical comparisons of groups required converting negative numbers to positive numbers because it was necessary to statistically analyze differences from a reference point. Statistical significance was set at $p < 0.05$.

3. Results
3.1. Demographic Data

All demographic, clinical, and operative data, including sex, age, body mass index (BMI), bone mineral density (BMD), symptom duration, main diagnosis of LSDs, spinal stenosis grade on MRI, fusion levels, and Kellgren-Lawrence grade were summarized in Table 1. In preoperative TKA group, mean interval between TKA and spinal fusion was 1.2 years. The mean age in the non-TKA and preoperative TKA groups was 68.4 years and 72.1 years, respectively ($p = 0.110$). Mean BMI in the non-TKA and preoperative TKA groups was 26 and 25.5, respectively ($p = 0.602$). Mean BMD in non-TKA and preoperative TKA groups was −0.7 and −1.1 at the spine as well as −1.1 and −1.4 at the femur. There were no significant differences in BMD of the spine and femur between the two groups ($p = 0.696$, $p = 0.284$). In total, 58% and 59.2 of patients had a symptom duration of more than 5 years in the non-TKA and preoperative TKA groups, respectively. A severe grade of spinal stenosis was presented in 52% and 54.5% of the non-TKA and preoperative TKA groups, respectively. The fusion levels in non-TKA and preoperative TKA group were not significant different ($p = 0.409$). Spondylolisthesis was presented in 26% of the non-TKA group and 45% of the preoperative TKA group for the main diagnosis of LSDs. All KOA were bilateral, which showed more than Kellgren-Lawrence grade III. There were no significant differences in demographic and operative data between the two groups (Table 1).

Table 1. Demographic and operative data for spinal fusion only and preoperative TKA with spinal fusion groups.

Variables	Non-TKA (n = 50)	Preoperative TKA (n = 22)	p-Value
Sex (M:F)	9:41	3:18	0.268 [†]
Age (years)	68.4 ± 7.9 *	72.1 ± 8.1 *	0.110
Height (cm)	155.4 ± 6.3 *	155.9 ± 5.1 *	0.787
Weight (kg)	62.7 ± 8.9 *	62.0 ± 10.1 *	0.786

Table 1. Cont.

Variables	Non-TKA (n = 50)	Preoperative TKA (n = 22)	p-Value
BMI (kg/m^2)	26.0 ± 3.5 *	25.5 ± 3.6 *	0.602
BMD (T-score)			
Spine	−0.7 ± 1.0 *	−0.8 ± 1.2 *	0.695
Femur	−1.1 ± 1.0 *	−1.4 ± 0.9 *	0.284
Symptom duration (n)			
6 months–1 year	10	2	
1–5 years	11	7	0.303 †
>5 years	29	13	
Main diagnosis of LSD (n)			
Spinal stenosis	37	12	0.205 †
Spondylolisthesis with spinal stenosis	13	10	
Spinal stenosis grade on MRI (n)			
Moderate	14	6	
Moderate to severe	10	4	0.806 †
Severe	26	12	
Fusion levels (n)			
1 level	22	12	0.409 †
2 levels	28	10	
Kellgren-Lawrence grade (n, Right:Left)			
Grade III	28:30	-	
Grade IV	22:20	-	

$p < 0.05$ is significant. * All values are expressed as mean ± standard deviation. p values were calculated by independent t-test for parametric data and Mann Whitney U test for non-parametric data. † p-values were calculated by chi-square test for parametric data and Fisher's exact test for non-parametric data. n = number; TKA = Total knee arthroplasty; M = Male; F = Female; BMI = Body mass index; BMD = Bone mineral density; LSDs = Lumbar spinal diseases; MRI = Magnetic resonance imaging.

3.2. Radiological Outcomes

Regarding the regional and global parameters of radiological outcomes, preoperative LL was significantly lower in the preoperative TKA group (32°) than the non-TKA group (23°) (p = 0.045). The 2-year follow-up LL was lower in the non-TKA group (35.3°) than the preoperative TKA group (27.1°) with statistical significance (p = 0.041). Preoperative SVA was 51.6 mm in the non-TKA group and 72.5 mm in the preoperative TKA group, with no significance (p = 0.066). Immediate postoperative (40 mm, 47.2 mm) and 2-year follow-up (41.2 mm, 47 mm) SVA in non-TKA and preoperative TKA groups was distributed within an age-adjusted target (about 54.5 mm from 65 to 74 years) with no significance (p = 0.455, 0.561) [3]. All TPAs were greater than 20° and those in the preoperative TKA group were higher than non-TKA group, but statistical difference was not significant. Regional and global parameters demonstrated worse outcomes in the preoperative TKA group than the non-TKA group. Only the preoperative and 2-year follow-up LL showed statistically significant differences (Table 2).

Regarding the coronal parameters, Cobb's angle preoperatively, immediate postoperative, and at 2-year follow-up was within 10° in both groups (all p > 0.05). All coronal balance values preoperatively, immediate postoperatively and at 2-year follow-up evaluations were within 20 mm and showed statistical insignificance between the two groups (all p > 0.05). For sagittal spinopelvic parameters, preoperative PI was significantly higher in the preoperative TKA group (62.8°) than the non-TKA group (53.5°) (p = 0.041). However, after spinal fusion, there were no significance differences between immediate postoperative (p = 0.398) and 2-year follow-up (p = 0.729) PI. All values of PI/LL mismatch were more than 11°. Preoperative PI/LL mismatch was significantly higher in the preoperative TKA group (39.8°) than the non-TKA group (21.5°) with statistical significance (p = 0.013). However, there were no significant difference observed in immediate postoperative (p = 0.286) and 2-year follow-up (p = 0.265) PI/LL mismatch. PT was greater at more than 22° and was higher in the preoperative TKA group (30.7°) than the non-TKA group (24°). Only preoperative PT showed a statistically difference ($p = 0.011$). All sacral slopes were greater in the preoperative TKA group than in the non-TKA group but without statistical significance (all $p > 0.05$) (Table 3).

Table 2. Comparison of regional and global parameters between spinal fusion only and preoperative TKA with spinal fusion groups.

Variables	Non-TKA ($n = 50$)	Preoperative TKA ($n = 22$)	p-Value
Regional parameters			
Lumbar lordosis (°)			
Preoperative	32.0 ± 16.0	23.0 ± 13.5	0.045
Immediate postoperative	34.1 ± 13.5	29.9 ± 12.6	0.274
2-year follow-up	35.3 ± 13.7	27.1 ± 13.6	0.041
Thoracic kyphosis (°)			
Preoperative	28.9 ± 12.6	24.4 ± 11.7	0.213
Immediate postoperative	28.9 ± 11.0	27.4 ± 9.5	0.643
2-year follow-up	28.9 ± 10.9	26.7 ± 11.4	0.5
Cervical lordosis (°)			
Preoperative	20.9 ± 10.2	18.1 ± 7.5	0.326
Immediate postoperative	21.0 ± 10.2	19.3 ± 8.6	0.572
2-year follow-up	21.6 ± 10.1	18.6 ± 7.5	0.28
Global parameters			
Sagittal Vertical Axis (mm)			
Preoperative	51.6 ± 30.8	72.5 ± 56.4	0.066
Immediate postoperative	40.0 ± 32.5	47.2 ± 30.9	0.455
2-year follow-up	41.2 ± 34.0	47.0 ± 30.9	0.561
T1 pelvic angle (°)			
Preoperative	26.3 ± 7.6	28.9 ± 7.3	0.247
Immediate postoperative	24.0 ± 7.0	22.1 ± 6.0	0.343
2-year follow-up	24.6 ± 7.3	22.6 ± 2.4	0.425

Data represent mean ± standard deviation values for each group. In the case of the sagittal vertical axis, the statistical analysis between groups was performed by converting negative numbers to positive numbers to analyze how the difference from the reference point. p-values were calculated by independent t-test for parametric data and Mann Whitney U test for non-parametric data. Significant differences were accepted for $p < 0.05$. n = number; TKA = Total knee arthroplasty.

3.3. Clinical Outcomes

ODI and VAS were used for assessing clinical outcomes preoperatively, immediate postoperatively, and at 6-month follow-up. The mean preoperative ODI was significantly worse in the preoperative TKA group (62.4) than the non-TKA group (50.4) ($p = 0.001$). However, after spinal fusion, the mean immediate postoperative ODI was 45.4 in the non-TKA group and 37.6 in the preoperative TKA group ($p = 0.008$). Mean 6-month follow-up ODI was 45.8 in the non-TKA group and 34.1 in the preoperative TKA group ($p < 0.001$). Mean preoperative VAS of the back was 7.57 in the non-TKA group and 8.44 in the preoperative TKA group. Mean immediate postoperative VAS of the back was 4.00 in the non-TKA group and 4.44 in the preoperative TKA group. Mean 6-month follow-up VAS of the back was 3.19 in the non-TKA group and 3.33 in the preoperative TKA group. None of these back VAS values were significantly different between groups (all $p > 0.05$). Preoperative VAS of the leg was close to 7.2 in the non-TKA group and 7.3 in the preoperative TKA ($p = 0.965$). Mean immediate postoperative VAS of the leg was 6.1 in the non-TKA group and 3 in the preoperative TKA group ($p < 0.001$). Six-month follow-up VAS of the leg was 6 in the non-TKA group and 2.7 in the preoperative TKA group, a significant difference ($p < 0.001$) (Table 4).

Table 3. Comparison of coronal and sagittal spinopelvic parameters between spinal fusion only and preoperative TKA with spinal fusion groups.

Variables	Non-TKA (n = 50)	Preoperative TKA (n = 22)	p-Value
Coronal parameters			
Cobb's angle (°)			
Preoperative	7.4 ± 5.4	8.5 ± 9.6	0.551
Immediate postoperative	6.3 ± 5.4	6.1 ± 5.0	0.887
2-year follow-up	6.6 ± 5.9	5.9 ± 5.3	0.67
Coronal balance (mm)			
Preoperative	9.1 ± 8.2	9.8 ± 8.8	0.783
Immediate postoperative	6.2 ± 4.9	9.7 ± 10.3	0.07
2-year follow-up	5.4 ± 4.4	12.9 ± 28.9	0.093
Sagittal spinopelvic parameters			
Pelvic incidence (°)			
Preoperative	53.5 ± 16.2	62.8 ± 13.1	0.041
Immediate postoperative	56.9 ± 16.9	61.3 ± 21.0	0.398
2-year follow-up	61.0 ± 16.2	59.5 ± 15.0	0.729
PI/LL mismatch			
Preoperative	21.5 ± 25.8	39.8 ± 21.7	0.013
Immediate postoperative	23.7 ± 10.3	31.1 ± 15.6	0.286
2-year follow-up	25.7 ± 20.1	32.3 ± 22.2	0.265
Pelvic tilt (°)			
Preoperative	24.0 ± 8.4	30.7 ± 10.2	0.011
Immediate postoperative	26.4 ± 9.9	27.8 ± 9.2	0.609
2-year follow-up	29.3 ± 11.7	29.6 ± 11.5	0.935
Sacral slope (°)			
Preoperative	29.5 ± 8.0	32.1 ± 9.6	0.286
Immediate postoperative	30.5 ± 7.5	33.4 ± 17.7	0.349
2-year follow-up	31.7 ± 6.8	29.8 ± 7.5	0.37

Data represent mean ± standard deviation values for each group. In the case of coronal balance, the statistical analysis between groups was performed by converting negative numbers to positive numbers to analyze how the difference from the reference point. p values were calculated by independent t-test for parametric data and Mann Whitney U test for non-parametric data. Significant differences were accepted for $p < 0.05$. n = number; TKA = Total Knee Arthroplasty; PI/LL mismatch = Pelvic incidence minus lumbar lordosis.

Table 4. Comparison for clinical outcomes between spinal fusion only and preoperative TKA with spinal fusion.

Clinical Outcomes	Non-TKA (n = 50)	Preoperative TKA (n = 22)	p-Value
ODI			
Preoperative	50.4 ± 9.0	62.4 ± 5.5	0.001
Immediate postoperative	45.4 ± 10.7	37.6 ± 5.3	0.008
6-month follow-up	45.8 ± 8.8	34.1 ± 4.7	<0.001
VAS Back			
Preoperative	7.6 ± 1.6	8.4 ± 1.2	0.193
Immediate postoperative	4.0 ± 0.8	4.4 ± 1.1	0.642
6-month follow-up	3.2 ± 0.8	3.3 ± 1.0	0.79
VAS Leg			
Preoperative	7.2 ± 1.7	7.3 ± 2.0	0.965
Immediate postoperative	6.1 ± 1.5	3.0 ± 0.7	<0.001
6-month follow-up	6.0 ± 1.1	2.7 ± 0.7	<0.001

Data represent mean ± standard deviation values for each group. p-values were calculated by independent t-test for parametric data and Mann–Whitney U test for non-parametric data. Significant differences were accepted for $p < 0.05$. n = number; TKA = Total knee arthroplasty; ODI = Oswestry Disability Index; VAS = Visual Analog Scale.

The ODI differences between preoperative and immediate postoperative was 5.0 ± 4.7 in non-TKA and 24.9 ± 6.2 in preoperative TKA with statistical significance ($p < 0.001$). VAS leg differences between preoperative and immediate postoperative was 1.0 ± 0.9 in non-TKA and 4.3 ± 1.9 in preoperative TKA with statistical significance ($p < 0.001$). However, ODI differences and VAS leg differences between immediate postoperative and 6-month follow-up showed not statistical insignificance ($p = 0.780$).

4. Discussion

Degenerative diseases including osteoarthritis and spinal stenosis are serious public health concerns globally because of the severe pain and disability they cause [14]. Specifically, lower back pain and osteoarthritis were the first ranked and 12th ranked, respectively, global burden of diseases that cause disability from a systemic analysis in 2016 [15]. Moreover, these chronic conditions lead to multi-morbidity, which limit function and cause pain and disability [14,15]. However, the impact of multi-morbid conditions has not been extensively studied yet [14]. In an arthroplasty study, the impact of total hip arthroplasty in spinal fusion was reported in hip-spine syndrome, but there is a relative lack of evidence for that of TKA [4]. Therefore, this study aimed to identify the impact of preoperative TKA in spinal fusion for patients with concurrent severe KOA and degenerative LSD.

Regarding preoperative radiological parameters, our results showed that LL and sagittal spinopelvic parameters were worse in the TKA group. There were attempts to elucidate the association between radiological factors of the spine and flexibility of the knee [6,16,17]. Flexion contracture of the knee was associated with not only loss of LL, but also poor sagittal spinopelvic parameters [16,17]. Kim et al. suggested that lumbar flexibility is important for spinal and lower limb alignment following TKA [7]. However, the studies reported that removal of flexion contracture by TKA could not compensate for sagittal global imbalances [5,6]. The results have similar preoperative aspects of worse LL and sagittal spinopelvic parameters, which support the finding that TKA does not compensate for these parameters. Our results suggest the patients that require both TKA and spinal fusion have relatively worse preoperative radiological outcomes in LL and sagittal spinopelvic parameters. Therefore, sagittal spinopelvic parameters could consider one of the factors for surgical decision-making in the patients with severe KOA and degenerative LSDs.

The pelvic morphology, which is influenced by sagittal malalignment, was significantly different in elderly patients with concurrent KOA and degenerative LSDs compared to patients with LSD only [18]. Increased sagittal malalignment with a lack of LL was caused by double-level listhesis (i.e., spondylolisthesis and/or retrolisthesis) and greater knee flexion [19]. Although decompression with short-segment fusion at less than three levels can yield improvement of clinical outcomes, corrective lumbar surgery alone may be insufficient for radiological outcomes because of greater pelvic retroversion (high PT) and, worse sagittal spinopelvic alignment [20,21]. Kohno et al. reported that surgical strategies in concurrent degenerative knee and LSDs may be necessary to restore sagittal spinopelvic alignment, followed by decreased pelvic retroversion [18]. In our study, patients with preoperative TKA exhibited greater pelvic retroversion than patients with KOA, and more often required fusion surgery for correction of sagittal spinopelvic alignment. The optimal values of sagittal spinopelvic parameters that need to be corrected was under-estimated by compensatory mechanism of spine from knee stiffness in non-TKA group. Therefore, preoperative TKA could be a benefit for in proper correction of sagittal spinopelvic alignment by spinal fusion.

Schwab et al. showed a PI/LL mismatch that reflected the disharmony between spine and pelvis correlate with increase in ODI [22]. From our result, the preoperative TKA group (i.e., the patients who needs to both spinal fusion and TKA) showed worse ODI values. Because TKA with worse sagittal spinopelvic parameters is associated with poor range of motion, it led to dissatisfaction and did not improve disability [6]. For significant improvement of ODI in the TKA group, preoperative TKA may have contributed to more vigorous activity by resolution of neurogenic claudication. The most important thing in our study was that complementing compensatory mechanisms by preoperative TKA gave a chance for better correction of sagittal spinopelvic parameters, which has a significant impact on improving disability. The value of ODI reflects pain as well as activities of daily living affected by knee discomfort [4]. Lee et al. reported that the presence of preoperative KOA and multi-level fusion were poor prognostic factors in lumbar spinal surgery, and Lee et al. also showed worse ODI scores in the patients who underwent TKA before spinal fusion on retrospective case analysis [23]. However, considering that our study included patients with spinal fusion at less than three levels, preoperatively worse spinopelvic sagittal parameters as well as lower lumbar lordosis contributed to a higher ODI level in the preoperative TKA group compared to the non-TKA group [24]. If the case of long-level spinal fusion and instrumentation, this can clearly affect balancing and lumbar spine alignment by nonunion and/or instrumentation failure. Therefore, in order to minimize this effect and evaluate the impact of preoperative TKA, we assessed only the patents who underwent spinal fusion at less than three-level (i.e., short-level fusion). Preoperative TKA in spinal fusion at less than three levels could be helpful for predicting disability and pain in the case of worse sagittal spinopelvic parameters.

Lower back pain is affected by various factors, and has a broad spectrum of symptoms that requires differential diagnosis based on degenerative, congenital, and traumatic causes [25]. Escobar et al. reported the preoperative absence of lower back pain in TKA as a predictor of a good quality of life in a multi-center prospective study conducted in 2007 [26]. Pivec et al. also suggested that the presence of spinal stenosis was associated with worse clinical outcomes following TKA [27]. However, little is known about the clinical relevance between back pain and preoperative TKA for fusion surgery in patients with KOA. In our study, back VAS was not significantly different between the two groups, which indicates that preoperative TKA in spinal fusion does not seem to have much impact on lower back pain. Preoperative TKA in spinal fusion showed better clinical outcomes in terms of leg VAS, which means significantly improved pain. Lumbar radiculopathy by nerve root compression from L3 to L5 is a typical clinical presentation of spinal stenosis, which share the same portion in anterior knee pain by joint degeneration [28]. Furthermore, the origin of pain from knee and/or spine could be impact on determining clinical outcomes [29]. Therefore, preoperative TKA in the case of short-level spinal fusion significantly impacts improvement by eradicating the pain source.

There were several limitations to our study. First, the number of patients was relatively small and we used a retrospective design. Future trials would be needed by large sample in multicenter study and/or meta-analysis. Secondly, this study did not reflect the morphology and clinical scales of the knee. It also included the limitation of being a retrospective study, which suggests the need to evaluate radiological factors and clinical function of the knee in future trials. However, our study focused on comparing radiological factors, function, and pain measures limited to the spine. Large multi-center prospective studies should be needed to perform to confirm our results. Nonetheless, our study suggested that preoperative TKA in spinal fusion (less than three levels) have significantly impact on lumbar radiculopathy and disability.

5. Conclusions

Preoperative TKA could be a benefit for in proper correction of sagittal spinopelvic alignment by spinal fusion. Therefore, preoperative TKA could be considered a preceding surgical option for patients with severe sagittal spinopelvic parameters in concurrent KOA and degenerative LSD.

Author Contributions: Conceptualization, H.J.K., J.H.Y. and D.-G.C.; methodology, H.J.K., J.H.Y. and S.W.S.; validation, H.J.K., J.H.Y., S.-I.K., K.-S.S. and W.C.; investigation, H.J.K.; data curation, H.J.K. and H.J.; writing—original draft preparation, H.J.K., J.H.Y. and D.-G.C.; writing—review and editing, H.J.K., J.H.Y. and D.-G.C.; visualization, J.H.Y. and S.W.S.; supervision, D.-G.C.; project administration, D.-G.C. All authors have read and agreed to the published version of the manuscript.

Funding: This research received no external funding.

Institutional Review Board Statement: The study was conducted according to the guidelines of the Declaration of Helsinki, and approved by the Institutional Review Board of of Inje University Sanggye Paik Hospital (IRB number: 2021-03-012).

Informed Consent Statement: Patient consent was waived due to retrospective design.

Data Availability Statement: Data collected for this study, including individual patient data, will not be made available.

Conflicts of Interest: The authors declare no conflict of interest.

References

1. Deyo, R.A.; Gray, D.T.; Kreuter, W.; Mirza, S.; Martin, B.I. United States Trends in Lumbar Fusion Surgery for Degenerative Conditions. *Spine* **2005**, *30*, 1441–1445. [CrossRef]
2. Lee, B.H.; Moon, S.-H.; Suk, K.-S.; Kim, H.-S.; Yang, J.-H.; Lee, H.-M. Lumbar Spinal Stenosis: Pathophysiology and Treatment Principle: A Narrative Review. *Asian Spine J.* **2020**, *14*, 682–693. [CrossRef]
3. Kim, H.J.; Yang, J.H.; Chang, D.-G.; Suk, S.-I.; Suh, S.W.; Song, K.-S.; Park, J.-B.; Cho, W. Adult Spinal Deformity: Current Concepts and Decision-Making Strategies for Management. *Asian Spine J.* **2020**, *14*, 886–897. [CrossRef] [PubMed]
4. Goodman, S.B.; Lachiewicz, P.F.; Liu, N.; Wood, K.B. Knee or Spine Surgery First? A Survey of Treatment Order for Patients with Concurrent Degenerative Knee and Lumbar Spinal Disorders. *J. Arthroplast.* **2020**, *35*, 2039–2043. [CrossRef]
5. Kitagawa, A.; Yamamoto, J.; Toda, M.; Hashimoto, Y. Spinopelvic Alignment and Low Back Pain before and after Total Knee Arthroplasty. *Asian Spine J.* **2021**, *15*, 9–16. [CrossRef]
6. Vigdorchik, J.M.; Sharma, A.K.; Feder, O.I.; Buckland, A.J.; Mayman, D.J.; Carroll, K.M.; Sculco, P.K.; Long, W.J.; Jerabek, S.A. Stiffness After Total Knee Arthroplasty: Is It a Result of Spinal Deformity? *J. Arthroplast.* **2020**, *35*, S330–S335. [CrossRef] [PubMed]
7. Kim, S.C.; Kim, J.S.; Choi, H.G.; Kim, T.W.; Lee, Y.S. Spinal Flexibility Is an Important Factor for Improvement in Spinal and Knee Alignment after Total Knee Arthroplasty: Evaluation Using a Whole Body EOS System. *J. Clin. Med.* **2020**, *9*, 3498. [CrossRef]
8. Jalai, C.M.; Cruz, D.L.; Diebo, B.G.; Poorman, G.; Lafage, R.; Bess, S.; Ramchandran, S.; Day, L.M.; Vira, S.; Liabaud, B.; et al. Full-Body Analysis of Age-Adjusted Alignment in Adult Spinal Deformity Patients and Lower-Limb Compensation. *Spine* **2017**, *42*, 653–661. [CrossRef] [PubMed]
9. Katz, J.N.; Arant, K.R.; Loeser, R.F. Diagnosis and Treatment of Hip and Knee Osteoarthritis: A Review. *JAMA* **2021**, *325*, 568–578. [CrossRef]
10. Ethgen, O.; Bruyère, O.; Richy, F.; Dardennes, C.; Reginster, J.-Y. Health-related quality of life in total hip and total knee arthroplasty. A qualitative and systematic review of the literature. *J. Bone Jt. Surg.-Am.* **2004**, *86*, 963–974. [CrossRef]
11. Jakola, A.S.; Sørlie, A.; Gulati, S.; Nygaard, P.; Lydersen, S.; Solberg, T. Clinical outcomes and safety assessment in elderly patients undergoing decompressive laminectomy for lumbar spinal stenosis: A prospective study. *BMC Surg.* **2010**, *10*, 34. [CrossRef]
12. Rampersaud, Y.R.; Lewis, S.J.; Davey, J.R.; Gandhi, R.; Mahomed, N.N. Comparative outcomes and cost-utility after surgical treatment of focal lumbar spinal stenosis compared with osteoarthritis of the hip or knee–part 1: Long-term change in health-related quality of life. *Spine J.* **2014**, *14*, 234–243. [CrossRef]
13. Lee, G.Y.; Lee, J.W.; Choi, H.S.; Oh, K.J.; Kang, H.S. A new grading system of lumbar central canal stenosis on MRI: An easy and reliable method. *Skeletal Radiol.* **2011**, *40*, 1033–1039. [CrossRef]
14. Young, J.J.; Hartvigsen, J.; Jensen, R.K.; Roos, E.M.; Ammendolia, C.; Juhl, C.B. Prevalence of multimorbid degenerative lumbar spinal stenosis with knee and/or hip osteoarthritis: Protocol for a systematic review and meta-analysis. *Syst. Rev.* **2020**, *9*, 232. [CrossRef]
15. Vos, T.; Abajobir, A.A.; Abate, K.H.; Abbafati, C.; Abbas, K.M.; Abd-Allah, F.; Abdulkader, R.S.; Abdulle, A.M.; Abebo, T.A.; Abera, S.F.; et al. Global, regional, and national incidence, prevalence, and years lived with disability for 328 diseases and injuries for 195 countries, 1990–2016: A systematic analysis for the Global Burden of Disease Study 2016. *Lancet* **2017**, *390*, 1211–1259. [CrossRef]
16. Lee, S.-M.; Yoon, M.G.; Moon, M.-S.; Lee, B.-J.; Lee, S.-R.; Seo, Y.H. Effect of Correction of the Contractured Flexed Osteoarthritic Knee on the Sagittal Alignment by Total Replacement. *Asian Spine J.* **2013**, *7*, 204–211. [CrossRef] [PubMed]
17. Murata, Y.; Takahashi, K.; Yamagata, M.; Hanaoka, E.; Moriya, H. The knee-spine syndrome. Association between lumbar lordosis and extension of the knee. *J Bone Joint Surg Br.* **2003**, *85*, 95–99. [CrossRef] [PubMed]
18. Kohno, M.; Iwamura, Y.; Inasaka, R.; Akiyama, G.; Higashihira, S.; Kawai, T.; Niimura, T.; Inaba, Y. Influence of comorbid knee osteoarthritis on surgical outcome and sagittal spinopelvic/lower-extremity alignment in elderly patients with degenerative lumbar spondylolisthesis undergoing transforaminal lumbar interbody fusion. *J. Neurosurg. Spine* **2020**, *32*, 850–858. [CrossRef] [PubMed]
19. Diebo, B.G.; Ferrero, E.; Lafage, R.; Challier, V.; Liabaud, B.; Liu, S. Recruitment of compensatory mechanisms in sagittal spinal malalignment is age and regional deformity dependent: A full-standing axis analysis of key radiographical parameters. *Spine* **2015**, *40*, 642–649. [CrossRef] [PubMed]

20. Kawakami, M.; Tamaki, T.; Ando, M.; Yamada, H.; Hashizume, H.; Yoshida, M. Lumbar Sagittal Balance Influences the Clinical Outcome After Decompression and Posterolateral Spinal Fusion for Degenerative Lumbar Spondylolisthesis. *Spine* **2002**, *27*, 59–64. [CrossRef]
21. Kim, M.K.; Lee, S.-H.; Kim, E.-S.; Eoh, W.; Chung, S.-S.; Lee, C.-S. The impact of sagittal balance on clinical results after posterior interbody fusion for patients with degenerative spondylolisthesis: A Pilot study. *BMC Musculoskelet. Disord.* **2011**, *12*, 69. [CrossRef] [PubMed]
22. Schwab, F.; Dubey, A.; Gamez, L.; El Fegoun, A.B.; Hwang, K.; Pagala, M.; Farcy, J.-P. Adult Scoliosis: Prevalence, SF-36, and Nutritional Parameters in an Elderly Volunteer Population. *Spine* **2005**, *30*, 1082–1085. [CrossRef] [PubMed]
23. Lee, B.H.; Kim, T.-H.; Chong, H.-S.; Lee, S.-H.; Park, J.-O.; Kim, H.-S.; Shim, D.-W.; Lee, H.-M.; Moon, S.-H. Prognostic Factors for Surgical Outcomes Including Preoperative Total Knee Replacement and Knee Osteoarthritis Status in Female Patients with Lumbar Spinal Stenosis. *J. Spinal Disord. Tech.* **2015**, *28*, 47–52. [CrossRef] [PubMed]
24. Cervera Irimia, J.; Tome-Bermejo, F.; Pinera-Parrilla, A.R.; Benito Gallo, M.; Bisaccia, M.; Fernandez-Gonzalez, M. Spinal fusion achieves similar two-year improvement in HRQoL as total hip and total knee replacement. A prospective, multicentric and observational study. *SICOT J.* **2019**, *5*, 26. [CrossRef] [PubMed]
25. Zileli, M.; Crostelli, M.; Grimaldi, M.; Mazza, O.; Anania, C.; Fornari, M.; Costa, F. Natural Course and Diagnosis of Lumbar Spinal Stenosis: WFNS Spine Committee Recommendations. *World Neurosurg. X* **2020**, *7*, 100073. [CrossRef] [PubMed]
26. Escobar, A.; Quintana, J.M.; Bilbao, A.; Azkarate, J.; Guenaga, J.I.; Arenaza, J.C.; Gutierrez, L.F. Effect of patient characteristics on reported outcomes after total knee replacement. *Rheumatology* **2007**, *46*, 112–119. [CrossRef]
27. Pivec, R.; Johnson, A.J.; Naziri, Q.; Issa, K.; Bonutti, P.M.; Mont, M.A. Lumbar Spinal Stenosis Impairs Function Following Total Knee Arthroplasty. *J. Knee Surg.* **2012**, *26*, 059–064. [CrossRef]
28. McNabb, D.C.; Olcott, C.W.; Del Gaizo, D.J.; Vaughn, B.K.; Lim, M.R. Lumbar Radiculopathy Confounded: Total Knee Arthroplasty Diminishes the Patellar Tendon Reflex. *Spine* **2015**, *40*, E1239–E1243. [CrossRef]
29. March, L.; Cross, M.; Tribe, K.; Lapsley, H.; Courtenay, B.; Brooks, P. Two knees or not two knees? Patient costs and outcomes following bilateral and unilateral total knee joint replacement surgery for OA. *Osteoarthr. Cartil.* **2004**, *12*, 400–408. [CrossRef]

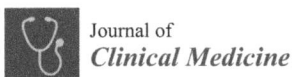

Article

Association between Severity of Diffuse Idiopathic Skeletal Hyperostosis and Ossification of Other Spinal Ligaments in Patients with Ossification of the Posterior Longitudinal Ligament

Soraya Nishimura [1], Takashi Hirai [2], Narihito Nagoshi [1,*], Toshitaka Yoshii [2], Jun Hashimoto [2], Kanji Mori [3], Satoshi Maki [4], Keiichi Katsumi [5], Kazuhiro Takeuchi [6], Shuta Ushio [2], Takeo Furuya [4], Kei Watanabe [5], Norihiro Nishida [7], Takashi Kaito [8], Satoshi Kato [9], Katsuya Nagashima [10], Masao Koda [10], Hiroaki Nakashima [11], Shiro Imagama [11], Kazuma Murata [12], Yuji Matsuoka [12], Kanichiro Wada [13], Atsushi Kimura [14], Tetsuro Ohba [15], Hiroyuki Katoh [16], Masahiko Watanabe [16], Yukihiro Matsuyama [17], Hiroshi Ozawa [18], Hirotaka Haro [15], Katsushi Takeshita [14], Yu Matsukura [2], Hiroyuki Inose [2], Masashi Yamazaki [10], Kota Watanabe [1], Morio Matsumoto [1], Masaya Nakamura [1], Atsushi Okawa [2] and Yoshiharu Kawaguchi [19] on behalf of the Japanese Organization of the Study for Ossification of Spinal Ligament (JOSL)

1. Department of Orthopedic Surgery, Keio University School of Medicine, Shinjuku-ku, Tokyo 160-8582, Japan; soraya.nishimura@gmail.com (S.N.); kw197251@keio.jp (K.W.); morio@a5.keio.jp (M.M.); masa@a8.keio.jp (M.N.)
2. Department of Orthopedic Surgery, Tokyo Medical and Dental University, Bunkyo-ku, Tokyo 113-8510, Japan; hirai.orth@tmd.ac.jp (T.H.); yoshii.orth@tmd.ac.jp (T.Y.); 0123456789jun@gmail.com (J.H.); ushiorth20@gmail.com (S.U.); matsukura.orth@tmd.ac.jp (Y.M.); inose.orth@tmd.ac.jp (H.I.); okawa.orth@tmd.ac.jp (A.O.)
3. Department of Orthopaedic Surgery, Shiga University of Medical Science, Ōtsu 520-2192, Japan; kanchi@belle.shiga-med.ac.jp
4. Department of Orthopedic Surgery, Chiba University Graduate School of Medicine, Chiba-shi 260-0856, Japan; satoshi.maki@chiba-u.jp (S.M.); takeo251274@yahoo.co.jp (T.F.)
5. Department of Orthopedic Surgery, Niigata University Medical and Dental General Hospital, Niigata-shi 951-8520, Japan; kkatsu_os@yahoo.co.jp (K.K.); keiwatanabe_39jp@live.jp (K.W.)
6. Department of Orthopedic Surgery, National Hospital Organization Okayama Medical Center, Okayama-shi 701-1192, Japan; takeuchi@okayamamc.jp
7. Department of Orthopedic Surgery, Yamaguchi University Graduate School of Medicine, Ube 755-8505, Japan; nishida3@yamaguchi-u.ac.jp
8. Department of Orthopaedic Surgery, Osaka University Graduate School of Medicine, Suita 565-0871, Japan; takashikaito@gmail.com
9. Department of Orthopedic Surgery, Graduate School of Medical Sciences, Kanazawa University, Kanazawa 920-8641, Japan; skato323@gmail.com
10. Department of Orthopedic Surgery, Faculty of Medicine, University of Tsukuba, Tsukuba 305-8577, Japan; katsu_n103@yahoo.co.jp (K.N.); masaokod@gmail.com (M.K.); masashiy@md.tsukuba.ac.jp (M.Y.)
11. Department of Orthopaedics, Nagoya University Graduate School of Medicine, 65 Tsurumai, Shouwa-ku, Nagoya 464-8601, Japan; hirospine@med.nagoya-u.ac.jp (H.N.); imagama@med.nagoya-u.ac.jp (S.I.)
12. Department of Orthopedic Surgery, Tokyo Medical University, Shinjuku, Tokyo 160-8402, Japan; kaz.mur26@gmail.com (K.M.); yuji_kazu77@yahoo.co.jp (Y.M.)
13. Department of Orthopaedic Surgery, Hirosaki University Graduate School of Medicine, Hirosaki 036-8562, Japan; wadak39@hirosaki-u.ac.jp
14. Department of Orthopedics, Jichi Medical University, Shimotsuke 329-0498, Japan; akimura@jichi.ac.jp (A.K.); dtstake@gmail.com (K.T.)
15. Department of Orthopedic Surgery, University of Yamanashi, Chuo 409-3898, Japan; tooba@yamanashi.ac.jp (T.O.); haro@yamanashi.ac.jp (H.H.)
16. Department of Orthopedic Surgery, Surgical Science, Tokai University School of Medicine, Isehara 259-1193, Japan; hero@tokai-u.jp (H.K.); masahiko@is.icc.u-tokai.ac.jp (M.W.)
17. Department of Orthopedic Surgery, Hamamatsu University School of Medicine, Hamamatsu 431-3125, Japan; spine-yu@hama-med.ac.jp
18. Department of Orthopaedic Surgery, Tohoku Medical and Pharmaceutical University, Sendai 981-8558, Japan; hozawa@med.tohoku.ac.jp
19. Department of Orthopedic Surgery, Faculty of Medicine, University of Toyama, Toyama-shi 930-0194, Japan; zenji@med.u-toyama.ac.jp
* Correspondence: nagoshi@2002.jukuin.keio.ac.jp; Tel.: +81-3-5363-3812

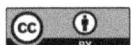

Abstract: Background: Although diffuse idiopathic skeletal hyperostosis (DISH) is known to coexist with the ossification of spinal ligaments (OSLs), details of the radiographic relationship remain unclear. Methods: We prospectively collected data of 239 patients with symptomatic cervical ossification of the posterior longitudinal ligament (OPLL) and analyzed the DISH severity on whole-spine computed tomography images, using the following grades: grade 0, no DISH; grade 1, DISH at T3–T10; grade 2, DISH at both T3–T10 and C6–T2 and/or T11–L2; and grade 3, DISH beyond C5 and/or L3. Ossification indices were calculated as the sum of vertebral and intervertebral levels with OSL for each patient. Results: DISH was found in 107 patients (44.8%), 65 (60.7%) of whom had grade 2 DISH. We found significant associations of DISH grade with the indices for cervical OPLL ($r = 0.45$, $p < 0.0001$), thoracic ossification of the ligamentum flavum (OLF; $r = 0.41$, $p < 0.0001$) and thoracic ossification of the supra/interspinous ligaments (OSIL; $r = 0.53$, $p < 0.0001$). DISH grade was also correlated with the index for each OSL in the whole spine (OPLL: $r = 0.29$, $p < 0.0001$; OLF: $r = 0.40$, $p < 0.0001$; OSIL: $r = 0.50$, $p < 0.0001$). Conclusion: The DISH grade correlated with the indices of OSL at each high-prevalence level as well as the whole spine.

Keywords: cervical ossification of the posterior longitudinal ligament; diffuse idiopathic skeletal hyperostosis; whole-spine computed tomography; grading system; multicenter study

1. Introduction

Ossification of the posterior longitudinal ligament (OPLL) is a well-known cause of severe myelopathy and radiculopathy, especially in East Asian countries [1,2]. Patients with OPLL often experience the ossification of spinal ligaments (OSLs). Previous reports suggest that the co-morbidity rate for diffuse idiopathic skeletal hyperostosis (DISH) and OPLL is around 25–50%, which is relatively high [3–6]. Given that DISH is usually found as a benign radiological condition that does not compress the spinal cord [7–10], this pathology has been considered clinically innocuous. However, patients with DISH are at higher risk for late-onset paralysis following ankylosing spinal fractures with minor trauma, especially in cases with spinal cord compression due to OPLL [11–13]. In addition, myelopathy frequently results from a concentration of stress factors—when spinal stenosis along with OSL is present above or below the ankylosing spine in DISH [14]. Therefore, assessing the degree of DISH is important in patients with cervical OPLL.

Despite the potentially devastating consequences of comorbid DISH and an additional OSL, such as cervical OPLL, a correlation remains to be determined between DISH severity and a predisposition to other OSL. To address this question, a tool is urgently needed for evaluating the spread of DISH. Previous studies have reported the degree of DISH according to the number of consecutive vertebral bodies involved, or the width and/or thickness of ossification on plain radiographs [15–17]; however, neither of these grading methods can accurately assess the development of ossified lesions.

In a previous study, we retrospectively examined the DISH distribution pattern in whole-spine computed tomography (CT) images for patients with cervical OPLL [6] and found that DISH developed at the thoracic level initially and extended to the cervical and/or lumbar spine over time. Therefore, we developed a novel four-point grading system that can evaluate the age-related progression of DISH (grade 0, DISH anywhere in the spine; grade 1, DISH at T3–T10; grade 2, DISH extending to the cervicothoracic junction (C6–T2) and/or thoracolumbar junction (T11–L2); grade 3, DISH extending to the cervical and/or lumbar spine beyond C5 and/or L3; Figure 1). At the Japanese Multicenter Research Organization for Ossification of the Spinal Ligament (JOSL), we established a nationwide patient registry to prospectively collect clinical and radiological data, including whole-spine CT scans of OPLL patients, with the aim of clarifying associations with the presence of each type of OSL. Accordingly, the aim of the present study was to investigate the relationship between the severity of DISH (the DISH grade [6]) and all other types of OSL based on the data collected in the patient registry.

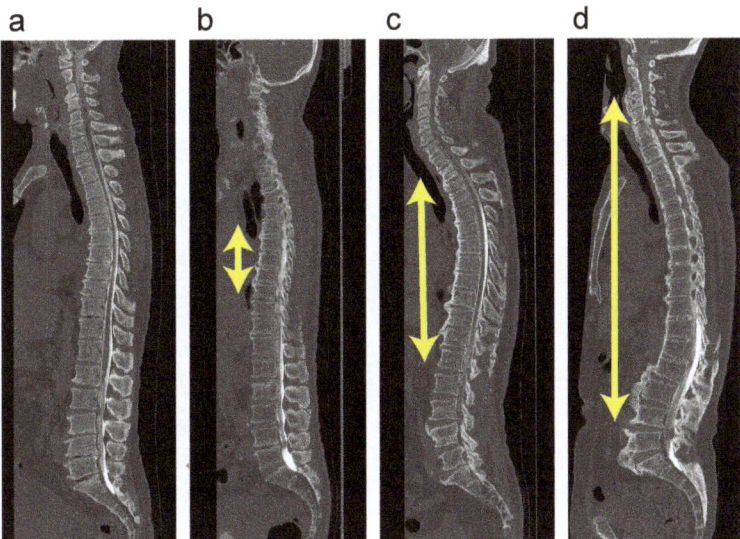

Figure 1. Representative sagittal computed tomography image for DISH grades 0–3. (**a**) Grade 0 (no DISH); (**b**) Grade 1 (DISH at T3–T10); (**c**) Grade 2 (DISH at both T3–T10 and C6–T2 and/or T11–L2); (**d**) Grade 3 (DISH extending beyond C5 and/or L3). DISH, diffuse idiopathic skeletal hyperostosis.

2. Materials and Methods

2.1. Patients and Methods

This multicenter prospective observational cross-sectional study was performed by the JOSL with the assistance of the Japanese Ministry of Health, Labour, and Welfare. The inclusion criteria were as follows: over 20 years of age; diagnosis of cervical OPLL on plain radiographs; symptoms such as neck pain, numbness in the upper or lower extremities, clumsiness, or gait disturbance; presentation to 1 of 16 institutions affiliated with the JOSL between September 2015 and December 2017; and whole-spine CT images available. Patients were excluded if they had undergone surgery to treat OPLL. The study included 239 Japanese subjects (163 men and 76 women). Basic clinical data for age, sex, body mass index (BMI), presence or absence of diabetes mellitus (DM), family history (FH) of OPLL, trauma history (TH), patients with or without surgical treatment, surgical methods and perioperative complications were obtained from patient records held at participating institutions. The study was approved by the institutional review board of each participating institution and was conducted in accordance with all relevant guidelines and regulations.

2.2. Radiographic Examinations

Six senior spine surgeons (S.U., K.M., S.M., K.K., N.N. and K.T.) independently determined the incidence of OPLL, ossification of the ligamentum flavum (OLF), ossification of the supra/interspinous ligaments (OSIL), ossification of the anterior longitudinal ligament (OALL), and ossification of the nuchal ligament (ONL) in whole-spine mid-sagittal CT images (Figure 2). Before the evaluation, inter-observer agreement was determined by assessing the incidence of OPLL and OALL, using CT images from the same 10 patients. The average kappa (κ) coefficients of inter-observer agreement for OPLL and OALL were 0.83 and 0.78, respectively. The prevalence rate of ONL was calculated for DISH grades 0 to 3, as described below. We recorded the presence of OPLL, OLF and OSIL for all vertebral bodies and intervertebral disc levels of the whole spine. An ossification index was calculated according to the number of levels with OPLL (OPLL index), OLF (OLF index), or OSIL (OSIL index), as described previously [6,18–20]. OALL was considered DISH if it completely bridged at least four contiguous adjacent vertebral bodies in the thoracic spine, according to the criteria established by Resnick and Niwayama (Figure 2) [21]. DISH was classified as follows: grade 0, no DISH at any spine level; grade 1, DISH at T3–T10; grade 2, DISH at both T3–T10 and C6–T2 and/or T11–L2; grade 3, DISH extending beyond C5 and/or L3.

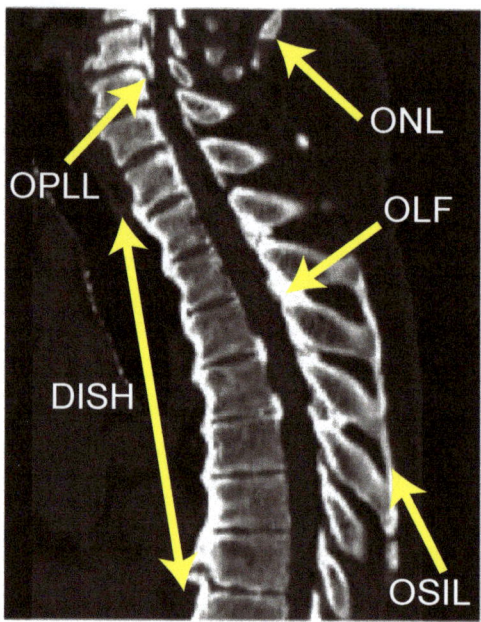

Figure 2. Representative sagittal computed tomography image for DISH, OPLL, OLF, OSIL and ONL. DISH, diffuse idiopathic skeletal hyperostosis; OLF, ossification of the ligamentum flavum; ONL, ossification of the nuchal ligament; OPLL, ossification of the posterior longitudinal ligament; and OSIL, ossification of the supra/interspinous ligaments.

2.3. Statistical Analysis

All data are presented as the mean ± standard deviation. Correlations between DISH grade and age, BMI, OPLL index, OLF index, and OSIL index were analyzed using the Pearson's correlation coefficient. The chi-squared test was used to examine differences in the prevalence rate of ONL, sex distribution, the presence of DM, FH of OPLL, TH, the number of patients treated surgically, the rate of each surgical method, and each complication rate. A p-value of <0.01 was considered statistically significant.

3. Results
3.1. Demographic Data and Surgery-Related Data According to DISH Grade

DISH was observed in 82 men and 25 women with cervical OPLL, with a co-morbidity rate of 44.8% (107/239; Table 1). Our grading system evaluation revealed that when DISH was present, grade 2 was the most common (65/107, 60.7%), followed by grade 1 (23/107, 21.5%) and grade 3 (19/107, 17.8%). There was a slight, yet significant, correlation of DISH grade with age (r = 0.30, $p < 0.0001$; Table 1) but not with sex, BMI, or the prevalence rate of DM, FH of OPLL or TH. Only one case was found in which the bridging of OALL over four adjacent vertebral bodies was localized in the cervical spine. This case was, therefore, excluded from the analysis of patients with DISH because it did not exhibit similar bridging in the thoracic spine.

Table 1. Demographic data and surgery-related data for each DISH grade.

	Grade 0	Grade 1	Grade 2	Grade 3	p-Value
Patients, n	132	23	65	19	
Mean age (years)	60.9 ± 11.6	65.4 ± 12.7	66.9 ± 12.3	72.8 ± 9.9	<0.0001
Male sex (%)	61.4	78.3	75.4	78.9	0.09
Body mass index	26.1 ± 4.7	25.7 ± 5.0	25.9 ± 3.7	24.7 ± 4.9	0.32
DM (%)	21.2	30.4	32.3	15.8	0.25
FH of OPLL (%)	3.03	4.35	3.08	5.26	0.95
Trauma history (%)	6.82	0.00	7.69	10.5	0.53
Cervical level					
Patients treated surgically, n (%)	74 (56.1)	8 (34.5)	37 (56.9)	10 (52.6)	0.27
Surgical Method					
Laminoplasty (%)	40.5	62.5	51.4	60.0	0.40
Laminectomy (%)	1.35	0.00	0.00	0.00	0.86
ADF (%)	29.7	25.0	13.5	0.00	0.08
PDF (%)	27.0	12.5	32.4	30.0	0.71
APF (%)	1.35	0.00	2.70	10.0	0.37
Perioperative complication (%)	14.9	0.00	32.4	0.20	0.07
Neurological deterioration (%)	1.35	0.00	2.70	0.00	0.89
C5 palsy (%)	8.11	0.00	13.5	0.10	0.63
CSF leakage (%)	1.35	0.00	2.70	0.00	0.89
Surgical site infection (%)	0.00	0.00	5.41	0.00	0.17
Screw loosening (%)	1.35	0.00	0.00	0.00	0.86
Screw malposition (%)	1.35	0.00	0.00	0.00	0.86
Dysphasia (%)	0.00	0.00	2.70	0.10	0.10
Deep vein thrombosis (%)	0.00	0.00	2.70	0.00	0.47
Heart failure (%)	1.35	0.00	0.00	0.00	0.86
Delirium (%)	0.00	0.00	2.70	0.00	0.47
Thoracic level					
Patients treated surgically, n (%)	11 (8.33)	4 (17.4)	9 (13.8)	2 (10.5)	0.48
Surgical Method					
Laminectomy (%)	36.4	0.00	22.2	50.0	0.46
PDF (%)	54.5	75.0	66.7	50.0	0.86
PF (%)	9.09	25.0	11.1	0.00	0.79
Perioperative complication (%)	36.4	0.00	22.2	0.00	0.41
Neurological deterioration (%)	27.3	0.00	0.00	0.00	0.20
Surgical site infection (%)	9.09	0.00	11.1	0.00	0.88
Wound dehiscence (%)	0.00	0.00	11.1	0.00	0.58
Lumbar level					
Patients treated surgically, n (%)	6 (4.55)	2 (8.70)	3 (4.62)	0 (0.00)	0.62
Surgical Method					
Laminectomy (%)	33.3	50.0	66.7	0.00	0.63
PDF (%)	66.7	0.00	33.3	0.00	0.23
PF (%)	0.00	50.0	0.00	0.00	0.08
Perioperative complication (%)	0.00	0.00	0.00	0.00	-

ADF, anterior decompression with fusion; APF, anterior and posterior decompression with fusion; CSF, cerebrospinal fluid; DISH, diffuse idiopathic skeletal hyperostosis; DM, diabetes mellitus; FH, family history; OPLL, ossification of the posterior longitudinal ligament; PDF, posterior decompression with fusion; PF posterior fusion.

Surgical treatment was performed in 59.4% of all cases (142/239; Table 1) in at least one of the spinal levels. The cervical spine was the most frequently treated level (129/239, 54.0%), followed by the thoracic (26/239, 10.9%) and lumbar spine (11/239, 4.6%). There was no significant difference in the rate of surgical treatment between each grade at any spinal level. Laminoplasty was the most common surgical procedure performed on the cervical spine (60/129, 46.5%) whereas posterior decompression with fusion (PDF) was more common at the thoracic spine (16/26, 61.5%). On the other hand, laminectomy and PDF were equally common at the lumbar spine (5/11, 45.5%). No remarkable differences were found in the rates of these procedures between each grade. Furthermore, all the incidences of perioperative complication were not statistically different among the grades.

3.2. Association between DISH Grade and OSL

Next, we calculated the correlation coefficient between the DISH grade and OSL for each spinal level. At the cervical level, the DISH grade was moderately correlated with the OPLL index ($r = 0.45$, $p < 0.0001$; Figure 3a); however, there was no correlation between DISH grade and the OLF index ($r = 0.14$, $p = 0.03$; Figure 3b). Moreover, the prevalence of ONL was significantly associated with DISH grade ($p = 0.003$, chi-squared test; Figure 3c). At the thoracic spine, the DISH grade was moderately correlated with the OLF and OSIL indices (OLF: $r = 0.41$, $p < 0.0001$, Figure 4b; OSIL: $r = 0.53$, $p < 0.0001$; Figure 4c), but not with OPLL ($r = 0.12$, $p = 0.06$; Figure 4a). There was no significant correlation of DISH grade with any OSL at the lumbar spine (OPLL: $r = -0.02$, $p = 0.78$, OLF: $r = 0.11$, $p = 0.11$, OSIL: $r = 0.14$, $p = 0.03$; Figure 5a–c). Finally, there were moderate to weak correlations between DISH grade and OPLL, OLF and OSIL indices in the whole spine (OPLL: $r = 0.29$, $p < 0.0001$, OLF: $r = 0.40$, $p < 0.0001$, OSIL: $r = 0.50$, $p < 0.0001$; Figure 6a–c).

3.3. Case Presentation

A 66-year-old man presented to one of our institutions with difficulty walking. Whole-spine CT imaging showed continuous-type cervical OPLL at C3–C7, with a cervical OPLL index of 10. In addition, extensive thoracic OLF was found, with a thoracic OLF index of 9. Grade 3 DISH was distributed from C4 to L2. The level of maximum compression in the spinal canal was C3/4 with OPLL (Figure 7). Therefore, we decided to perform a two-stage surgery for cervical OPLL. First, anterior decompression with fusion (ADF) was performed from C2 to C5 with grafted bone harvested from the fibula. Two weeks after the initial surgery, an additional posterior fixation was performed from C2 to C7. Five years after the surgeries, the man's neurological symptoms have shown satisfactory improvement.

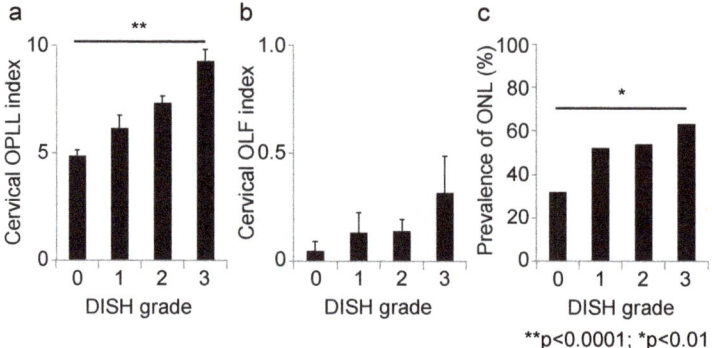

Figure 3. Correlation between DISH grade and OSL at the cervical spine. (**a**) Cervical OPLL index; (**b**) cervical OLF index; (**c**) prevalence of ONL. DISH, diffuse idiopathic skeletal hyperostosis; OLF, ossification of the ligamentum flavum; ONL, ossification of the nuchal ligament; OPLL, ossification of the posterior longitudinal ligament; OSL, ossification of the spinal ligaments.

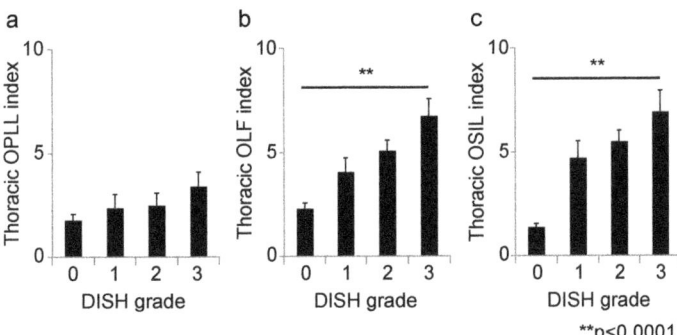

Figure 4. Correlation between DISH grade and OSL at the thoracic level. (**a**) Thoracic OPLL index; (**b**) thoracic OLF index; (**c**) thoracic OSIL index. DISH, diffuse idiopathic skeletal hyperostosis; OLF, ossification of the ligamentum flavum; OPLL, ossification of the posterior longitudinal ligament; OSIL, ossification of the supra/interspinous ligaments; OSL, ossification of the spinal ligaments.

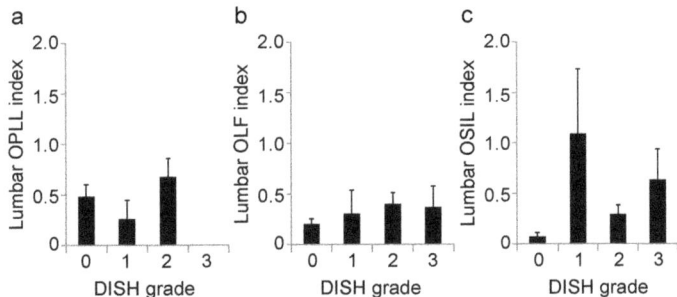

Figure 5. Correlation between DISH grade and OSL at the lumbar level. (**a**) Lumbar OPLL index; (**b**) lumbar OLF index; (**c**) lumbar OSIL index. DISH, diffuse idiopathic skeletal hyperostosis; OLF, ossification of the ligamentum flavum; OPLL, ossification of the posterior longitudinal ligament; OSIL, ossification of the supra/interspinous ligaments; OSL, ossification of the spinal ligaments.

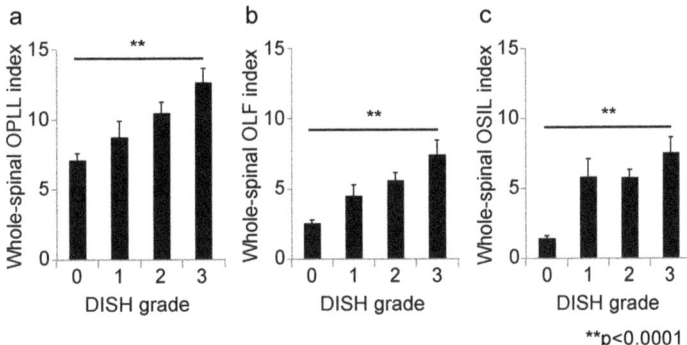

Figure 6. Correlation between DISH grade and OSL in the whole spine. (**a**) Whole-spine OPLL index; (**b**) whole-spine OLF index; (**c**) whole-spine OSIL index. DISH, diffuse idiopathic skeletal hyperostosis; OLF, ossification of the ligamentum flavum; OPLL, ossification of the posterior longitudinal ligament; OSIL, ossification of the supra/interspinous ligaments; OSL, ossification of the spinal ligaments.

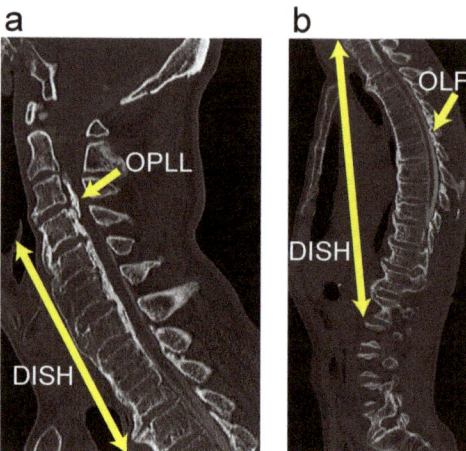

Figure 7. Illustrative case of grade 3 DISH. (**a**) Sagittal cervical CT imaging; (**b**) Sagittal thoracolumbar CT imaging. CT, computed tomography; DISH, diffuse idiopathic skeletal hyperostosis; OLF, ossification of the ligamentum flavum; OPLL, ossification of the posterior longitudinal ligament.

4. Discussion

In a previous study, we reported on the distribution of DISH in patients with cervical OPLL by cluster analysis [6]. In that study, DISH was found to be gradually distributed from the thoracic to the cervical and lumbar spine, and rarely extended beyond C5 and L3 [6]. Based on these findings, we defined DISH found only in the thoracic spine as a mild case, with C5 and L3 indicating the boundaries between moderate and severe cases. The present study found a weak but significant correlation between DISH grade and age. In addition, there was only one case in which bridging of OALL over four or more vertebral bodies was found in the cervical spine but not in the thoracic spine. These findings support the rationale of our grade, that DISH mainly develops from the thoracic spine to the cervical and lumbar spine over time; therefore, our DISH grade might be a reliable tool for evaluating the severity of this pathology. However, our grade may present challenges in the clinical setting. For example, there are exceptional cases in which bridging of OALL is found outside the thoracic spine. In addition, the clinical significance of this grading system is unclear. Thus, our future research will investigate the association between DISH grade and the incidence of vertebral body fractures.

The DISH grade is correlated with the cervical OPLL index and with the thoracic OLF and OSIL indices, all of which have frequently been detected in clinical settings [5,10,22,23]. Moreover, the progression of the DISH grade correlates moderately or slightly with various OSL indices, even in the whole spine. Thus, the severity of DISH might be correlated with that of OSL in other areas in the spine in patients with cervical OPLL. Okada et al. reported that surgery was performed in about 85% of cases exhibiting a spinal fracture with DISH, of which approximately 80% underwent conventional, open posterior fixation. In addition, the presence of OPLL was associated with residual neurological paralysis at the final follow-up [12]. In contrast, Yoshii et al. analyzed data from 2353 cases with cervical OPLL, of which 1333 cases underwent ADF and 1020 cases underwent PDF. Their report revealed that at least one local complication, such as cerebrospinal fluid leakage or surgical site infection, occurred in about 6.5% and 4.7% of anterior and posterior cases, respectively [24]. In cases with symptomatic cervical OPLL and/or DISH, including those with complications, the surgical outcomes were sometimes unsatisfactory; therefore, it is necessary to carefully monitor for neurological deterioration caused by the combination of multiple OSLs.

In this study, DISH was observed in nearly 40% of subjects and the most common grade was grade 2. This is because this study targeted patients with symptomatic cervical OPLL, and the range of DISH in the spine progressed with age. In contrast, fewer patients had grade 1. Although DISH is frequently comorbid with cervical OPLL [6,25], Fujimori et al. demonstrated that healthy subjects without OPLL may occasionally have DISH [5]. Therefore, our present findings and those of previous studies indicate that patients with grade 1 DISH can be broadly divided into two categories: those with and those without cervical OPLL. Our study focused specifically on patients with OPLL which could explain why a minority of the population had grade 1 DISH. Similarly, grade 3 DISH was an uncommon finding in our study population. As our results demonstrate, OSL may progress in patients with advanced DISH, and these patients usually need to be treated surgically. However, the present study did not include patients who had undergone spinal surgery, so the number of subjects with a grade 3 DISH was relatively small.

Ankylosing spondylitis (AS) is a spinal ankylosing condition similar to DISH. The radiological hallmark of DISH is ossification flowing along the spine similarly to "melting candle wax" [26–28], whereas AS is characterized by thinner and finer syndesmophytes connecting between adjacent vertebral bodies, which is known as "bamboo spine" [26,27,29]. Although experienced spine surgeons can easily distinguish between these two ossification disorders, it is uncertain whether all diagnoses are accurate. Moreover, these two pathologies occasionally show a degree of overlap [30]. Therefore, it is possible that our subjects diagnosed as having DISH constituted a heterogeneous population that consisted mainly of cases of DISH alone but may have also included some cases with AS or both conditions.

Spinal ossification is potentially associated with various metabolic diseases. In particular, DM is frequently comorbid with OSLs [31,32]; however, no significant correlation was found between the DISH grade and the prevalence rate of DM in the present study. A previous study found that the prevalence rate of DM was neither associated with the ossification types of OPLL nor the occupying ratio of OPLL in the spinal canal [33]. Thus, the presence or absence of DM might not be related to the radiographic progression of ossification.

This study has several limitations. First, our subjects were patients with symptomatic cervical OPLL who may have been predisposed to ossification in the whole spine. Further research is necessary to clarify whether our findings apply to asymptomatic patients with DISH found incidentally. Second, our study performed evaluations using CT imaging, which is associated with the problem of radiation exposure; therefore, it would be preferable to use plain radiography rather than CT. Finally, the study had a cross-sectional design, resulting in a lower level of evidence. Thus, a longitudinal study is needed to confirm whether the severity of OSL progresses with DISH simultaneously.

5. Conclusions

DISH was found in nearly 40% of patients with symptomatic cervical OPLL, about 60% of whom had a grade 2 DISH, using our classification system. Our DISH grade correlated with age and the indices of OSL in other areas at each high-prevalence level as well as the whole spine. Patients with cervical OPLL and severe DISH might also have a simultaneous severe OSL. In patients with symptomatic cervical OPLL, DISH extending to the cervical or lumbar spine is a radiographic sign suggesting a tendency toward diffuse ossification in the whole spine.

Author Contributions: Conceptualization, S.N., T.H., N.N. (Narihito Nagoshi), T.Y., K.M. (Kanji Mori), S.U., S.M., K.K., N.N. (Norihiro Nishida) and Y.K.; Methodology, S.N.; Software, S.N., T.H and N.N. (Narihito Nagoshi); Validation, S.N., T.H., N.N. (Narihito Nagoshi), T.Y., K.M. (Kanji Mori), S.M. and K.K. Formal Analysis, S.N. and N.N. (Narihito Nagoshi); Investigation, K.M. (Kanji Mori), T.Y., T.H., N.N. (Narihito Nagoshi), S.N., K.T. (Kazuhiro Takeuchi), S.M. and K.K.; Resources, M.Y., M.M. and A.O.; Data Curation, S.N., T.H., N.N. (Narihito Nagoshi), T.Y., K.M. (Kanji Mori), S.U., S.M., K.K., M.M., M.N., K.W. (Kota Watanabe) and Y.K. designed the study; S.N., T.H., N.N. (Narihito Nagoshi), T.Y., S.U., J.H., K.M. (Kanji Mori), S.M., K.K., K.T. (Katsushi Takeshita), T.F., K.W.

(Kei Watanabe), K.W. (Kota Watanabe), T.K., S.K., K.N., M.K., H.N., S.I., Y.M. (Yuji Matsuoka), K.W. (Kanichiro Wada), A.K., T.O., H.K., H.O., K.M. (Kazuma Murata), Y.M. (Yu Matsukura), H.I. and Y.K.; Writing—Original Draft Preparation, S.N., T.H., N.N. (Narihito Nagoshi), H.H., Y.M. (Yukihiro Matsuyama), K.T. (Katsushi Takeshita), H.O., A.O. and Y.K.; Writing—Review and Editing, S.N., T.H., N.N. (Narihito Nagoshi), T.Y., S.U., K.M. (Kanji Mori), S.M., K.K., K.T. (Kazuhiro Takeuchi), T.F., K.W. (Kei Watanabe), N.N. (Norihiro Nishida), K.W. (Kota Watanabe), T.K., S.K., K.N., M.K., H.N., S.I., Y.M. (Yukihiro Matsuyama), K.W. (Kanichiro Wada), A.K., T.O., H.K., H.O. and Y.K.; Visualization, S.N., T.H., N.N. (Narihito Nagoshi), K.M. (Kanji Mori) and S.U.; Supervision, M.M., M.W., M.N., M.Y., A.O. and Y.K.; Project Administration, T.H. and Y.K. Funding Acquisition, M.M., M.Y. and A.O. All authors have read and agreed to the published version of the manuscript.

Funding: This research was funded by a Health and Labour Science Research grant (grant number 201610008B) and by the Japan Agency for Medical Research and Development (grant number 16ek0109136h0002).

Institutional Review Board Statement: The study was conducted according to the guidelines of the Declaration of Helsinki, and approved by the institutional review board of each participating institution (protocol code 28–34; 14 March 2017).

Informed Consent Statement: Informed consent was obtained from all subjects involved in the study.

Acknowledgments: We thank Nobuko Nakajima, Tomomi Kobayashi, Namiko Katayama and Yukiko Oya for data collection.

Conflicts of Interest: The authors declare no conflict of interest. The funders had no role in the design of the study; in the collection, analyses, or interpretation of data; in the writing of the manuscript, or in the decision to publish the results.

References

1. Matsunaga, S.; Sakou, T. Ossification of the posterior longitudinal ligament of the cervical spine: Etiology and natural history. *Spine* **2012**, *37*, E309–E314. [CrossRef]
2. Stetler, W.R.; La Marca, F.; Park, P. The genetics of ossification of the posterior longitudinal ligament. *Neurosurg. Focus* **2011**, *30*, E7. [CrossRef]
3. Ehara, S.; Shimamura, T.; Nakamura, R.; Yamazaki, K. Paravertebral ligamentous ossification: DISH, OPLL and OLF. *Eur. J. Radiol.* **1998**, *27*, 196–205. [CrossRef]
4. Epstein, N.E. Simultaneous cervical diffuse idiopathic skeletal hyperostosis and ossification of the posterior longitudinal ligament resulting in dysphagia or myelopathy in two geriatric North Americans. *Surg. Neurol.* **2000**, *53*, 427–431, discussion 431. [CrossRef]
5. Fujimori, T.; Watabe, T.; Iwamoto, Y.; Hamada, S.; Iwasaki, M.; Oda, T. Prevalence, concomitance, and distribution of ossification of the spinal ligaments: Results of whole spine CT scans in 1500 Japanese patients. *Spine* **2016**, *41*, 1668–1676. [CrossRef]
6. Nishimura, S.; Nagoshi, N.; Iwanami, A.; Takeuchi, A.; Hirai, T.; Yoshii, T.; Takeuchi, K.; Mori, K.; Yamada, T.; Seki, S.; et al. Prevalence and distribution of diffuse idiopathic skeletal hyperostosis on whole-spine computed tomography in patients with cervical ossification of the posterior longitudinal ligament: A multicenter study. *Clin. Spine Surg.* **2018**, *31*, E460–E465. [CrossRef] [PubMed]
7. Kagotani, R.; Yoshida, M.; Muraki, S.; Oka, H.; Hashizume, H.; Yamada, H.; Enyo, Y.; Nagata, K.; Ishimoto, Y.; Teraguchi, M.; et al. Prevalence of diffuse idiopathic skeletal hyperostosis (DISH) of the whole spine and its association with lumbar spondylosis and knee osteoarthritis: The ROAD study. *J. Bone Miner. Metab.* **2015**, *33*, 221–229. [CrossRef] [PubMed]
8. Mori, K.; Kasahara, T.; Mimura, T.; Nishizawa, K.; Nakamura, A.; Imai, S. Prevalence of thoracic diffuse idiopathic skeletal hyperostosis (DISH) in Japanese: Results of chest CT-based cross-sectional study. *J. Orthop. Sci.* **2017**, *22*, 38–42. [CrossRef] [PubMed]
9. Toyoda, H.; Terai, H.; Yamada, K.; Suzuki, A.; Dohzono, S.; Matsumoto, T.; Nakamura, H. Prevalence of diffuse idiopathic skeletal hyperostosis in patients with spinal disorders. *Asian Spine J.* **2017**, *11*, 63–70. [CrossRef] [PubMed]
10. Liang, H.; Liu, G.; Lu, S.; Chen, S.; Jiang, D.; Shi, H.; Fei, Q. Epidemiology of ossification of the spinal ligaments and associated factors in the Chinese population: A cross-sectional study of 2000 consecutive individuals. *BMC Musculoskelet. Disord.* **2019**, *20*, 253. [CrossRef]
11. Chaudhary, B.R.; Fehlings, M.G. Ankylosing spinal disorders–falls, flawed flexibility, and fixations. *World Neurosurg.* **2015**, *83*, 724–726. [CrossRef]
12. Okada, E.; Yoshii, T.; Yamada, T.; Watanabe, K.; Katsumi, K.; Hiyama, A.; Watanabe, M.; Nakagawa, Y.; Okada, M.; Endo, T.; et al. Spinal fractures in patients with Diffuse idiopathic skeletal hyperostosis: A nationwide multi-institution survey. *J. Orthop. Sci.* **2019**, *24*, 601–606. [CrossRef]

13. Westerveld, L.A.; Verlaan, J.J.; Oner, F.C. Spinal fractures in patients with ankylosing spinal disorders: A systematic review of the literature on treatment, neurological status and complications. *Eur. Spine J.* **2009**, *18*, 145–156. [CrossRef] [PubMed]
14. Guo, Q.; Ni, B.; Yang, J.; Zhu, Z.; Yang, J. Simultaneous ossification of the posterior longitudinal ligament and ossification of the ligamentum flavum causing upper thoracic myelopathy in DISH: Case report and literature review. *Eur. Spine J.* **2011**, *20*, S195–S201. [CrossRef] [PubMed]
15. Bloom, R.A. The prevalence of ankylosing hyperostosis in a Jerusalem population–with description of a method of grading the extent of the disease. *Scand. J. Rheumatol.* **1984**, *13*, 181–189. [CrossRef] [PubMed]
16. Fornasier, V.L.; Littlejohn, G.; Urowitz, M.B.; Keystone, E.C.; Smythe, H.A. Spinal entheseal new bone formation: The early changes of spinal diffuse idiopathic skeletal hyperostosis. *J. Rheumatol.* **1983**, *10*, 939–947.
17. Haller, J.; Resnick, D.; Miller, C.W.; Schils, J.P.; Kerr, R.; Bielecki, D.; Sartoris, D.J.; Gundry, C.R. Diffuse idiopathic skeletal hyperostosis: Diagnostic significance of radiographic abnormalities of the pelvis. *Radiology* **1989**, *172*, 835–839. [CrossRef]
18. Hirai, T.; Yoshii, T.; Iwanami, A.; Takeuchi, K.; Mori, K.; Yamada, T.; Wada, K.; Koda, M.; Matsuyama, Y.; Takeshita, K.; et al. Prevalence and distribution of ossified lesions in the whole spine of patients with cervical ossification of the posterior longitudinal ligament a multicenter study (JOSL CT study). *PLoS ONE* **2016**, *11*, e0160117. [CrossRef]
19. Mori, K.; Yoshii, T.; Hirai, T.; Iwanami, A.; Takeuchi, K.; Yamada, T.; Seki, S.; Tsuji, T.; Fujiyoshi, K.; Furukawa, M.; et al. Prevalence and distribution of ossification of the supra/interspinous ligaments in symptomatic patients with cervical ossification of the posterior longitudinal ligament of the spine: A CT-based multicenter cross-sectional study. *BMC Musculoskelet. Disord.* **2016**, *17*, 492. [CrossRef]
20. Yoshii, T.; Hirai, T.; Iwanami, A.; Nagoshi, N.; Takeuchi, K.; Mori, K.; Yamada, T.; Seki, S.; Tsuji, T.; Fujiyoshi, K.; et al. Co-existence of ossification of the nuchal ligament is associated with severity of ossification in the whole spine in patients with cervical ossification of the posterior longitudinal ligament—A multi-center CT study. *J. Orthop. Sci.* **2019**, *24*, 35–41. [CrossRef]
21. Resnick, D.; Niwayama, G. Radiographic and pathologic features of spinal involvement in diffuse idiopathic skeletal hyperostosis (DISH). *Radiology* **1976**, *119*, 559–568. [CrossRef] [PubMed]
22. Kawaguchi, Y.; Nakano, M.; Yasuda, T.; Seki, S.; Hori, T.; Suzuki, K.; Makino, H.; Kimura, T. Characteristics of ossification of the spinal ligament; incidence of ossification of the ligamentum flavum in patients with cervical ossification of the posterior longitudinal ligament—Analysis of the whole spine using multidetector CT. *J. Orthop. Sci.* **2016**, *21*, 439–445. [CrossRef] [PubMed]
23. Mori, K.; Kasahara, T.; Mimura, T.; Nishizawa, K.; Murakami, Y.; Matsusue, Y.; Imai, S. Prevalence, distribution, and morphology of thoracic ossification of the yellow ligament in Japanese: Results of CT-based cross-sectional study. *Spine* **2013**, *38*, E1216–E1222. [CrossRef] [PubMed]
24. Yoshii, T.; Morishita, S.; Inose, H.; Yuasa, M.; Hirai, T.; Okawa, A.; Fushimi, K.; Fujiwara, T. Comparison of perioperative complications in anterior decompression with fusion and posterior decompression with fusion for cervical ossification of the posterior longitudinal ligament: Propensity score matching analysis using a nation-wide inpatient database. *Spine* **2020**, *45*, E1006–E1012. [CrossRef] [PubMed]
25. Yoshimura, N.; Nagata, K.; Muraki, S.; Oka, H.; Yoshida, M.; Enyo, Y.; Kagotani, R.; Hashizume, H.; Yamada, H.; Ishimoto, Y.; et al. Prevalence and progression of radiographic ossification of the posterior longitudinal ligament and associated factors in the Japanese population: A 3-year follow-up of the ROAD study. *Osteoporos. Int.* **2014**, *25*, 1089–1098. [CrossRef]
26. Latourte, A.; Charlon, S.; Etcheto, A.; Feydy, A.; Allanore, Y.; Dougados, M.; Molto, A. Imaging findings suggestive of axial spondyloarthritis in diffuse idiopathic skeletal hyperostosis. *Arthritis Care Res.* **2018**, *70*, 145–152. [CrossRef] [PubMed]
27. Mader, R.; Baraliakos, X.; Eshed, I.; Novofastovski, I.; Bieber, A.; Verlaan, J.-J.; Kiefer, D.; Pappone, N.; Atzeni, F. Imaging of diffuse idiopathic skeletal hyperostosis (DISH). *RMD Open* **2020**, *6*, e001151. [CrossRef] [PubMed]
28. Mori, K.; Yayama, T.; Nishizawa, K.; Nakamura, A.; Mimura, T.; Imai, S. Aortic pulsation prevents the development of ossification of anterior longitudinal ligament toward the aorta in patients with diffuse idiopathic skeletal hyperostosis (DISH) in Japanese: Results of chest CT-based cross-sectional study. *J. Orthop. Sci.* **2019**, *24*, 30–34. [CrossRef] [PubMed]
29. Olivieri, I.; D'Angelo, S.; Palazzi, C.; Padula, A.; Mader, R.; Khan, M.A. Diffuse idiopathic skeletal hyperostosis: Differentiation from ankylosing spondylitis. *Curr. Rheumatol. Rep.* **2009**, *11*, 321–328. [CrossRef]
30. Kuperus, J.S.; Waalwijk, J.F.; Regan, E.A.; van der Horst-Bruinsma, I.E.; Oner, F.C.; de Jong, P.A.; Verlaan, J.-J. Simultaneous occurrence of ankylosing spondylitis and diffuse idiopathic skeletal hyperostosis: A systematic review. *Rheumatology* **2018**, *57*, 2120–2128. [CrossRef]
31. Kobashi, G.; Washio, M.; Okamoto, K.; Sasaki, S.; Yokoyama, T.; Miyake, Y.; Sakamoto, N.; Ohta, K.; Inaba, Y.; Tanaka, H. High body mass index after age 20 and diabetes mellitus are independent risk factors for ossification of the posterior longitudinal ligament of the spine in Japanese subjects: A case-control study in multiple hospitals. *Spine* **2004**, *29*, 1006–1010. [CrossRef]
32. Akune, T.; Ogata, N.; Seichi, A.; Ohnishi, I.; Nakamura, K.; Kawaguchi, H. Insulin secretory response is positively associated with the extent of ossification of the posterior longitudinal ligament of the spine. *J. Bone Jt. Surg. Am.* **2001**, *83*, 1537–1544. [CrossRef]
33. Nagoshi, N.; Watanabe, K.; Nakamura, M.; Matsumoto, M.; Li, N.; Ma, S.; He, D.; Tian, W.; Jeon, H.; Lee, J.J.; et al. Does diabetes affect the surgical outcomes in cases with cervical ossification of the posterior longitudinal ligament? A multicenter study from Asia pacific spine study group. *Glob. Spine J.* **2021**, *10*, 2192568221996300. [CrossRef]

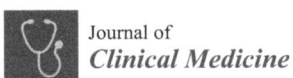

Article

Comparison of Lateral Lumbar Interbody Fusion and Posterior Lumbar Interbody Fusion as Corrective Surgery for Patients with Adult Spinal Deformity—A Propensity Score Matching Analysis

Yu Matsukura [1], Toshitaka Yoshii [1,*], Shingo Morishita [1], Kenichiro Sakai [2], Takashi Hirai [1], Masato Yuasa [1], Hiroyuki Inose [1], Atsuyuki Kawabata [1], Kurando Utagawa [1], Jun Hashimoto [1], Masaki Tomori [2], Ichiro Torigoe [2], Tsuyoshi Yamada [3], Kazuo Kusano [3], Kazuyuki Otani [3], Satoshi Sumiya [4], Fujiki Numano [4], Kazuyuki Fukushima [5], Shoji Tomizawa [6], Satoru Egawa [1], Yoshiyasu Arai [2], Shigeo Shindo [3] and Atsushi Okawa [1]

[1] Department of Orthopaedic Surgery, Graduate School of Medical and Dental Sciences, Tokyo Medical and Dental University, 1-5-45 Yushima, Bunkyo-ku, Tokyo 113-8510, Japan; matsukura.orth@tmd.ac.jp (Y.M.); morsorth@tmd.ac.jp (S.M.); hirai.orth@tmd.ac.jp (T.H.); yuasa.orth@tmd.ac.jp (M.Y.); inose.orth@tmd.ac.jp (H.I.); 060211ms@gmail.com (A.K.); utag.orth@tmd.ac.jp (K.U.); 0123456789jun@gmail.com (J.H.); egawa.orth@tmd.ac.jp (S.E.); okawa.orth@tmd.ac.jp (A.O.)

[2] Department of Orthopaedic Surgery, Saiseikai Kawaguchi General Hospital, 5-11-5 Nishikawaguchi, Kawaguchi 332-8558, Japan; kenitiro1122@gmail.com (K.S.); masaki0803.197571@gmail.com (M.T.); tori@zj8.so-net.ne.jp (I.T.); arai.orth@gmail.com (Y.A.)

[3] Department of Orthopaedic Surgery, Kudanzawa Hospital, 1-6-12 Kudanminami, Chiyoda-ku, Tokyo 102-0074, Japan; yamada.orth@tmd.ac.jp (T.Y.); kz_kusano@yahoo.co.jp (K.K.); ootani_k@kudanzaka.com (K.O.); shindo_s@kudanzaka.com (S.S.)

[4] Department of Orthopaedic Surgery, Yokohama City Minato Red Cross Hospital, 3-12-1 Shinyamashita, Naka-ku, Yokohama 231-8682, Japan; sumiya.orth.7077@gmail.com (S.S.); fnumano@js6.so-net.ne.jp (F.N.)

[5] Department of Orthopaedic Surgery, Saku General Hospital, 3400-28 Nakagomi, Saku 385-0051, Japan; kaz.fuku0628@gmail.com

[6] Department of Orthopaedic Surgery, Tokyo Bay Urayasu Ichikawa Medical Center, 3-4-32 Toudaijima, Urayasu 279-0001, Japan; shoji.tomizawa@gmail.com

* Correspondence: yoshii.orth@tmd.ac.jp; Tel.: +81-3-5803-5272; Fax: +81-3-5803-5281

Abstract: Lateral lumbar interbody fusion (LLIF) is increasingly performed as corrective surgery for patients with adult spinal deformity (ASD). This paper compares the surgical results of LLIF and conventional posterior lumbar interbody fusion (PLIF)/transforaminal lumbar interbody fusion (TLIF) in ASD using a propensity score matching analysis. We retrospectively reviewed patients with ASD who received LLIF and PLIF/TLIF, and investigated patients' backgrounds, radiographic parameters, and complications. The propensity scores were calculated from patients' characteristics, including radiographic parameters and preoperative comorbidities, and one–to-one matching was performed. Propensity score matching produced 21 matched pairs of patients who underwent LLIF and PLIF/TLIF. All radiographic parameters significantly improved in both groups at the final follow-up compared with those of the preoperative period. The comparison between both groups demonstrated no significant difference in terms of postoperative pelvic tilt, lumbar lordosis (LL), or pelvic incidence–LL at the final follow-up. However, the sagittal vertical axis tended to be smaller in the LLIF at the final follow-up. Overall, perioperative and late complications were comparable in both procedures. However, LLIF procedures demonstrated significantly less intraoperative blood loss and a smaller incidence of postoperative epidural hematoma compared with PLIF/TLIF procedures in patients with ASD.

Keywords: adult spinal deformity (ASD); posterior lumbar interbody fusion; lateral lumbar interbody fusion; sagittal correction; perioperative complications; surgical invasiveness; degenerative adult deformity

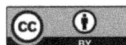

1. Introduction

Adult spinal deformity (ASD) is a disease defined as the deviation of the alignment of the spinal column that presents during adulthood. ASD is caused by a variety of conditions, such as de novo scoliosis, progressive adolescent idiopathic scoliosis, degenerative disc disease, iatrogenic kyphosis, and post-traumatic kyphosis [1–3]. Moreover, ASD causes a substantial and increasing burden on elderly patients and healthcare systems, as patients with ASD have a disability and a poor health-related quality of life (HR-QOL) [4,5]. Therefore, recognizing the importance of restoring sagittal balance in the surgical treatment of ASD has recently increased [3]. Thus, the goal of surgical treatment for patients with ASD is to achieve ideal sagittal alignment and balance, which are closely associated with pain and disability [6,7]. However, because of the high risk of perioperative complications despite the advances in surgical techniques and implant selection, surgical treatment for ASD remains challenging [8,9].

ASD has various surgical treatments (e.g., posterior interbody fusion (PLIF), transforaminal interbody fusion (TLIF), lateral lumbar interbody fusion (LLIF), and three-column osteotomy) [10,11]. A correction at the interbody space (e.g., LLIF and PLIF/TLIF) is a reasonable surgical method in patients with ASD and degenerative disc with kyphosis [1]. The current application of LLIF has increased in ASD patients [11–13]. Minimally invasive LLIF techniques are expected to reduce the risk of intraoperative bleeding and neurological damage, and thus LLIF may reduce the perioperative complications in the corrective surgery for ASD. Furthermore, a large interbody cage may have the potential to enhance spinal alignment correction in patients with ASD. However, few studies have investigated the surgical outcomes and risks for complications in comparison with LLIF and conventional PLIF/TLIF for patients with ASD [14].

Information regarding the surgical results of these treatment options is important in surgeons' decision-making. Therefore, we investigated the results of radiographic parameters and surgical complications after LLIF and PLIF/TLIF for ASD patients in an elderly Japanese population. A propensity score matching analysis was conducted to minimize the selection bias of surgical procedures when comparing the surgical results of LLIF and PLIF/TLIF.

2. Materials and Methods

This multicenter study retrospectively reviewed ASD patients who were surgically treated between 1 January 2010 and 31 December 2016, at the hospital of this study and seven other affiliated hospitals. Institutional review board approval was obtained at each hospital for data collection. The inclusion criteria consisted of being ≥21 years of age at the time of surgery, a minimum follow-up period of 1 year with sufficient radiographic data, a surgery that included posterior instrumentation of ≥4 levels, and lower instrumented vertebra surgery of the pelvis with iliac screws or S2 ala-iliac screws in addition to S1 pedicle screws. The etiologies included degenerative kyphosis/kyphoscoliosis and post lumbar surgery. Patients with ASD caused by vertebral fractures were excluded.

Demographic data included age, sex, body mass index (BMI), medical comorbidities, location of the upper instrumented vertebra, number of intervertebral fusion levels, radiographic parameters, surgical procedure (i.e., LLIF, PLIF/TLIF, three-column osteotomy, or others), surgical invasiveness (intraoperative blood loss and surgical time), and incidence of surgical complications. Medical comorbidities (e.g., diabetes, renal dysfunction, cerebrovascular disease, cardiovascular disease, and respiratory disease) were registered. Radiographic parameters included the sagittal vertical axis (SVA), lumbar lordosis (LL), pelvic tilt (PT), pelvic incidence (PI), and spinopelvic harmony, which are evaluated by determining the PI minus LL (PI−LL) before surgery, 4 weeks after surgery, and at the final follow-up in standing position. Surgical complications are classified into perioperative and late complications. Perioperative complications are classified into surgery-related complications (e.g., epidural hematoma, postoperative neurological deficits, and surgical site infection) and systemic complications (e.g., cardiovascular events and deep vein thrombosis), which are usually observed soon after, or during, the operation. Late complications included proximal junction kyphosis (PJK), distal junction kyphosis, pseudarthrosis, rod breakage, or newly occurred vertebral fracture, which were generally caused by the stress on the implant or vertebra.

2.1. Surgical Procedures

This study investigated two surgical procedures, the LLIF and PLIF/TLIF. In the LLIF group in this study, first, multilevel LLIF was performed using the oblique lateral interbody fusion (OLIF, Medtronic, Minneapolis, MN, USA) or extreme lateral interbody fusion (XLIF, NuVasive Inc., San Diego, CA, USA) from L1–2 or L2–3 to L4–5, followed by posterior instrumentation. Schwab grade 1 or 2 osteotomies [15] were performed from L1–2 to L5–S1 using the posterior approach. L5–S1 PLIF/TLIF was then routinely performed using large lordotic cages, and lumbar lordosis was restored using a rod cantilever and compression technique. The instrumentation was performed from the lower thoracic spine/thoracolumbar junction to the sacrum/ilium. In the PLIF/TLIF group in this study, multilevel PLIF/TLIF combined with Schwab grade 1 or 2 osteotomies [15] were performed from L1–2 or L2–3 to L5–S1, and lumbar lordosis was restored using a rod cantilever and compression technique. The instrumentation was similarly performed from the lower thoracic spine/thoracolumbar junction to the sacrum/ilium with iliac screws or S2 ala-iliac screws, in addition to S1 pedicle screws. A hard brace was generally used for 3–6 months after surgery, regardless of the surgical procedures. The surgical procedure selection was determined at the discretion of each surgeon. Generally, surgeons were more likely to choose PLIF/TLIF when patients had histories of abdominal surgery or diseases, vascular abnormality, and difficulties in lateral access because of a high riding psoas muscle, high iliac crest, etc. LLIF tended to be chosen for patients who did not have the above factors, especially when surgeons wanted to avoid greater surgical invasiveness.

2.2. Statistics Analysis

Propensity score matching analysis was conducted to minimize the selection bias of surgical procedures by adjusting known confounding variables [16–18]. Furthermore, propensity scores for the surgical procedure (i.e., LLIF or PLIF/TLIF) were calculated with the following variables: the patient's age and sex, BMI, medical comorbidities, number of intervertebral fusion levels, and radiographic parameters (SVA, LL, PI, and PI-LL at preoperation). The procedure was performed using a logistic regression model. The C-statistic suggested that the fitting was 0.77, which is a fairly good state. One-to-one matching of LLIF and PLIF/TLIF patients was performed based on propensity scores on the condition that the caliper was <0.4. After the matching, postoperative radiographic parameters, surgical invasiveness, perioperative complications, and late complications were compared between the two surgical procedures in the matched cases using a Mann–Whitney U test or chi-squared test. All statistical analyses were conducted using the Stata/MP version 14 (StataCorp, College Station, TX, USA), and p-values of <0.05 were considered as statistically significant.

3. Results

This study included 91 patients with full preoperative and postoperative radiographic data with a minimum 1 year follow-up. The cohort included 76 women and 15 men (mean age, 73.2 years; mean follow-up period, 24.2 months). Of the patients, 22 underwent LLIF and 69 underwent PLIF/TLIF. Propensity score matching resulted in 21 pairs of patients undergoing LLIF and PLIF/TLIF. Consequently, biases between the treatment groups diminished after the propensity score matching. The patients' ages and sexes, BMIs, number of intervertebral fusion levels, and radiographic parameters before operation were adjusted (Table 1).

Table 1. Patient characteristics in the lateral lumbar interbody fusion (LLIF) group and the posterior lumbar interbody fusion (PLIF)/transforaminal lumbar interbody fusion (TLIF) group after the matching.

Parameter	LLIF (N = 21)	PLIF/TLIF (N = 21)	*p*-Value
Age at surgery (years)	74.0 ± 7.6	73.2 ± 7.3	0.687
Sex (male/female: cases)	2/19	2/19	1.000
BMI	21.7 ± 4.0	22.1 ± 3.3	0.823
Medical comorbidity (yes/no)	8/13	5/16	0.317
SVA (mm)	153.7 ± 78.9	148.3 ± 48.6	0.763
LL (deg.)	1.1 ± 12.6	1.6 ± 12.1	0.930
PI (deg.)	51.6 ± 9.1	50.0 ± 9.1	0.496
PI-LL (deg.)	50.5 ± 14.5	48.4 ± 11.9	0.660
PT (deg.)	37.1 ± 15.4	32.1 ± 7.7	0.162
TK (T4-12) (deg.)	28.4 ± 16.7	20.9 ± 16.5	0.290
No. of fixed levels	8.4 ± 1.9	7.7 ± 1.52	0.548
Type of anchor for pelvis (iliac screw/S2-ala-iliac screw: cases)	15/6	19/2	0.116

Mean ± standard deviation; LLIF, lateral lumbar interbody fusion; PLIF, posterior lumbar interbody fusion; TLIF, transforaminal lumbar interbody fusion; BMI, body mass index; SVA, sagittal vertical axis; LL, lumbar lordosis; PI, pelvic incidence; PT, pelvic tilt; TK, thoracic kyphosis; deg., degree; No., number.

The LLIF group had significantly lower intraoperative blood loss (849 vs. 2359 mL). However, total surgical time was significantly longer in the LLIF group (536 vs. 421 min; Table 2). All parameters were significantly improved at 4 weeks after surgery and at the final follow-up compared with those at the preoperative period in both groups (Table 3). Consequently, most of the radiographic parameters were not significantly different between the two groups postoperatively. However, SVA tended to be smaller in the LLIF group at the final follow-up (Table 3).

Table 2. Surgical invasion in the LLIF group and the PLIF/TLIF group.

Parameter	LLIF (N = 21)	PLIF/TLIF (N = 21)	*p*-Value
Surgical time (min)	535.9 ± 123.1	426.8 ± 96.2	<0.001 *
Estimated blood loss (grams)	848.7 ± 477.1	2358.6 ± 1911.6	<0.001 *

Mean LLIF, lateral lumbar interbody fusion; PLIF, posterior lumbar interbody fusion; TLIF, transforaminal lumbar interbody fusion; ± standard deviation; LLIF, lateral lumbar interbody fusion; PLIF, posterior lumbar interbody fusion; TLIF, transforaminal lumbar inter-body fusion; *, $p < 0.05$.

Table 3. The comparison of the LLIF group and the PLIF/TLIF group for radiographic parameters at each follow-up time.

Parameter	LLIF (N = 21)	PLIF/TLIF (N = 21)	*p*-Value
At 4 weeks after surgery			
SVA (mm)	24.1 ± 41.7	33.8 ± 41.4	0.279
ΔSVA (mm)	−129.6 ± 76.9	−114.5 ± 51.6	0.725
LL (deg.)	45.2 ± 7.8	41.0 ± 10.9	0.268
ΔLL (deg.)	44.1 ± 15.1	39.4 ± 15.5	0.473
PI-LL (deg.)	6.4 ± 8.9	9.1 ± 13.9	0.920
ΔPI-LL (deg.)	−44.1 ± 15.1	−39.0 ± 15.5	0.473
PT (deg.)	21.5 ± 15.4	21.4 ± 6.1	0.890
ΔPT (deg.)	−15.6 ± 9.2	−11.0 ± 5.4	0.057
TK (T4-12) (deg.)	36.7 ± 11.8	32.3 ± 13.2	0.473
ΔTK (T4-12) (deg.)	8.3 ± 13.3	11.4 ± 13.1	0.562

Table 3. Cont.

Parameter	LLIF (N = 21)	PLIF/TLIF (N = 21)	p-Value
At final follow-up			
SVA (mm)	23.2 ± 37.6	52.4 ± 41.4	0.044 *
ΔSVA (mm)	−130.4 ± 84.2	−95.9 ± 45.0	0.097
LL (deg.)	43.9 ± 9.4	40.1 ± 10.1	0.420
ΔLL (deg.)	42.8 ± 15.6	38.5 ± 18.3	0.513
PI-LL (deg.)	7.8 ± 9.4	9.9 ± 16.3	0.753
PT (deg.)	25.1 ± 14.7	21.6 ± 7.5	0.092
ΔPT (deg.)	−12.0 ± 12.3	−11.0 ± 6.9	0.705
TK (T4-12) (deg.)	42.8 ± 15.6	36.7 ± 14.9	0.273
ΔTK (T4-12) (deg.)	16.7 ± 13.1	15.8 ± 15.1	0.830
Loss of correction from 4 weeks postoperatively at last observation			
SVA (mm)	−0.1 ± 49.1	18.6 ± 31.0	0.326
LL (deg.)	1.3 ± 3.1	0.9 ± 4.0	0.638
PT (deg.)	3.6 ± 11.1	0.3 ± 5.9	0.289
TK (T4-12) (deg.)	6.0 ± 6.7	4.4 ± 7.7	0.434

Mean ± standard deviation; LLIF, lateral lumbar interbody fusion; PLIF, posterior lumbar interbody fusion; TLIF, transforaminal lumbar inter-body fusion; SVA, sagittal vertical axis; LL, lumbar lordosis; PI, pelvic incidence; PT, pelvic tilt; TK, thoracic kyphosis; deg., degrees; *, $p < 0.05$.

Table 4 shows the incidence of surgical complications in both groups. No significant difference in the incidence of either overall local or systemic complications was observed in terms of perioperative complications. However, the incidence of epidural hematoma was significantly lower in the LLIF than in the PLIF/TLIF group (0.0% vs. 19.0%; $p = 0.035$). Moreover, the incidence of late complications was not significantly different between the two groups.

Table 4. Surgical complications of the LLIF group and the PLIF/TLIF group.

Parameter	LLIF (N = 21)	PLIF/TLIF (N = 21)	p-Value
Perioperative complications			
Local complications (yes/no)	4/17 (19.0%)	6/15 (28.6%)	0.454
Neurological deficit (yes/no)	4/17 (19.0%)	3/18 (14.3%)	0.679
Epidural hematoma (yes/no)	0/21 (0.0%)	4/17 (19.0%)	0.035 *
Surgical site infection (yes/no)	1/20 (4.8%)	0/21 (0.0%)	0.261
Systemic complications (yes/no)	1/20 (4.8%)	1/20 (4.8%)	1.000
	Cerebrovascular events: 1	Deep vein thrombosis: 1	
Total (yes/no)	5/16 (23.8%)	7/14 (33.3%)	0.482
Late complications			
Implant failure (yes/no)	1/20 (4.8%)	1/20 (4.8%)	1.000
Proximal junctional kyphosis (yes/no)	5/16 (31.3%)	5/16 (31.3%)	1.000
Newly occurred vertebral fracture (yes/no)	3/18 (14.3%)	3/18 (14.3%)	1.000
Total (yes/no)	7/14 (33.3%)	6/15 (28.6%)	0.739
Revision surgery	2/19 (9.5%)	1/20 (4.8%)	0.549

Mean *: $p < 0.05$.

4. Discussion

The surgical invasiveness and the associated risks of complications in ASD surgeries remain problematic. Recently, the minimally invasive LLIF technique has been increasingly performed to potentially reduce the surgical risks of ASD surgeries [12,19–21]. However, insufficient information exists on whether LLIF indeed decreases the surgical invasiveness and the incidence of surgical compilations in ASD patients. Therefore, the use of PLIF/TLIF and the recently increased use of LLIF were compared, both of which are intervertebral corrections for the treatment of ASD. Furthermore, the propensity matching method was used to compare the surgical results in the two procedures. As surgical treatment for

ASD is generally a high-risk surgery [8,9], conducting a randomized trial is difficult. The propensity score is a balancing score calculated by logistic regression analysis, which makes the distribution of measured baseline covariates similar between the two treatment groups [22]. In the current study, all of the covariates were successfully adjusted after one-to-one propensity score matching (Table 1), indicating no selection bias in the baseline characteristics between the LLIF and PLIF/TLIF groups.

Both the LLIF and PLIF/TLIF groups in this study resulted in favorable sagittal alignment correction, with significant improvements in SVA, LL, and PT, as well as PI−LL mismatch, compared with the preoperative parameters. In the comparison between the LLIF and PLIF/TLIF groups, SVA was smaller and the improvement in SVA from the preoperative value tended to be larger at the final follow-up in the LLIF group. However, we did not find marked differences between the two groups in terms of postoperative LL and PI−LL at 4 weeks after surgery and at the final follow-up. Previous studies have reported that LLIF is better able to correct sagittal imbalance than posterior corrective fusion in ASD patients. However, the surgical procedure of the posterior approach in these studies was the posterior spinal fusion with interbody fusion only at L5/S1, not multilevel PLIF/TLIF [11,23,24]. In this study, four-level interbody fusion (L2/3–5/S) was conducted in both the LLIF and PLIF/TLIF groups. In the LLIF procedure, interbody space can be lifted up using large cages, and may potentially have greater ability to restore segmental alignment. However, if the procedure is performed at multiple segments, the tightness of the anterior longitudinal ligament (ALL) limits the degree of lift-up and the correction of lumbar lordosis. Thus, the correction angle of LL in the LLIF group was slightly higher but not significant compared with that of the PLIF/TLIF group (LLIF, $44.1° \pm 15.1°$; PLIF/TLIF, $39.4° \pm 15.5°$). The release of ALL in addition to the LLIF procedure (anterior column realignment technique) would make a more radical correction [25,26], although the potential risk of vascular injury exists.

Since ASD mostly affects the elderly population, surgical invasiveness for ASD patients is a major problem [23,24]. Intraoperative blood loss is one of the major factors related to surgical invasiveness. Thus, this study demonstrated that the intraoperative blood loss of the LLIF group was reduced to one-third compared with the PLIF/TLIF group. In the PLIF/TLIF group, access to the intervertebral disc space was performed through the epidural space, and therefore, bleeding from the epidural venous plexus was inevitable at multilevel intervertebral discs. However, the LLIF group showed minimized epidural bleeding because access to the intervertebral disc space was performed through the retroperitoneal approach, except access to the L5/S level. Previous studies also reported the benefits of utilizing the lateral approach in reducing intraoperative blood loss [23,24]. Consequently, the total operation time in the LLIF group averaged 100 min longer than that in the PLIF/TLIF group. The PLIF/TLIF group was performed in this study through a single posterior approach, whereas the LLIF group was performed through the combined approach: the lateral oblique approach for anterior interbody fusion, and the subsequent posterior approach for pedicle screw fixation. Thus, the combined approach makes the total operating time much longer in the LLIF group. Previous reports have shown that blood loss is a risk factor for perioperative complications in lumbar fusion surgery; however, surgical time was not a significant factor [27–29]. Despite the longer operating time, LLIF procedures may have the benefit of reducing the bleeding and surgical risks through the combined approach. Additionally, two-stage surgery (performing anterior and posterior approaches on a separate day) can be selected for high-risk patients in LLIF procedures. Thus, the LLIF procedure is considered to be a good option for safe, corrective surgery for elderly ASD patients because patients with ASD are commonly older in age. Percutaneous posterior fixation, which is applicable for flexible patients, would further reduce surgical invasiveness [30–34].

The overall incidence of perioperative complications, including local and systemic complications, was not significantly different between the two groups in the present study. However, the incidence of epidural hematoma was significantly higher in the PLIF/TLIF group than in the LLIF group. The possible reasons for the reduced hematoma incidence are that the LLIF group in this study required minimal epidural manipulation, and that surgery-related bleeding occurred significantly less in the LLIF group compared to the PLIF/TLIF group. Previous studies reported that the abundant intraoperative blood loss was a significant risk factor for early perioperative complications in the fusion and instrumentation of degenerative lumbar scoliosis [27–29]. Therefore, the LLIF procedure may potentially reduce surgical risks for ASD patients. In terms of late complications, no differences were noted in overall incidence, implant failure, PJK, or newly occurred vertebral fractures between the two groups. This result is similar to previous reports of comparisons between LLIF and single posterior approaches in surgical treatments for ASD [11,23,24,35]. We generally use hard braces after the surgery for 3–6 months. However, the long-term use of hard braces is reported to cause complications in elderly patients [36]. It was also reported that bracing after deformity-correction surgery did not effectively reduce PJK [37]. At the final stages, shifting from a hard brace, to a soft brace, or a dynamic brace [38] may be important for avoiding brace-related complications, preserving back muscle strength and improving QOL.

This study has several limitations. The main limitations are the small number of patients and their short-term follow-up. Further studies should involve a larger sample size and a longer follow-up period. In addition, HR-QOL was not investigated in this study. Previous studies have reported that lumbar spinal fusions and corrective surgeries are effective in improving QOL [6,24,39–41]. Further studies should be conducted using HR-QOL evaluations, such as the Oswestry Disability Index, SRS-22, and SF-36. Lastly, the choice of surgical approaches was not randomized in this study. A propensity score matching analysis was conducted to minimize the selection bias of the surgical procedures.

Despite these limitations, this is the first study that compared multilevel LLIF and PLIF/TLIF procedures for ASD patients using propensity score matching methods, clearly showing that intraoperative bleeding and postoperative hematoma were reduced in the LLIF procedures.

5. Conclusions

In comparison with LLIF and PLIF/TLIF procedures for the correction of ASD, the majority of the radiographic parameters were not significantly different between the two groups postoperatively. However, SVA tended to be smaller in the LLIF group at the final follow-up. Overall perioperative complications were comparable in LLIF and PLIF/TLIF for patients with ASD. However, LLIF procedures demonstrated significantly less intraoperative blood loss and a smaller incidence of postoperative epidural hematoma.

Author Contributions: Conceptualization, Y.M., T.Y. (Toshitaka Yoshii), K.S., T.H., M.T., T.Y. (Tsuyoshi Yamada), K.O., S.S. (Satoshi Sumiya), Y.A., S.S. (Shigeo Shindo), and A.O.; methodology, Y.M., T.Y. (Toshitaka Yoshii), S.M., K.S., T.H., M.T., T.Y. (Tsuyoshi Yamada), K.K., K.O., S.S. (Satoshi Sumiya), S.T., S.E., Y.A., and S.S. (Shigeo Shindo); collected data, Y.M., K.S., A.K., K.U., J.H., M.Y., I.T., T.Y. (Tsuyoshi Yamada), K.K., S.S. (Satoshi Sumiya), F.N., K.F., and S.T.; data analysis and interpre-tation, Y.M. and T.Y. (Toshitaka Yoshii); writing of initial draft, Y.M. and T.Y. (Toshitaka Yoshii); statistical analyses, Y.M., T.Y. (Toshitaka Yoshii), and S.M.; manuscript revision, T.Y. (Toshitaka Yoshii), T.H., H.I., and A.O.; supervision, T.H., K.O., Y.A., S.S. (Shigeo Shindo), and A.O. All authors have read and agreed to the published version of the manuscript.

Funding: This research received no external funding.

Institutional Review Board Statement: The study was conducted according to the guidelines of the Declaration of Helsinki, and approved by the institutional review board of each participating institution (protocol code M2017-115, 25 September 2017).

Informed Consent Statement: Informed consent was obtained from all subjects involved in the study.

Data Availability Statement: The datasets generated during and/or analyzed during the current study are available from the corresponding author on reasonable request.

Acknowledgments: We greatly thank Nobuko Nakajima and Yukiko Oya for data collection.

Conflicts of Interest: The authors declare no conflict of interest.

References

1. Youssef, J.A.; Orndorff, D.O.; Patty, C.A.; Scott, M.A.; Price, H.L.; Hamlin, L.F.; Williams, T.L.; Uribe, J.S.; Deviren, V. Current status of adult spinal deformity. *Glob. Spine J.* **2013**, *3*, 051–062. [CrossRef]
2. Aebi, M. The adult scoliosis. *Eur. Spine J.* **2005**, *14*, 925–948. [CrossRef]
3. Smith, J.S.; Shaffrey, C.I.; Bess, S.; Shamji, M.F.; Brodke, D.; Lenke, L.G.; Fehlings, M.G.; Lafage, V.; Schwab, F.; Vaccaro, A.R.; et al. Recent and emerging advances in spinal deformity. *Clin. Neurosurg.* **2017**, *80*, S77–S85. [CrossRef]
4. Schwab, F.J.; Blondel, B.; Bess, S.; Hostin, R.; Shaffrey, C.I.; Smith, J.S.; Boachie-Adjei, O.; Burton, D.C.; Akbarnia, B.A.; Mundis, G.M.; et al. Radiographical spinopelvic parameters and disability in the setting of adult spinal deformity: A prospective multicenter analysis. *Spine* **2013**, *38*, 803–812. [CrossRef]
5. Scheer, J.K.; Hostin, R.; Robinson, C.; Schwab, F.; Lafage, V.; Burton, D.C.; Hart, R.A.; Kelly, M.P.; Keefe, M.; Polly, D.; et al. Operative management of adult spinal deformity results in significant increases in QALYs gained compared to nonoperative management. *Spine* **2018**, *43*, 339–347. [CrossRef] [PubMed]
6. Daubs, M.D.; Lenke, L.G.; Bridwell, K.H.; Kim, Y.J.; Hung, M.; Cheh, G.; Koester, L.A. Does correction of preoperative coronal imbalance make a difference in outcomes of adult patients with deformity? *Spine* **2013**, *38*, 476–483. [CrossRef] [PubMed]
7. Glassman, S.D.; Bridwell, K.; Dimar, J.R.; Horton, W.; Berven, S.; Schwab, F. The impact of positive sagittal balance in adult spinal deformity. *Spine* **2005**, *30*, 2024–2029. [CrossRef]
8. Charosky, S.; Guigui, P.; Blamoutier, A.; Roussouly, P.; Chopin, D. Complications and risk factors of primary adult scoliosis surgery: A multicenter study of 306 patients. *Spine* **2012**, *37*, 693–700. [CrossRef] [PubMed]
9. Soroceanu, A.; Burton, D.C.; Oren, J.H.; Smith, J.S.; Hostin, R.; Shaffrey, C.I.; Akbarnia, B.A.; Ames, C.P.; Errico, T.J.; Bess, S.; et al. Medical complications after adult spinal deformity surgery incidence, risk factors, and clinical impact. *Spine* **2016**, *41*, 1718–1723. [CrossRef]
10. Zanirato, A.; Damilano, M.; Formica, M.; Piazzolla, A.; Lovi, A.; Villafañe, J.H.; Berjano, P. Complications in adult spine deformity surgery: A systematic review of the recent literature with reporting of aggregated incidences. *Eur. Spine J.* **2018**, *27*, 2272–2284. [CrossRef]
11. Bae, J.; Theologis, A.A.; Strom, R.; Tay, B.; Burch, S.; Berven, S.; Mummaneni, P.V.; Chou, D.; Ames, C.P.; Deviren, V. Comparative analysis of 3 surgical strategies for adult spinal deformity with mild to moderate sagittal imbalance. *J. Neurosurg. Spine* **2018**, *28*, 40–49. [CrossRef] [PubMed]
12. Ozgur, B.M.; Aryan, H.E.; Pimenta, L.; Taylor, W.R. Extreme Lateral Interbody Fusion (XLIF): A novel surgical technique for anterior lumbar interbody fusion. *Spine J.* **2006**, *6*, 435–443. [CrossRef]
13. Acosta, F.L.; Liu, J.; Slimack, N.; Moller, D.; Fessler, R.; Koski, T. Changes in coronal and sagittal plane alignment following minimally invasive direct lateral interbody fusion for the treatment of degenerative lumbar disease in adults: A radiographic study-Clinical article. *J. Neurosurg. Spine* **2011**, *15*, 92–96. [CrossRef] [PubMed]
14. Iwamae, M.; Matsumura, A.; Namikawa, T.; Kato, M.; Hori, Y.; Yabu, A.; Sawada, Y.; Hidaka, N.; Nakamura, H. Surgical outcomes of multilevel posterior lumbar interbody fusion versus lateral lumbar interbody fusion for the correction of adult spinal deformity: A comparative clinical study. *Asian Spine J.* **2020**, *14*, 421–429. [CrossRef] [PubMed]
15. Schwab, F.; Blondel, B.; Chay, E.; Demakakos, J.; Lenke, L.; Tropiano, P.; Ames, C.; Smith, J.S.; Shaffrey, C.I.; Glassman, S.; et al. The comprehensive anatomical spinal osteotomy classification. *Neurosurgery* **2014**, *74*, 112–120. [CrossRef] [PubMed]
16. Rosenbaum, P.R.; Rubin, D.B. The central role of the propensity score in observational studies for causal effects. *Matched Sampl. Causal Eff.* **2006**, 170–184. [CrossRef]
17. Chikuda, H.; Yasunaga, H.; Takeshita, K.; Horiguchi, H.; Kawaguchi, H.; Ohe, K.; Fushimi, K.; Tanaka, S. Mortality and morbidity after high-dose methylprednisolone treatment in patients with acute cervical spinal cord injury: A propensity-matched analysis using a nationwide administrative database. *Emerg. Med. J.* **2014**, *31*, 201–206. [CrossRef]
18. Kato, S.; Chikuda, H.; Ohya, J.; Oichi, T.; Matsui, H.; Fushimi, K.; Takeshita, K.; Tanaka, S.; Yasunaga, H. Risk of infectious complications associated with blood transfusion in elective spinal surgery-a propensity score matched analysis. *Spine J.* **2016**, *16*, 55–60. [CrossRef]
19. Silvestre, C.; Mac-Thiong, J.M.; Hilmi, R.; Roussouly, P. Complications and morbidities of mini-open anterior retroperitoneal lumbar interbody fusion: Oblique lumbar interbody fusion in 179 patients. *Asian Spine J.* **2012**, *6*, 89–97. [CrossRef]
20. Fujibayashi, S.; Hynes, R.A.; Otsuki, B.; Kimura, H.; Takemoto, M.; Matsuda, S. Effect of indirect neural decompression through oblique lateral interbody fusion for degenerative lumbar disease. *Spine* **2015**, *40*, E175–E182. [CrossRef]
21. Ohtori, S.; Mannoji, C.; Orita, S.; Yamauchi, K.; Eguchi, Y.; Ochiai, N.; Kishida, S.; Kuniyoshi, K.; Aoki, Y.; Nakamura, J.; et al. Mini-open anterior retroperitoneal lumbar interbody fusion: Oblique lateral interbody fusion for degenerated lumbar spinal kyphoscoliosis. *Asian Spine J.* **2015**, *9*, 565–572. [CrossRef]
22. Kato, S.; Nouri, A.; Wu, D.; Nori, S.; Tetreault, L.; Fehlings, M.G. Comparison of anterior and posterior surgery for degenerative cervical myelopathy. *J. Bone Jt. Surg.* **2017**, *99*, 1013–1021. [CrossRef]
23. Park, H.Y.; Ha, K.Y.; Kim, Y.H.; Chang, D.G.; Kim, S., II; Lee, J.W.; Ahn, J.H.; Kim, J.B. Minimally invasive lateral lumbar interbody fusion for adult spinal deformity. *Spine* **2018**, *43*, E813–E821. [CrossRef] [PubMed]

24. Strom, R.G.; Bae, J.; Mizutani, J.; Valone, F.; Ames, C.P.; Deviren, V. Lateral interbody fusion combined with open posterior surgery for adult spinal deformity. *J. Neurosurg. Spine* **2016**, *25*, 697–705. [CrossRef] [PubMed]
25. Wewel, J.T.; Godzik, J.; Uribe, J.S. The utilization of minimally invasive surgery techniques for the treatment of spinal deformity. *J. Spine Surg.* **2019**, *5*, S84–S90. [CrossRef] [PubMed]
26. Hosseini, P.; Mundis, G.M.; Eastlack, R.K.; Bagheri, R.; Vargas, E.; Tran, S.; Akbarnia, B.A. Preliminary results of anterior lumbar interbody fusion, anterior column realignment for the treatment of sagittal malalignment. *Neurosurg. Focus* **2017**, *43*, 1–7. [CrossRef]
27. Bianco, K.; Norton, R.; Schwab, F.; Smith, J.S.; Klineberg, E.; Obeid, I.; Mundis, G., Jr.; Shaffrey, C.I.; Kebaish, K.; Hostin, R.; et al. Complications and intercenter variability of three-column osteotomies for spinal deformity surgery: A retrospective review of 423 patients. *Neurosurg. Focus* **2014**, *36*. [CrossRef] [PubMed]
28. Cho, K.J.; Suk, S., II; Park, S.R.; Kim, J.H.; Kim, S.S.; Choi, W.K.; Lee, K.Y.; Lee, S.R. Complications in posterior fusion and instrumentation for degenerative lumbar scoliosis. *Spine* **2007**, *32*, 2232–2237. [CrossRef] [PubMed]
29. Olsen, M.A.; Nepple, J.J.; Riew, K.D.; Lenke, L.G.; Bridwell, K.H.; Mayfield, J.; Fraser, V.J. Risk factors for surgical site infection following orthopaedic spinal operations. *J. Bone Jt. Surg. Ser. A* **2008**, *90*, 62–69. [CrossRef] [PubMed]
30. Medici, A.; Meccariello, L.; Falzarano, G. Non-operative vs. percutaneous stabilization in magerl's A1 or A2 thoracolumbar spine fracture in adults: Is it really advantageous for A good alignment of the spine? preliminary data from a prospective study. *Eur. Spine J.* **2014**, *23*, S677–S683. [CrossRef]
31. Caruso, L.; Bisaccia, M.; Rinonapoli, G.; Caraffa, A.; Pace, V.; Bisaccia, O.; Morante, C.A.; Prada-Cañizares, A.; Pichierri, P.; Pica, G.; et al. Short segment fixation of thoracolumbar fractures with pedicle fixation at the level of the fracture. *EuroMediterr. Biomed. J.* **2018**, *13*, 132–136. [CrossRef]
32. Hussain, I.; Fu, K.M.; Uribe, J.S.; Chou, D.; Mummaneni, P.V. State of the art advances in minimally invasive surgery for adult spinal deformity. *Spine Deform.* **2020**, *8*, 1143–1158. [CrossRef] [PubMed]
33. Ishihara, M.; Taniguchi, S.; Adachi, T.; Kushida, T.; Paku, M.; Ando, M.; Saito, T.; Kotani, Y.; Tani, Y. Rod contour and overcorrection are risk factors of proximal junctional kyphosis after adult spinal deformity correction surgery. *Eur. Spine J.* **2021**, *30*, 1208–1214. [CrossRef] [PubMed]
34. Than, K.D.; Mummaneni, P.V.; Bridges, K.J.; Tran, S.; Park, P.; Chou, D.; La Marca, F.; Uribe, J.S.; Vogel, T.D.; Nunley, P.D.; et al. Complication rates associated with open versus percutaneous pedicle screw instrumentation among patients undergoing minimally invasive interbody fusion for adult spinal deformity. *Neurosurg. Focus* **2017**, *43*, 1–7. [CrossRef]
35. Sembrano, J.N.; Yson, S.C.; Horazdovsky, R.D.; Santos, E.R.G.; Polly, D.W. Radiographic comparison of lateral lumbar interbody fusion versus traditional fusion approaches: Analysis of sagittal contour change. *Int. J. Spine Surg.* **2015**, *9*. [CrossRef]
36. Yee, A.J.; Yoo, J.U.; Marsolais, E.B.; Carlson, G.; Poe-Kochert, C.; Bohlman, H.H.; Emery, S.E. Use of a postoperative lumbar corset after lumbar spinal arthrodesis for degenerative conditions of the spine. A prospective randomized trial. *J. Bone Jt. Surg. Ser. A* **2008**, *90*, 2062–2068. [CrossRef] [PubMed]
37. Lord, E.L.; Ayres, E.; Woo, D.; Vasquez-Montes, D.; Parekh, Y.; Jain, D.; Buckland, A.; Protopsaltis, T. The Impact of Global Alignment and Proportion Score and Bracing on Proximal Junctional Kyphosis in Adult Spinal Deformity. *Glob. Spine J.* **2021**. [CrossRef]
38. Meccariello, L.; Muzii, V.F.; Falzarano, G.; Medici, A.; Carta, S.; Fortina, M.; Ferrata, P. Dynamic corset versus three-point brace in the treatment of osteoporotic compression fractures of the thoracic and lumbar spine: A prospective, comparative study. *Aging Clin. Exp. Res.* **2017**, *29*, 443–449. [CrossRef] [PubMed]
39. Irimia, J.C.; Tomé-Bermejo, F.; Piñera-Parrilla, A.R.; Benito Gallo, M.; Bisaccia, M.; Fernández-González, M.; Villar-Pérez, J.; Fernández-Carreira, J.M.; Orovio De Elizaga, J.; Areta-Jiménez, F.J.; et al. Spinal fusion achieves similar two-year improvement in HRQoL as total hip and total knee replacement. A prospective, multicentric and observational study. *SICOT J.* **2019**, *5*. [CrossRef]
40. Bridwell, K.H.; Glassman, S.; Horton, W.; Shaffrey, C.; Schwab, F.; Zebala, L.P.; Lenke, L.G.; Hilton, J.F.; Shainline, M.; Baldus, C.; et al. Does treatment (nonoperative and operative) improve the two-year quality of life in patients with adult symptomatic lumbar scoliosis: A prospective multicenter evidence-based medicine study. *Spine* **2009**, *34*, 2171–2178. [CrossRef]
41. Smith, J.S.; Klineberg, E.; Schwab, F.; Shaffrey, C.I.; Moal, B.; Ames, C.P.; Hostin, R.; Fu, K.M.G.; Burton, D.; Akbarnia, B.; et al. Change in classification grade by the srs-schwab adult spinal deformity classification predicts impact on health-related quality of life measures; prospective analysis of operative and nonoperative treatment. *Spine* **2013**, *38*, 1663–1671. [CrossRef] [PubMed]

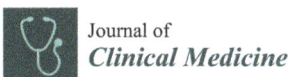
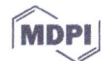

Article

Anterior Cervical Corpectomy with Fusion versus Anterior Hybrid Fusion Surgery for Patients with Severe Ossification of the Posterior Longitudinal Ligament Involving Three or More Levels: A Retrospective Comparative Study

Takashi Hirai [1,*], Toshitaka Yoshii [1], Kenichiro Sakai [2], Hiroyuki Inose [1], Masato Yuasa [1], Tsuyoshi Yamada [1], Yu Matsukura [1], Shuta Ushio [1], Shingo Morishita [1], Satoru Egawa [1], Hiroaki Onuma [1], Yutaka Kobayashi [1], Kurando Utagawa [1], Jun Hashimoto [1], Atsuyuki Kawabata [1], Tomoyuki Tanaka [1], Takayuki Motoyoshi [1], Takuya Takahashi [1], Motonori Hashimoto [1], Kentaro Sakaeda [1], Tsuyoshi Kato [1], Yoshiyasu Arai [2], Shigenori Kawabata [1] and Atsushi Okawa [1]

Citation: Hirai, T.; Yoshii, T.; Sakai, K.; Inose, H.; Yuasa, M.; Yamada, T.; Matsukura, Y.; Ushio, S.; Morishita, S.; Egawa, S.; et al. Anterior Cervical Corpectomy with Fusion versus Anterior Hybrid Fusion Surgery for Patients with Severe Ossification of the Posterior Longitudinal Ligament Involving Three or More Levels: A Retrospective Comparative Study. J. Clin. Med. 2021, 10, 5315. https://doi.org/10.3390/jcm10225315

Academic Editor: Emmanuel Andrès

Received: 5 October 2021
Accepted: 12 November 2021
Published: 15 November 2021

Publisher's Note: MDPI stays neutral with regard to jurisdictional claims in published maps and institutional affiliations.

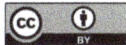

Copyright: © 2021 by the authors. Licensee MDPI, Basel, Switzerland. This article is an open access article distributed under the terms and conditions of the Creative Commons Attribution (CC BY) license (https://creativecommons.org/licenses/by/4.0/).

[1] Department of Orthopedic Surgery, Tokyo Medical and Dental University, 1-5-45 Yushima, Bunkyo-ku, Tokyo 113-8510, Japan; yoshii.orth@tmd.ac.jp (T.Y.); inose.orth@tmd.ac.jp (H.I.); yuaorth@tmd.ac.jp (M.Y.); yamada.orth@tmd.ac.jp (T.Y.); Matsukura.orth@tmd.ac.jp (Y.M.); ushiorth20@gmail.com (S.U.); morsorth@tmd.ac.jp (S.M.); egawa.orth@tmd.ac.jp (S.E.); onuma.orj@tmd.ac.jp (H.O.); kobayashi.orth@tmd.ac.jp (Y.K.); utag.orth@tmd.ac.jp (K.U.); 0123456789jun@gmail.com (J.H.); 060211ms@gmail.com (A.K.); the.tomo.rrow@gmail.com (T.T.); motoyoshi.orth@tmd.ac.jp (T.M.); tttt841000@gmail.com (T.T.); hmoto95@gmail.com (M.H.); sakaeda.orth@tmd.ac.jp (K.S.); katoorth@gmail.com (T.K.); kawabata.orth@tmd.ac.jp (S.K.); okawa.orth@tmd.ac.jp (A.O.)

[2] Department of Orthopedic Surgery, Saitamaken-Saiseikai Kawaguchi General Hospital, 5-11-5 Nishikawaguchu, Kawaguchi City 332-8558, Japan; kenitiro1122@gmail.com (K.S.); arai.orth@gmail.com (Y.A.)

* Correspondence: hirai.orth@tmd.ac.jp; Tel.: +81-35803-5279

Abstract: Various studies have found a high incidence of early graft dislodgement after multilevel corpectomy. Although a hybrid fusion technique was developed to resolve implant failure, the hybrid and conventional techniques have not been clearly compared in terms of perioperative complications in patients with severe ossification of the posterior longitudinal ligament (OPLL) involving three or more levels. The purpose of this study was to compare clinical and radiologic outcomes between anterior cervical corpectomy with fusion (ACCF) and anterior hybrid fusion for the treatment of multilevel cervical OPLL. We therefore retrospectively reviewed the clinical and radiologic data of 53 consecutive patients who underwent anterior fusion to treat cervical OPLL: 30 underwent ACCF and 23 underwent anterior hybrid fusion. All patients completed 2 years of follow-ups. Implant migration was defined as subsidence > 3 mm. There were no significant differences in demographics or clinical characteristics between the ACCF and hybrid groups. Early implant failure occurred significantly more frequently in the ACCF group (5 cases, 16.7%) compared with the hybrid group (0 cases, 0%). The fusion rate was 80% in the ACCF group and 100% in the hybrid group. Although both procedures can achieve satisfactory neurologic outcomes for multilevel OPLL patients, hybrid fusion likely provides better biomechanical stability than the conventional ACCF technique.

Keywords: anterior cervical corpectomy and fusion; hybrid fusion; ossification of the posterior longitudinal ligament; implant failure; graft subsidence; complications; perioperative outcomes; fusion rate; segmental paralysis; mechanical stability

1. Introduction

Ossification of the posterior longitudinal ligament (OPLL) is a heterotopic ossification of spinal ligaments and a unique degenerative spine disease that causes neurologic disorders in middle and old age [1,2]. Although the prevalence of OPLL in Asian countries is reported to range from 1.9% to 4.3% [2], a majority of patients with OPLL seem to have no neurologic symptoms [3]. However, ossified lesions that develop in the spinal canal compress the spinal cord and nerve roots, causing myelopathy or radiculopathy [4]. Surgical treatment should be provided for patients with progressive myelopathy [5,6], whereas conservative treatment is suitable for minimally symptomatic patients [7].

Surgical strategies have evolved as options for treating OPLL based on various studies. Posterior decompression with fusion was demonstrated to provide indirect decompression and stabilize the spinal structure in multiple segments [8]. However, it is also known that sufficient decompression cannot be achieved via a posterior approach in patients with massive OPLL who have kyphosis, and outcomes are relatively poor in posterior decompression with fusion even after eliminating the dynamic factor [9]. Anterior cervical corpectomy and fusion (ACCF) is a key strategy for achieving adequate decompression in patients with cervical OPLL [6]. However, implant failure often occurs in patients treated with anterior cervical corpectomy, and other complications also frequently occur, such as respiratory problems and dysphagia [10]. It was also reported that ACCF results in higher perioperative complication rates compared with anterior cervical discectomy and fusion (ACDF) [11]. Graft dislodgement immediately after ACCF requires emergent salvage surgery; therefore, posterior surgery is widely used by spine surgeons and neurosurgeons even for the treatment of patients with massive ossification or sagittal malalignment [12]. To overcome these issues, an anterior hybrid technique of combined ACCF and ACDF was developed for patients with multiple segmental OPLL [13,14]. This technique allows for more screws to be placed to stabilize the anterior strut, and it is thought to provide better postoperative stability of the fused segments compared with ACCF for patients with multi-level OPLL [15]. However, no investigations have compared traditional ACCF and hybrid ACCF to perform a detailed verification of the structural stability of constructs in these two surgeries, and no studies have focused exclusively on patients with severe OPLL involving three or more segments. Therefore, we conducted this retrospective study to compare the clinical and radiologic outcomes of anterior decompression with traditional ACCF and hybrid ACCF in patients with severe OPLL.

2. Materials and Methods

2.1. Patients and Methods

This single-center retrospective cohort study was carried out in accordance with the STROBE guidelines [16] and compared ACCF and hybrid fusion for treatment of patients with OPLL involving ≥3 levels. Patients with a history of previous cervical spine surgery or injury were excluded. The study involved consecutive patients in whom anterior surgery was required to treat severe myelopathy due to a compressive lesion involving at least 3 segments, regardless of the duration of symptoms, in our hospital from 2007 to 2018. We previously performed traditional ACCF for all patients until 2011, and thereafter we performed anterior hybrid fusion where possible for patients in whom the vertebral body in the lesion could be preserved. In principle, anterior cervical surgery was performed in patients with OPLL occupying 50% or more of the anteroposterior diameter of the spinal canal. The level to be decompressed was decided based on the neurologic findings and the presence of spinal cord compression. In addition, we performed corpectomy in the levels that had the most compressive OPLL lesion and applied ACDF in the most proximal or distal segments that had relatively small compressive lesions in the anterior hybrid operation.

2.2. Operative Technique

2.2.1. Anterior Cervical Corpectomy with Fusion (ACCF Group)

The operative technique for this procedure was described previously [1]. The anterior decompression with fusion procedure includes partial removal of vertebral body and discs with a strut graft. Segments to be operated were diagnosed based on preoperative radiographic and clinical findings. The length of the bone graft was measured intraoperatively using X-calipers between the upper and lower endplates of vertebral bodies operated in a neutral cervical position. A strut graft collected from the iliac crest or made using artificial bone made from hydroxyapatite (Boneceram®; Olympus Corporation, Tokyo, Japan) was used for 2 corpectomies (3 segments), and fibula strut grafts were used for 3 or more corpectomies (4 or more segments). A semi-rigid plate was inserted in all cases. In principle, fixed screws were placed for the distal vertebrae and variable screws for the proximal vertebrae (VENTURE™ Anterior Cervical Plate System; Medtronic Sofamor Danek Inc., Memphis, TN; Figure 1a). This technique was performed by five senior spine surgeons. Patients basically wore a neck collar for 2–3 months postoperatively.

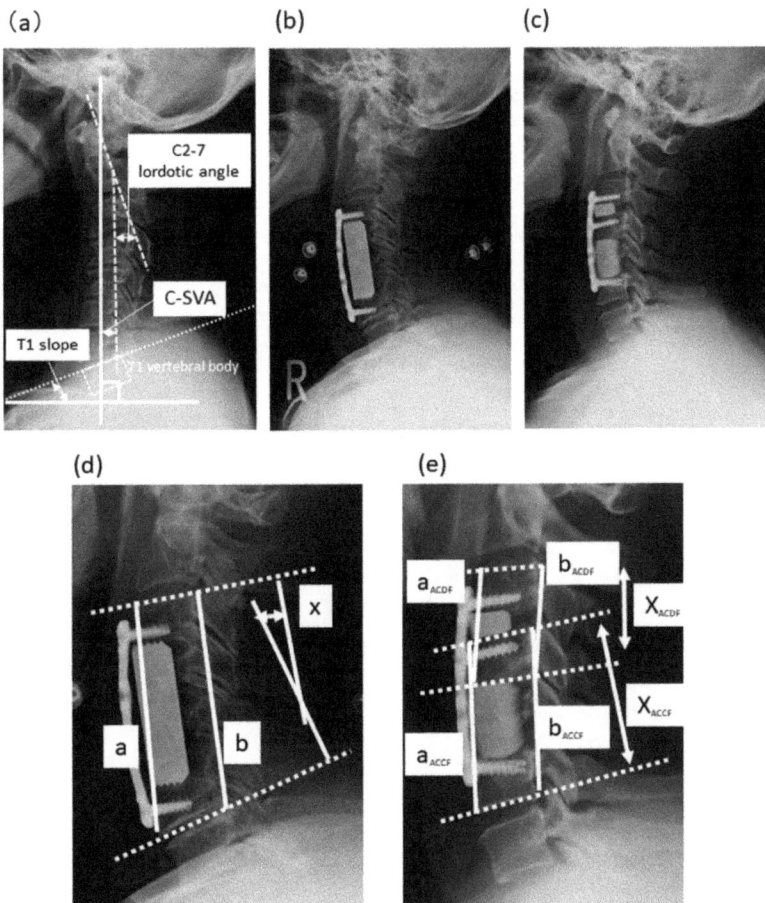

Figure 1. Long semi-constrained plate fixation with artificial bone graft. (**a**) Preoperative radiograph showing the C2–7 lordotic angle, C-SVA, and T1 slope. Postoperative radiographs (**b**) after dual-level corpectomy (C4–5) and ossification floating decompression and (**c**) with dual artificial bone graft after discectomy (C3/4) and single corpectomy (C5). (**d**) Postoperative radiograph showing fused segment angle and fused segment height in the ACCF group. (**e**) Postoperative radiograph showing fused segment angle and fused segment height in the hybrid group.

2.2.2. Anterior Hybrid Procedure (Corpectomy-Discectomy with Fusion, Hybrid Group)

The ≥2 levels that caused relatively severe cord compression were treated with corpectomy (as in the ACCF group), and the remaining disc level was treated with discectomy. Autograft or artificial bone graft (Boneceram®; Olympus Corporation, Tokyo, Japan) for segments treated with corpectomy and cervical fusion cage or artificial bone graft were placed with a plate and 6-screws fixation (Figure 1b). This technique was performed by four senior spine surgeons. Patients basically wore a neck collar for 2–3 months postoperatively.

2.3. Clinical Evaluations

Most of the patients visited at 3, 6, 12, 18, and 24 months for postoperative clinical and radiologic follow-up. All patients were followed up for 2 years at our institution. The degree of cervical myelopathy before and after surgery was assessed using the Japanese Orthopaedic Association (JOA) scoring system [5]. Briefly, this score comprises four items, including upper extremity motor function, lower extremity motor function, sensory function, and bladder function (Table 1). The JOA score is the sum of these items (I + II + III + IV in Table 1). The recovery rate of the JOA score was calculated to compare pre- and postoperative JOA scores as follows: Recovery rate (%) = (Postoperative score—Preoperative score) × 100/(17—Preoperative score). These clinical findings were recorded using electronic data capture (Claris FileMaker Pro 19; Claris International, Cupertino, CA) with security systems in place. The presence of dysphagia was defined as moderate or severe symptoms according to Bazaz score. The incidence of segmental paralysis (so-called C5 palsy), aspiration pneumonia, delirium, and deep venous thrombosis were recorded.

Table 1. Scoring system for cervical myelopathy (JOA score).

I Upper extremity motor function		
	0:	Unable to feed oneself with any tableware including chopsticks, spoon, or fork, and/or unable to fasten buttons of any size
	1:	Can manage to feed oneself with spoon and/or fork but not chopsticks
	2:	Either chopsticks feeding or writing is possible but not practical, and/or large buttons can be fastened
	3:	Either chopsticks feeding or writing is clumsy but practical, and/or cuff buttons can be fastened
	4:	Normal
II Lower extremity motor function		
	0:	Unable to stand up and walk by any means
	0.5:	Able to stand up but unable to walk
	1:	Unable to walk without a cane or other support on level ground
	1.5:	Able to walk without support but with a clumsy gait
	2:	Walks independently on level ground but needs support on stairs
	2.5:	Walks independently when going upstairs, but needs support when going downstairs
	3:	Capable of walking fast but clumsily
	4:	Normal
III Sensory function		
A. Upper extremity		
	0:	Complete loss of touch and pain sensation
	0.5:	50% or below of normal sensation and/or severe pain or numbness
	1:	Over 60% of normal sensation and/or moderate pain or numbness
	1.5:	Subjective numbness of a slight degree without any objective sensory deficit
	2:	Normal
B. Lower extremity		
		Same as A
C. Trunk		
		Same as A
IV Bladder function		
	0:	Urinary retention and/or incontinence
	1:	Sensory of retention, dribbling, thin stream and/or incomplete continence
	2:	Urinary retardation and/or pollakiuria
	3:	Normal

2.4. Radiologic Evaluations

Cervical sagittal alignment (C2–7 lordotic angle) was assessed using tangential lines drawn on the posterior edge of the C2 and C7 vertebral bodies on lateral radiographs acquired in a neutral standing position [10]. Preoperative center of the head—C7 sagittal vertical axis (C-SVA) [17] and T1 slope [18]—were also measured (Figure 1a). The fused segment angle (FSA) and fused segment height (FSH) were also determined. Briefly, FSA is the angle between lines drawn parallel to the cranial endplate of the cranial vertebrae of the fused segment and the caudal endplate of the caudal vertebrae of the fused segment, and FSH was determined as the mean value of the anterior and posterior vertebral body heights at the fused segments (Figure 1d,e) [19,20]. In the hybrid group, these parameters were independently calculated in the ACCF and ACDF segments. Additionally calculated were changes in both FSA (ΔFSA) and FSH (ΔFSH) between before and immediately after the operation, |ΔFSA| and |ΔFSH|. Graft migration was defined as subsidence >3 mm. Solid fusion was defined as the presence of continuous bone connecting the Luschka joints at the operated segments on X-ray. Radiologic measurements were performed by an independent assessor (M.H.). Formal analysis was performed by another independent assessor (T.H.). These two doctors are certified by the Japanese Society for Spine Surgery and Related Research to perform spine surgery.

2.5. Statistical Analysis

Differences between the two groups were assessed using one-way analysis of variance, the Mann Whitney U test, or the Chi-square test. Multivariate logistic regression with a forward stepwise procedure was performed to identify key risk factors for postoperative implant migration ($p < 0.1$ for entry), with occurrence of graft migration as the objective variable and age, sex, and radiographic parameters as explanatory variables. All statistical analyses were carried out using SPSS for Windows (version 20.0; IBM Corp., Armonk, NY, USA). A p-value of less than 0.05 was considered statistically significant.

3. Results
3.1. Demographic Data and Clinical Outcomes

Patients (41 men, 12 women; follow-up rate, 100%) completed at least 2 years of follow-ups (Table 2). Of these, 30 patients were categorized into the ACCF group and 23 into the hybrid group. Mean preoperative/postoperative JOA scores were 11.9/15.0 points and 11.1/14.6 points, respectively. The average number of fused segments was 3.3 levels in the ACCF group and 3.5 levels in the hybrid group. Mean estimated blood loss and operative time were 437 mL and 6.5 h in the ACCF group and 197 mL and 6.0 h in the hybrid group, respectively. Duration of intensive care unit (ICU) stay and timing of extubation were respectively 2.8 days and 0.5 days in the ACCF group and 3.3 days and 0.9 days in the hybrid group. Duration of hospitalization was 24.2 days and 29.3 days, respectively. There were no significant differences in demographic and clinical characteristics between the two groups.

The incidence of perioperative complications was similar between the groups (Table 3). In the ACCF group, there was persistent dysphagia in four cases categorized as moderate by their Bazaz score (13.3%), aspiration pneumonitis in three (10%), delirium in two (6.7%), segmental paralysis in two (6.7%), and deep vein thrombosis in one (3.3%). In one case, dysphagia did not resolve until 2 months after the operation. However, other complications were resolved during the hospital stay. In the hybrid group, there was one case each (4.3%) of dyspnea caused by internal hematoma, aspiration pneumonitis, delirium, and segmental paralysis.

Table 2. Demographic and clinical characteristics in the ACCF and hybrid groups.

	ACCF Group (n = 30)	Hybrid Group (n = 23)	p
Age (years)	61.7 ± 9.1	62.9 ± 10.5	0.71
Male:Female	24:6	17:6	0.74
Diabetes mellitus (%)	10 (33.3)	6 (26.1)	0.57
History of smoking (%)	12 (40)	7 (30.4)	0.47
Preoperative JOA score (points)	11.9 ± 2.1	11.1 ± 3.8	0.39
Postoperative JOA score (points)	15.0 ± 1.4	14.6 ± 2.3	0.50
Recovery rate of JOA score (%)	56.3 ± 32.1	70.4 ± 27.0	0.12
No. of fused segments	3.3 ± 0.6	3.5 ± 0.7	0.33
Graft type in ACCF part	Artificial bone 20 Fibular graft 6 Iliac graft 4	Artificial bone 20 Fibular graft 3	0.28
Graft type in ACDF part	-	Artificial bone 20 fusion cage 3	-
Estimated blood loss (mL)	437 ± 778	197 ± 151	0.20
Operating time (h)	6.5 ± 2.4	6.0 ± 2.4	0.40
Duration of ICU stay (days)	2.8 ± 1.4	3.3 ± 2.6	0.39
Time to postoperative extubation (days)	0.5 ± 1.1	0.9 ± 2.6	0.55
Hospital stay (days)	24.2 ± 10.7	29.3 ± 12.3	0.55

Data are shown as the mean ± standard deviation. ACCF, anterior cervical corpectomy with fusion; JOA, Japanese Orthopaedic Association; ICU, intensive care unit.

Table 3. Perioperative complications in the ACCF and hybrid groups.

	ACCF Group (n = 30)	Hybrid Group (n = 23)	p
Complications, n (%)			
Total	12 (40%)	4 (17.4%)	0.08
Dysphagia	4 (13.3%)	0 (0%)	0.07
Aspiration pneumonitis	3 (10%)	1 (4.3%)	0.44
Delirium	2 (6.7%)	1 (4.3%)	0.72
Segmental paralysis	2 (6.7%)	1 (4.3%)	0.72
DVT	1 (3.3%)	0 (0%)	0.37
Dyspnea (internal hematoma)	0 (0%)	1 (4.3%)	0.24
Revision surgery, n (%)			
Total	5 (16.7%)	1 (5.3%)	0.16
Graft dislodgement	5 (16.7%)	0 (0%)	0.04 *
Segmental paralysis	0 (0%)	1 (5.3%)	0.24

Data are shown as the mean ± standard deviation. ACCF, anterior cervical corpectomy with fusion; DVT, Deep vein thrombosis; * Statistically significant, $p < 0.05$.

Revision surgery for implant failure was performed in five cases (16.7%) in the ACCF group but in none in the hybrid group (Table 3). However, additional corpectomy was required for one patient who developed segmental motor dysfunction in the hybrid group. The incidence of reoperation, especially due to strut dislodgement immediately postoperatively, was significantly higher in the ACCF group compared with the hybrid group ($p = 0.04$, Table 3).

3.2. Radiographic Outcomes

Chronological changes on radiographs were evaluated. Mean C2–7 angle increased immediately postoperatively and was maintained in both groups (Figure 2a). C-SVA was increased immediately postoperatively, but it had gradually decreased by 6 months postoperatively in both groups (Figure 2b). T1 slope did not change during the follow-up period (Figure 2c). In the ACCF group, mean FSA was increased immediately postoperatively and was maintained. However, there was a gradual decrease with a loss of 0.7 degrees 1 year after the operation. In the hybrid group, mean FSA was increased in segments treated with either ACDF or ACCF after surgery and was unchanged at the 1-year follow-up (Figure 2d).

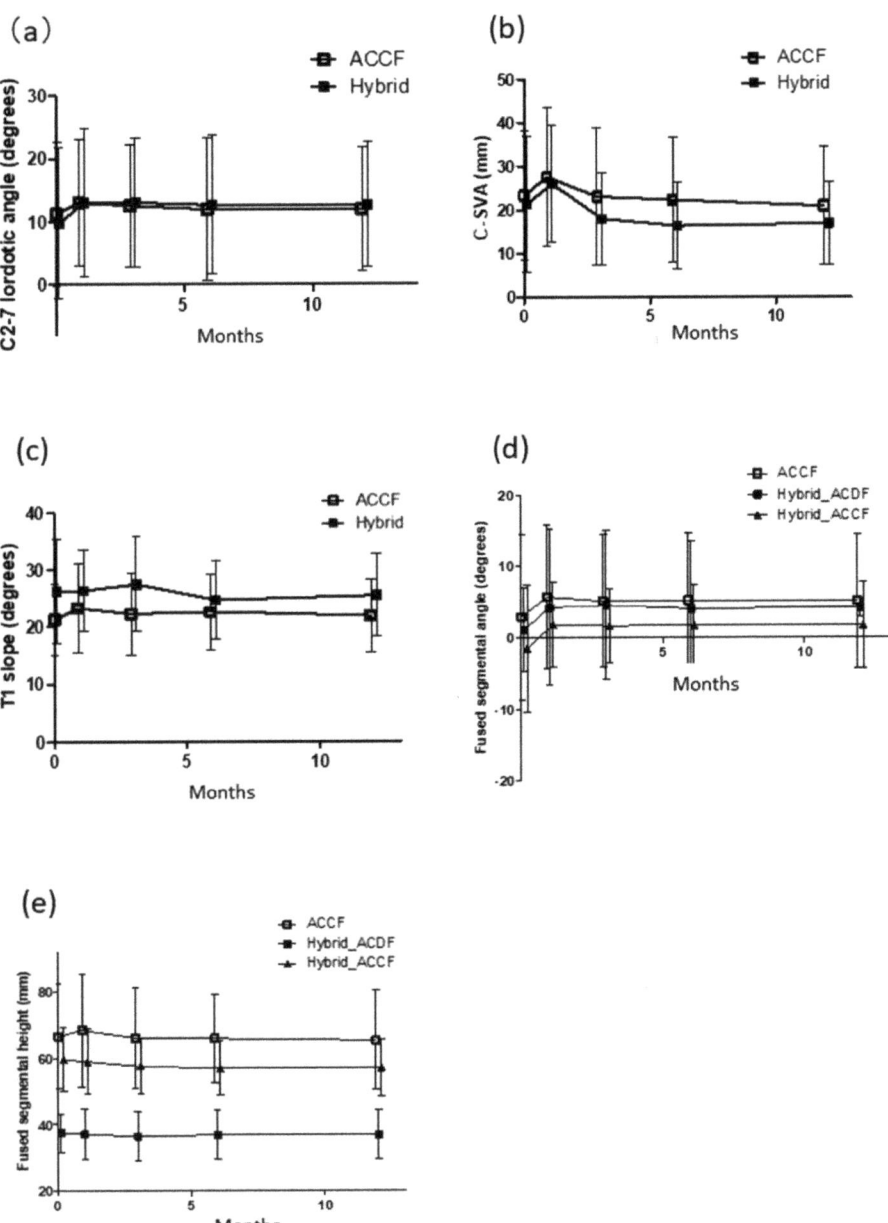

Figure 2. Radiographic measurement of (**a**) C2–7 angle; (**b**) C2–7 SVA; (**c**) T1 slope; (**d**) FSA; and (**e**) FSH in the ACCF and hybrid groups.

In the ACCF group, mean FSH was increased by 2 mm immediately postoperatively. However, there was a 2-mm decrease at 1 year postoperatively. In the hybrid group, mean FSH was unchanged postoperatively, even compared with preoperatively (Figure 2e). Strut subsidence was observed in eight cases (26.7%) in the ACCF group and three cases (13.0%) in the hybrid group (Table 4). Among patients with strut subsidence, secondary surgery was required for early implant dislodgement in four cases in the ACCF group, but no secondary surgeries were required in the hybrid group. The fusion rate was significantly higher in the hybrid group than in the ACCF group (100% vs. 80%).

Table 4. Radiologic outcomes in the ACCF and hybrid groups.

		ACCF Group (n = 30)	Hybrid Group (n = 23)				p
C2–7 angle (°)	Preoperative	11.2 ± 11.4	9.7 ± 12.0				0.76
	Immediate postoperative	13.0 ± 10.1	13.0 ± 11.7				0.94
	1 year	11.9 ± 9.8	12.6 ± 9.9				0.66
C-SVA (mm)	Preoperative	23.4 ± 14.9	21.4 ± 15.5				0.97
	Immediate postoperative	27.6 ± 16.0	26.0 ± 13.5				0.59
	1 year	20.9 ± 13.5	16.9 ± 9.5				0.39
T1 slope (°)	Preoperative	21.2 ± 6.3	26.2 ± 9.1				0.77
	Immediate postoperative	23.3 ± 7.8	26.4 ± 7.2				0.27
	1 year	21.9 ± 6.4	25.5 ± 7.3				0.61
		ACCF	ACDF part	ACCF part	Overall		
FSA (°)	Preoperative	2.9 ± 11.6	1.1 ± 5.9	−1.6 ± 8.9	1.9 ± 11.3		0.77 #
	Immediate postoperative	5.7 ± 10.0	4.2 ± 10.9	1.8 ± 6.0	4.7 ± 10.8		0.27 #
	1 year	5.1 ± 9.4	4.2 ± 1.3	1.7 ± 6.0	4.3 ± 10.4		0.36 #
FSH (mm)	Preoperative	66.6 ± 15.7	37.4 ± 5.8	59.6 ± 9.6	69.4 ± 16.3		0.66 #
	Immediate postoperative	68.4 ± 17.1	37.0 ± 7.7	59.0 ± 9.9	69.1 ± 15.4		0.54 #
	1 year	66.4 ± 15.0	36.8 ± 7.4	58.4 ± 8.6	68.8 ± 15.1		0.37 #
ΔC2–7 angle (°)		1.8 ± 8.2	3.3 ± 8.2				0.53
ΔFSA (°)		2.8 ± 7.9	2.6 ± 8.1	2.8 ± 7.5	2.8 ± 8.4		0.96 #
ΔFSH (mm)		3.2 ± 7.1 *	−0.4 ± 3.0	−0.6 ± 3.5	1.4 ± 7.7		0.23 #
Graft subsidence (cases)		8 (26.7%)	3 (13.0%)				0.22
Fusion rate		80%	100% *				0.02 *

Data are shown as the mean ± standard deviation. ACCF, anterior cervical corpectomy with fusion; ACDF, anterior cervical discectomy with fusion; C-SVA, cervical-sagittal vertical axis; FSA, fused segmental angle; FSH, fused segmental height. * Statistically significant, $p < 0.05$. # Compared between the ACCF group and all patients in the hybrid group.

3.3. Association of Change in FSH Immediately Postoperatively with Strut Subsidence in the ACCF Group

To identify postoperative structural changes in the fused segments, associations between the incidence of graft dislodgement and parameters including FSA and FSH were evaluated in the ACCF group. Graft subsidence was more likely to occur in those with ΔFSH > 5 mm (Figure 3a). Of note, early strut dislodgement that required secondary surgery occurred in three of four cases with ΔFSH >10 mm. Stepwise logistic regression analysis demonstrated that only |ΔFSH| was a key risk factor for postoperative graft subsidence (odds ratio 1.328, 95% confidence interval 1.017–1.733; $p = 0.04$; Figure 3b).

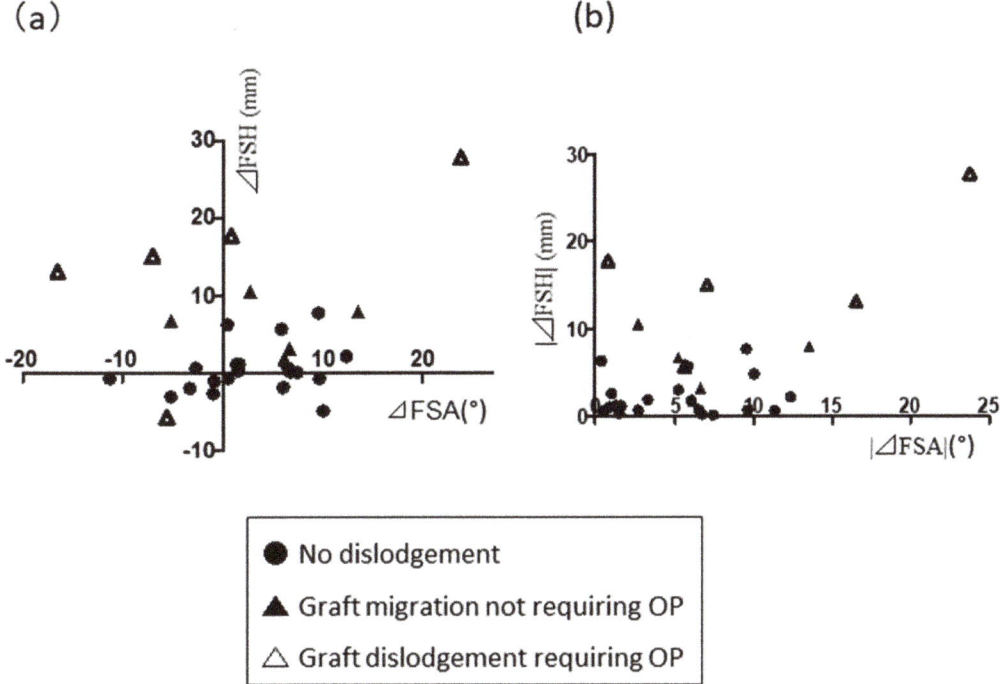

Figure 3. (a) Plot showing changes in FSA and FSH (ΔFSA and ΔFSH) and the incidence of graft subsidence; (b) Plot showing associations between absolute values of ΔFSA and ΔFSH and graft migration. A large |ΔFSH| is more closely linked with graft migration than |ΔFSA|.

4. Discussion

Various studies have discussed the superiority of certain surgical procedures for the treatment of patients with multilevel OPLL [5,6,8,9,21]. A meta-analysis revealed the anterior procedure provides more favorable results in terms of neurological recovery and postoperative cervical alignment [5]. Fujiyoshi et al. developed the K-line, which connects the midpoints of the spinal canal at C2 and C7 on neutral lateral radiographs, as a means of predicting poor clinical outcomes in patients with ossification of the posterior longitudinal ligament (OPLL) [22]. They classified OPLL patients into two groups, K-line (+) and K-line (−), and demonstrated that there was an insufficient posterior shift of the spinal cord and no neurologic improvement after posterior decompression surgery in patients in the K-line (−) group, in whom the anterior compression of OPLL exceeds the line. Notably, the classification is able to predict whether anterior compression of the spinal cord, which often impairs postoperative neural recovery [23], remains even after posterior decompression, and thus it is a very effective tool for deciding which surgical treatment—anterior or posterior—should be performed [8]. We also previously reported better outcomes after ACCF than after posterior procedures in patients who had severe OPLL with kyphotic alignment [9,21]. However, most comparative studies have shown that surgical complications were more frequent with anterior cervical surgery [6,21,24]. Of all complications after ACCF, airway obstruction and early graft migration are the most serious, often leading to emergency treatment and high reoperation rates [6,21,24]. For spine surgeons and neurosurgeons especially, it is important to recognize risk factors for predicting such perioperative complications.

This study also showed that the hybrid group had a relatively higher recovery rate in terms of JOA score (Table 1) and a lower incidence of complications (Table 2), although these differences did not reach significance. Additionally, no significant differences were found in terms of duration of ICU stay, the timing of postoperative extubation, hospital stay, or blood loss, although blood loss was certainly lower in the hybrid group. Fortunately, none of our patients needed a blood transfusion due to circulatory shock in this study. We speculate that corpectomy often violates the epidural venous plexus when decompressing the lateral portion of the spinal canal, thereby increasing the incidence of massive epidural bleeding in the ACCF procedure. Hospital stays were somewhat longer in the hybrid group than in the ACCF group, despite the lower complication rate in the hybrid group. Although there were more mechanical complications in the ACCF group, this finding suggests that the ACCF technique may be more invasive but may not affect the general condition of the patient as much as the hybrid procedure seems to.

Various studies have investigated the incidence of complications after anterior cervical surgery, which is reported to range from 11.3% to 64.3% [5,6,21,25–27]. Generally, it has been recognized that the hybrid procedure results in lower complication rates, ranging from 0% to 22.2%, and improved clinical outcomes compared with conventional ACCF, ranging from 6.2% to 43.6% [14,28,29]. In our study, the rate was 30.2% overall (ACCF, 40%; hybrid, 17.4%), relatively consistent with the results of previous studies. Of note, dysphagia occurred in four cases (13.3%) in the ACCF group, but did not occur in the hybrid group. A recent meta-analysis reviewed 38 studies and found an incidence of 16.8% after anterior cervical surgery [30]. Fortunately, the complication rate of dysphagia in this study was lower than previously reported. We speculate that because our institution is a high-volume center for cervical spine surgery, especially anterior cervical spine operation, the complication rate might be relatively low. Despite finding no significant difference between the two groups in our study, dysphagia caused by postoperative soft tissue swelling was likely lower in the hybrid group (0%) than in the ACCF group (13.3%). First, various surgical instruments, such as surgical osteotomes and retractors, were different between these two group because the patients categorized into the ACCF group underwent surgery in an earlier period than those in the hybrid group. Second, posterior cooling pads were placed on the anterior aspect of the neck immediately after surgery to prevent soft tissue swelling from 2012. In addition, we speculate that the superior laryngeal nerve and muscles related to swallowing might be less susceptible to mechanical damage in the hybrid group than in the ACCF group, likely because operative retractors can be loosened during decompression of the ossified lesions in the most compressed segment in the hybrid group, although they should be sufficiently expanded during decompression in the ACCF group. Because dysphagia can potentially develop even in patients treated with anterior hybrid fusion, it should be kept in mind postoperatively for both patients undergoing traditional ACCF and those undergoing hybrid fusion. Nevertheless, we believe that the hybrid technique could be a less invasive and more structurally stable strategy for treating severe OPLL compared with the conventional ACCF method.

It is known that multiple ACDF provides several advantages over multiple corpectomies [11]. ACDF is less invasive and is technically easier than ACCF. There is also less graft dislodgement, better correction of kyphotic deformity, and less need for postoperative immobilization because the screws are inserted into the preserved vertebral bodies [11]. However, there is some degree of difficulty involved in decompressing multilevel continuous lesions in the spinal canal and foramen using ACDF [8,20]. In patients with multilevel OPLL, corpectomy is often required to decompress the lesion entirely [20,21]. Vaccaro et al. reported that early graft dislodgement was seen in 9% of patients treated with 1-vertebra body corpectomy, and in as high as 50% of those receiving 2-vertebral body corpectomy [31]. Similarly, Okawa et al. reported that implant migration was observed in 30% of patients undergoing ACCF with average 3.8-level decompression [32]. The present study is the first to focus exclusively on severe OPLL affecting three or more levels and demonstrated that the incidence of reoperation for graft dislodgement was significantly higher in the ACCF group (16.7%) compared with the hybrid group (0%). In addition, mean FSH was decreased by 2 mm at 1 year after surgery in the ACCF group, whereas it was unchanged in the hybrid group (Table 3 and Figure 2e). Interestingly, mean FSH at 1 year returned to the preoperative value in the ACCF group. These findings suggest that the longer sized-graft bone could be applied to patients with ≥3 levels OPLL. As we previously reported, a postoperative increase in FSH can affect graft stability and lead to early implant migration [13]. The long lever arm created by long strut graft and fixation with four screws in the ACCF technique often stresses the screws and sometimes results in graft dislodgement [20]. A biomechanical study demonstrated that the hybrid technique was more effective for strengthening cervical stability and reconstructing sagittal alignment compared with the ACCF technique [33]. We also found that the fusion rate was significantly higher in the hybrid group at 1 year after the surgery. Taken together, our findings and previous findings indicate that the placement of two additional anchors in the hybrid technique can reduce stress on the proximal and distal screws and prevent loosening of the screws and graft dislodgement.

In this study, C2–7 lordotic angle and C-SVA were improved in both the ACCF and hybrid groups. Various studies have shown improvement and maintenance of cervical sagittal alignment after anterior cervical surgery [8,10,20,21]. This suggests that complete anterior decompression of ossified lesions may allow patients to assume a posture with more extension of the cervical spine. However, repeated micromotion can loosen the screws and could lead to severe reconstruction failure even while wearing a neck collar postoperatively. Particularly in cervical OPLL in patients with ankylosing spondylitis, reconstruction surgery with rigid fixation should be applied for the affected levels adjacent to the lesion. Interestingly, the prevalence of diffuse idiopathic skeletal hyperostosis (DISH) w shown to be approximately 45% in cervical OPLL patients [34,35]. Other observational studies have also demonstrated that multiple ossified lesions in the cervical spine often coexist with ossification of the spinal ligaments in the thoracolumbar spine [34,36–38]. In our study, of the four patients who underwent secondary surgery due to early implant failure in the ACCF group, three had DISH. Therefore, reconstruction surgery with rigid fixation and adequate structural alignments, such as hybrid fusion or anterior pedicle screw fixation [39], should be performed for cervical OPLL in patients with ankylosing thoracic spondylitis.

This study has several limitations. First, this was a retrospective study with a relatively small number of subjects and heterogeneity in terms of the implants used. Second, the degree of preservation of the cephalic and caudal endplates was not consistent in our series, although it was preserved as much as possible. Third, we could not assess factors associated with the location of the graft or screw angle and length. Fourth, these two techniques were performed by several independent surgeons. Fifth, the period was different between the two methods. Nevertheless, despite these limitations, our study highlights the fact that FSH should not be increased extremely after graft placement and plating should be carried out to prevent postoperative graft dislodgement in ACCF. Additionally, the hybrid fusion procedure is recommended for multilevel cervical OPLL in patients with ankylosing spondylitis to achieve sufficient stability of fused segments.

5. Conclusions

This study is the first to compare conventional ACCF and the hybrid fusion technique focusing exclusively on patients with severe OPLL involving three or more levels. Although both procedures can achieve satisfactory neurologic outcomes in patients with multilevel OPLL, hybrid fusion was superior to the conventional ACCF technique in terms of fusion rate and perioperative graft stability.

Author Contributions: Conceptualization, T.H., T.Y. (Toshitaka Yoshii), K.S. (Kenichiro Sakai) and A.O.; Data collection, H.I., M.Y., T.Y. (Tsuyoshi Yamada), Y.M., S.U., S.M., S.E., H.O., Y.K., K.U., J.H., A.K., T.T. (Tomoyuki Tanaka), T.M., T.T. (Takuya Takahashi), and M.H.; Formal Analysis, T.H., M.Y. and T.K.; Writing—Original Draft Preparation, T.H., H.I., Y.A. and A.O.; Software, Validation, T.H., T.Y. (Toshitaka Yoshii) T.H., T.Y. (Tsuyoshi Yamada), K.S. (Kentaro Sakaeda) and S.K., A.O.; T.Y (Toshitaka Yoshii) and Y.A.; Funding Acquisition, T.H., T.Y. (Tsuyoshi Yamada), T.K., K.S. (Kenichiro Sakai) and

A.O.; Writing—Review and Editing, T.H. and Y.A. All authors have read and agreed to the published version of the manuscript.

Funding: This research was supported by a Health and Labor Science Research grant (201610008B).

Institutional Review Board Statement: The study was conducted in accordance with the Declaration of Helsinki, and the study was approved by our institutional ethics committee (M2017-118).

Informed Consent Statement: Informed consent was obtained from all subjects involved in the study.

Data Availability Statement: Detailed data are available on request from corresponding author.

Acknowledgments: We thank Nobuko Nakajima, Yukiko Oya, Mika Morikawa and Namiko Katayama for data collection.

Conflicts of Interest: The authors declare no conflict of interest. The sponsors had no role in the design, execution, interpretation, or writing of the study.

References

1. Matsunaga, S.; Kukita, M.; Hayashi, K.; Shinkura, R.; Koriyama, C.; Sakou, T.; Komiya, S. Pathogenesis of myelopathy in patients with ossification of the posterior longitudinal ligament. *J. Neurosurg.* **2002**, *96*, 168–172. [CrossRef] [PubMed]
2. Matsunaga, S.; Sakou, T. Ossification of the posterior longitudinal ligament of the cervical spine: Etiology and natural history. *Spine (Phila Pa 1976)* **2012**, *37*, E309–E314. [CrossRef]
3. Sasaki, E.; Ono, A.; Yokoyama, T.; Wada, K.; Tanaka, T.; Kumagai, G.; Iwasaki, H.; Takahashi, I.; Umeda, T.; Nakaji, S.; et al. Prevalence and symptom of ossification of posterior longitudinal ligaments in the Japanese general population. *J. Orthop. Sci.* **2014**, *19*, 405–411. [CrossRef]
4. Nouri, A.; Martin, A.R.; Mikulis, D.; Fehlings, M.G. Magnetic resonance imaging assessment of degenerative cervical myelopathy: A review of structural changes and measurement techniques. *Neurosurg. Focus* **2016**, *40*, E5. [CrossRef] [PubMed]
5. Iwasaki, M.; Okuda, S.; Miyauchi, A.; Sakaura, H.; Mukai, Y.; Yonenobu, K.; Yoshikawa, H. Surgical strategy for cervical myelopathy due to ossification of the posterior longitudinal ligament: Part 1: Clinical results and limitations of laminoplasty. *Spine (Phila Pa 1976)* **2007**, *32*, 647–653. [CrossRef]
6. Iwasaki, M.; Okuda, S.; Miyauchi, A.; Sakaura, H.; Mukai, Y.; Yonenobu, K.; Yoshikawa, H. Surgical strategy for cervical myelopathy due to ossification of the posterior longitudinal ligament: Part 2: Advantages of anterior decompression and fusion over laminoplasty. *Spine (Phila Pa 1976)* **2007**, *32*, 654–660. [CrossRef] [PubMed]
7. Sumi, M. Updates on ossification of posterior longitudinal ligament. Conservative treatments for OPLL. *Clin. Calcium.* **2009**, *19*, 1480–1485. [CrossRef] [PubMed]
8. Yoshii, T.; Sakai, K.; Hirai, T.; Yamada, T.; Inose, H.; Kato, T.; Enomoto, M.; Tomizawa, S.; Kawabata, S.; Arai, Y.; et al. Anterior decompression with fusion versus posterior decompression with fusion for massive cervical ossification of the posterior longitudinal ligament with a ≥50% canal occupying ratio: A multicenter retrospective study. *Spine J.* **2016**, *16*, 1351–1357. [CrossRef]
9. Youssef, J.A.; Heiner, A.D.; Montgomery, J.R.; Tender, G.C.; Lorio, M.P.; Morreale, J.M.; Phillips, F.M. Outcomes of posterior cervical fusion and decompression: A systematic review and meta-analysis. *Spine J.* **2019**, *19*, 1714–1729. [CrossRef]
10. Hirai, T.; Okawa, A.; Arai, Y.; Takahashi, M.; Kawabata, S.; Kato, T.; Enomoto, M.; Tomizawa, S.; Sakai, K.; Torigoe, I.; et al. Middle-term results of a prospective comparative study of anterior decompression with fusion and posterior decompression with laminoplasty for the treatment of cervical spondylotic myelopathy. *Spine (Phila Pa 1976)* **2011**, *36*, 1940–1947. [CrossRef] [PubMed]
11. Katz, A.D.; Mancini, N.; Karukonda, T.; Cote, M.; Moss, I.L. Comparative and Predictor Analysis of 30-day Readmission, Reoperation, and Morbidity in Patients Undergoing Multilevel ACDF Versus Single and Multilevel ACCF Using the ACS-NSQIP Dataset. *Spine (Phila Pa 1976)* **2019**, *44*, E1379–E1387. [CrossRef] [PubMed]
12. Ashkenazi, E.; Smorgick, Y.; Rand, N.; Millgram, M.A.; Mirovsky, Y.; Floman, Y. Anterior decompression combined with corpectomies and discectomies in the management of multilevel cervical myelopathy: A hybrid decompression and fixation technique. *J. Neurosurg. Spine* **2005**, *3*, 205–209. [CrossRef] [PubMed]
13. Liu, Y.; Qi, M.; Chen, H.; Yang, L.; Wang, X.; Shi, G.; Gao, R.; Wang, C.; Yuan, W. Comparative analysis of complications of different reconstructive techniques following anterior decompression for multilevel cervical spondylotic myelopathy. *Eur. Spine J.* **2012**, *21*, 2428–2435. [CrossRef] [PubMed]
14. Wei-Bing, X.; Wun-Jer, S.; Gang, L.; Yue, Z.; Ming-Xi, J.; Lian-Shun, J. Reconstructive techniques study after anterior decompression of multilevel cervical spondylotic myelopathy. *J. Spinal Disord. Tech.* **2009**, *22*, 511–515. [CrossRef] [PubMed]
15. Badhiwala, J.H.; Leung, S.N.; Ellenbogen, Y.; Akbar, M.A.; Martin, A.R.; Jiang, F.; Wilson, J.R.F.; Nassiri, F.; Witiw, C.D.; Wilson, J.R.; et al. A comparison of the perioperative outcomes of anterior surgical techniques for the treatment of multilevel degenerative cervical myelopathy. *J. Neurosurg. Spine* **2020**, 1–8. [CrossRef]
16. von Elm, E.; Altman, D.G.; Egger, M.; Pocock, S.J.; Gøtzsche, P.C.; Vandenbroucke, J.P.; Initiative, S. The Strengthening the Reporting of Observational Studies in Epidemiology (STROBE) statement: Guidelines for reporting observational studies. *Lancet* **2007**, *370*, 1453–1457. [CrossRef]

17. Sakai, K.; Yoshii, T.; Hirai, T.; Arai, Y.; Torigoe, I.; Tomori, M.; Sato, H.; Okawa, A. Cervical sagittal imbalance is a predictor of kyphotic deformity after laminoplasty in cervical spondylotic myelopathy patients without preoperative kphotic alignment. *Spine (Phila Pa 1976)* **2016**, *41*, 299–305. [CrossRef]
18. Kim, T.H.; Lee, S.Y.; Kim, Y.C.; Park, M.S.; Kim, S.W. T1 slope as a predictor of kyphotic alignment change after laminoplasty in patients with cervical myelopathy. *Spine (Phila Pa 1976)* **2013**, *38*, E992–E997. [CrossRef]
19. Kim, M.K.; Kim, S.M.; Jeon, K.M.; Kim, T.S. Radiographic comparison of four anterior fusion procedures in two level cervical disc diseases: Autograft plate fixation versus cage plate fixation versus stand-alone cage fusion versus corpectomy and plate fixation. *J. Korean Neurosurg. Soc.* **2012**, *51*, 135–140. [CrossRef]
20. Hirai, T.; Yoshii, T.; Egawa, S.; Sakai, K.; Inose, H.; Yuasa, M.; Yamada, T.; Ushio, S.; Kato, T.; Arai, Y.; et al. Increased height of fused segments contributes to early-phase strut dislodgement after anterior cervical corpectomy with fusion for multilevel ossification of the posterior longitudinal ligament. *Spine Surg. Relat. Res.* **2020**, *4*, 294–299. [CrossRef]
21. Sakai, K.; Okawa, A.; Takahashi, M.; Arai, Y.; Kawabata, S.; Enomoto, M.; Kato, T.; Hirai, T.; Shinomiya, K. Five-year follow-up evaluation of surgical treatment for cervical myelopathy caused by ossification of the posterior longitudinal ligament: A prospective comparative study of anterior decompression and fusion with floating method versus laminoplasty. *Spine (Phila Pa 1976)* **2012**, *37*, 367–376. [CrossRef]
22. Fujiyoshi, T.; Yamazaki, M.; Kawabe, J.; Endo, T.; Furuya, T.; Koda, M.; Okawa, A.; Takahashi, K.; Konishi, H. A new concept for making decisions regarding the surgical approach for cervical ossification of the posterior longitudinal ligament: The K-line. *Spine (Phila Pa 1976)* **2008**, *33*, E990–E993. [CrossRef]
23. Hirai, T.; Kawabata, S.; Enomoto, M.; Kato, T.; Tomizawa, S.; Sakai, K.; Yoshii, T.; Sakaki, K.; Shinomiya, K.; Okawa, A. Presence of anterior compression of the spinal cord after laminoplasty inhibits upper extremity motor recovery in patients with cervical spondylotic myelopathy. *Spine (Phila Pa 1976)* **2012**, *37*, 377–384. [CrossRef] [PubMed]
24. Caspar, W.; Pitzen, T.; Papavero, L.; Geisler, F.H.; Johnson, T.A. Anterior cervical plating for the treatment of neoplasms in the cervical vertebrae. *J. Neurosurg.* **1999**, *90*, 27–34. [CrossRef]
25. Hou, Y.; Liang, L.; Shi, G.D.; Xu, P.; Xu, G.H.; Shi, J.G.; Yuan, W. Comparing effects of cervical anterior approach and laminoplasty in surgical management of cervical ossification of posterior longitudinal ligament by a prospective nonrandomized controlled study. *Orthop. Traumatol. Surg. Res.* **2017**, *103*, 733–740. [CrossRef] [PubMed]
26. Liu, H.; Li, Y.; Chen, Y.; Wu, W.; Zou, D. Cervical curvature, spinal cord MRIT2 signal, and occupying ratio impact surgical approach selection in patients with ossification of the posterior longitudinal ligament. *Eur. Spine J.* **2013**, *22*, 1480–1488. [CrossRef]
27. Tani, T.; Ushida, T.; Ishida, K.; Iai, H.; Noguchi, T.; Yamamoto, H. Relative safety of anterior microsurgical decompression versus laminoplasty for cervical myelopathy with a massive ossified posterior longitudinal ligament. *Spine (Phila Pa 1976)* **2002**, *27*, 2491–2498. [CrossRef]
28. Ryu, W.H.A.; Platt, A.; Deutsch, H. Hybrid decompression and reconstruction technique for cervical spondylotic myelopathy: Case series and review of the literature. *J. Spine Surg.* **2020**, *6*, 181–195. [CrossRef] [PubMed]
29. Liu, J.M.; Peng, H.W.; Liu, Z.L.; Long, X.H.; Yu, Y.Q.; Huang, S.H. Hybrid decompression technique versus anterior cervical corpectomy and fusion for treating multilevel cervical spondylotic myelopathy: Which one is better? *World Neurosurg.* **2015**, *84*, 2022–2029. [CrossRef] [PubMed]
30. Wang, T.; Tian, X.M.; Liu, S.K.; Wang, H.; Zhang, Y.-Z.; Ding, W.-Y. Prevalence of complications after surgery in treatment for cervical compressive myelopathy: A meta-analysis for last decade. *Medicine (Baltimore)* **2017**, *96*, e6421. [CrossRef]
31. Vaccaro, A.R.; Falatyn, S.P.; Scuderi, G.J.; Eismont, F.J.; McGuire, R.A.; Singh, K.; Garfin, S.R. Early failure of long segment anterior cervical plate fixation. *J. Spinal Disord.* **1998**, *11*, 410–415. [CrossRef] [PubMed]
32. Okawa, A.; Sakai, K.; Hirai, T.; Kato, T.; Tomizawa, S.; Enomoto, M.; Kawabata, S.; Takahashi, M.; Shinomiya, K. Risk factors for early reconstruction failure of multilevel cervical corpectomy with dynamic plate fixation. *Spine (Phila Pa 1976)* **2011**, *36*, E582–E587. [CrossRef] [PubMed]
33. Singh, K.; Vaccaro, A.R.; Kim, J.; Lorenz, E.P.; Lim, T.-H.; An, H.S. Enhancement of stability following anterior cervical corpectomy: A biomechanical study. *Spine (Phila Pa 1976)* **2004**, *29*, 845–849. [CrossRef]
34. Nishimura, S.; Nagoshi, N.; Iwanami, A.; Takeuchi, A.; Hirai, T.; Yoshii, T.; Takeuchi, K.; Mori, K.; Yamada, T.; Seki, S.; et al. Prevalence and Distribution of Diffuse Idiopathic Skeletal Hyperostosis on Whole-spine Computed Tomography in Patients With Cervical Ossification of the Posterior Longitudinal Ligament: A Multicenter Study. *Clin. Spine Surg.* **2018**, *31*, E460–E465. [CrossRef]
35. Hirai, T.; Nishimura, S.; Yoshii, T.; Nagoshi, N.; Hashimoto, J.; Mori, K.; Maki, S.; Katsumi, K.; Takeuchi, K.; Ushio, S.; et al. Associations between Clinical Findings and Severity of Diffuse Idiopathic Skeletal Hyperostosis in Patients with Ossification of the Posterior Longitudinal Ligament. *J. Clin. Med.* **2021**, *10*, 4137. [CrossRef]
36. Hirai, T.; Yoshii, T.; Iwanami, A.; Takeuchi, K.; Mori, K.; Yamada, T.; Wada, K.; Koda, M.; Matsuyama, Y.; Takeshita, K.; et al. Prevalence and distribution of ossified lesions in the whole spine of patients with cervical ossification of the posterior longitudinal ligament a multicenter study (JOSL CT study). *PLoS ONE* **2016**, *11*, e0160117. [CrossRef]
37. Mori, K.; Yoshii, T.; Hirai, T.; Iwanami, A.; Takeuchi, K.; Yamada, T.; Seki, S.; Tsuji, T.; Fujiyoshi, K.; Furukawa, M.; et al. Prevalence and distribution of ossification of the supra/interspinous ligaments in symptomatic patients with cervical ossification of the posterior longitudinal ligament of the spine: A CT-based multicenter cross-sectional study. *BMC Musculoskelet. Disord.* **2016**, *17*, 492. [CrossRef]

38. Yoshii, T.; Hirai, T.; Iwanami, A.; Nagoshi, N.; Takeuchi, K.; Mori, K.; Yamada, T.; Seki, S.; Tsuji, T.; Fujiyoshi, K.; et al. Co-existence of ossification of the nuchal ligament is associated with severity of ossification in the whole spine in patients with cervical ossification of the posterior longitudinal ligament -A multi-center CT study. *J. Orthop. Sci.* **2019**, *24*, 35–41. [CrossRef]
39. Aramomi, M.; Masaki, Y.; Koshizuka, S.; Kadota, R.; Okawa, A.; Koda, M.; Yamazaki, M. Anterior pedicle screw fixation for multilevel cervical corpectomy and spinal fusion. *Acta Neurochir.* **2008**, *150*, 575–582. [CrossRef] [PubMed]

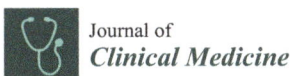

Article

Cervical Spinal Alignment Change Accompanying Spondylosis Exposes Harmonization Failure with Total Spinal Balance: A Japanese Cohort Survey Randomly Sampled from a Basic Resident Registry

Shota Ikegami [1,2], Masashi Uehara [1,*], Ryosuke Tokida [2], Hikaru Nishimura [2], Noriko Sakai [3], Hiroshi Horiuchi [1,2], Hiroyuki Kato [1] and Jun Takahashi [1]

[1] Department of Orthopaedic Surgery, Shinshu University School of Medicine, 3-1-1 Asahi, Matsumoto 390-8621, Nagano, Japan; sh.ikegami@gmail.com (S.I.); horiuchih@aol.com (H.H.); hirokato@shinshu-u.ac.jp (H.K.); jtaka@shinshu-u.ac.jp (J.T.)
[2] Rehabilitation Center, Shinshu University Hospital, 3-1-1 Asahi, Matsumoto 390-8621, Nagano, Japan; tryosuke@shinshu-u.ac.jp (R.T.); hikaru5@shinshu-u.ac.jp (H.N.)
[3] Department of Orthopaedic Surgery, New Life Hospital, Obuse, Nagano 381-0295, Kamitakai-gun, Japan; wpowaro@yahoo.co.jp
* Correspondence: masashi_u560613@yahoo.co.jp; Tel.: +81-263-37-2659; Fax: +81-263-35-8844

Abstract: The relationship between spinal posture and quality of life has garnered considerable attention with the increase in older community-dwelling residents. However, details of this association remain insufficient. A recent Japanese population cohort epidemiological locomotion survey (the Obuse study) revealed that the C2–C7 cervical sagittal vertical axis (CSVA) began to increase in males from their 60s, but not in females. This study aimed to clarify the pathology of these cervical spondylotic changes. A total of 411 participants (202 male and 209 female) aged between 50 and 89 years were selected by random sampling from a cooperating town's resident registry. All participants underwent lateral X-ray photography in a standing position for the measurement of several sagittal spinal alignment parameters, including CSVA, C2–C7 cervical lordosis (CL), T1 slope (T1S), and sagittal vertical axis (SVA). The presence of cervical spondylotic changes was also recorded. Associations of cervical sagittal spinal alignment with cervical spondylosis and between cervical and total sagittal spinal alignment were examined. The prevalence of cervical spondylosis was significantly higher in males (81%) than in females (70%) ($p = 0.01$). CL was significantly smaller in cervical spondylosis subjects when adjusted by age (3.4 degrees less; $p = 0.01$). T1S minus CL displayed a moderate positive correlation with CSVA in both males and females (r = 0.49 and 0.48, respectively, both $p < 0.01$). In males only, CSVA and CL showed weak positive correlations with SVA (r = 0.31 and 0.22, respectively, both $p < 0.01$) independently of age. Cervical spinal misalignment was more clearly associated with diminished SF-8™ scores in females than in males. In community-dwelling elderly residents, cervical sagittal spinal alignment change accompanying cervical spondylosis manifested as hypofunction to compensate for whole-spine imbalance.

Keywords: epidemiological study; resident cohort; resident registry; spinal alignment; spinal balance; cervical spine; aging; gender; adult spine

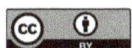

1. Introduction

Sagittal spinal alignment is more strongly correlated than coronal spinal alignment to health-related quality of life (HRQOL) [1] even for mild spinal deformity, which can be an important barometer of health status for ordinary citizens. Sagittal spinal alignment deteriorates with age in community-dwelling older people [2–4]. In addition, an increase in sagittal vertical axis (SVA; anteriorization of the center of gravity line of the cervical spine base) is associated with a decrease in lumbar lordosis [5]. Age-related changes in lumbo-pelvic condition are known to affect sagittal spinal alignment. Two epidemiological studies conducted in different regions corroborated the finding of a characteristic gender difference in the process of spinal alignment change with aging. Specifically, alignment changes over time in males were prominent in the cervical spine region, while females predominantly displayed changes in the lumbo-pelvic area [3,4]. However, no clear evidence has been presented on the reasons for such phenomena. Spinal alignment can be affected by a variety of factors, including activity level and profession. Age-related cervical spondylosis may contribute to poor alignment of the cervical spine [6]. This study aimed to clarify the pathomechanism of sagittal cervical alignment changes in community-dwelling older residents.

2. Materials and Methods

2.1. Creation of a Randomly Sampled Resident Cohort for Epidemiological Survey

In the establishment of a new population study of Japanese people, we employed random sampling from the basic resident registry of a cooperating town to minimize selection bias and obtain a cohort representative of the general population. Residents between the age of 50 and 89 years were randomly sampled from the basic resident registry of a town to construct a 415-participant cohort termed "the Obuse study" cohort. "Obuse" is the name of the cooperating town located in the central inland area of Japan, with a population of approximately 10,000 people. The Obuse study is a comprehensive investigation on the locomotion health of community-dwelling older people. In the Obuse study cohort, 411 individuals who were able to stand unassisted and whose cervical spinal alignment could be measured were subjected to analysis. According to participant interview results, 21 subjects with a history of thoracolumbar spondylosis and five with a history of rheumatoid arthritis were included. As they were not in such a condition that would cause them to lose their standing balance, they were added to the analysis. Individuals with spinal instrumentation surgery were not included, and those with diagnosed illnesses that significantly altered balance, such as adult spinal deformity and Parkinson's disease, were excluded as well.

2.2. X-ray Examination and Measurement of Spinal Alignment

All participants underwent lateral X-ray photography for the measurement of sagittal spinal alignment parameters, including C2–C7 sagittal vertical axis (CSVA; the distance between a plumb line from the center of the C2 vertebral body and posterior superior corner of C7), C2–C7 cervical lordosis (CL; the angle between the C2 inferior endplate and C7 inferior endplate), T1 slope (T1S), and SVA. The average values of measurements by two board-certified spine surgeons and a trained staff member were used for each parameter. The inter-rater reliability of each parameter was as follows: 0.96 for CSVA, 0.88 for CL, 0.88 for T1S, and 0.95 for SVA. The presence of cervical spondylotic changes was also recorded. The two spine surgeons independently determined the presence or absence of spondylotic changes, with cases determined as having spondylosis by both raters being regarded as spondylotic (inter-rater reliability: 0.95). Osteophyte formation around the vertebral endplates with a loss of intervertebral disc height as well as osteophyte formation and osteosclerotic change of the articular facet joints were defined as spondylotic changes.

2.3. HRQOL Assessments

SF-8™ Health Survey measures were determined for all participants for HRQOL evaluation. Results were calculated and expressed as two summary scores: physical component summary (PCS) and mental component summary (MCS).

2.4. Statistical Analysis

We compared cervical sagittal spinal alignment parameters between spondylotic and non-spondylotic groups using linear regression models. The response variable was the alignment parameter and the explanatory variables were the presence of cervical spondylosis and age. The Pearson correlation coefficient between T1S minus CL, which is also known as the residual lordotic compensation for subcervical anterior tilting [7], and CSVA were assessed for each gender. We examined the correlation between cervical and subcervical alignment parameters following age adjustment for each gender. For other analyses, Welch's t-test was used to compare quantitative variables, and Fisher's exact test was used to compare qualitative variables. Statistical analyses were carried out using the statistical package R, version 3.4.3 (available at http://www.r-project.org accessed on 26 November 2021). The level of significance was set at $p < 0.05$.

3. Results

Table 1 shows the baseline characteristics of the Obuse study cohort. The 411 participants were almost uniformly divided into every gender/age decade category. Tertiary industry workers represented the majority of Obuse town residents in their 50s, although this proportion decreased for subjects in their 60s, likely due to mandatory retirement. Table 2 shows the spinal alignment distributions by gender. Overall CSVA and T1S were significantly larger in males (both $p < 0.01$), with no remarkable gender differences for CL or SVA ($p = 0.54$ and $p = 0.96$, respectively). The prevalence of cervical spondylosis in males and females was 80.7% and 69.9% respectively (Table 2). Cervical spondylotic change was significantly more frequent in males ($p = 0.01$, Fisher's exact test). There were no remarkable differences for CSVA or CL in subjects with or without spondylosis. The odds ratios, 95% confidence intervals, and p-values for spinal parameters were as follows: CSVA, −0.6 (−3.8, 2.5), $p = 0.70$; and CL, −1.0 (−3.7, 1.6), $p = 0.45$. CL became significantly smaller in subjects with cervical spondylosis when adjusted by age (−3.4 (−6.1, −0.7), $p = 0.01$) (Figure 1).

Table 1. Baseline characteristics of the study cohort.

Gender	Age (Years)	Number	Height (cm)	Weight (kg)	BMI (kg/m^2)	Job (Pri; Sec; Ter; None)
Male	50s	50	171.8 (6.0)	67.1 (9.1)	22.7 (2.9)	3; 7; 40; 0
	60s	53	166.7 (4.7)	66.9 (7.7)	24.1 (2.7)	18; 5; 19; 11
	70s	54	163.1 (5.0)	59.9 (10.3)	22.4 (3.5)	22; 2; 7; 23
	80s	45	160.1 (5.7)	57.5 (8.5)	22.4 (2.8)	19; 0; 3; 23
	All	202	165.5 (6.8)	63.0 (9.8)	22.9 (3.1)	62; 14; 69; 57
Female	50s	47	158.1 (4.9)	55.4 (9.0)	22.2 (3.8)	5; 4; 29; 9
	60s	61	152.8 (5.4)	52.2 (7.6)	22.3 (2.8)	21; 4; 17; 19
	70s	53	149.8 (5.2)	50.7 (8.0)	22.5 (3.2)	16; 3; 8; 26
	80s	48	144.6 (5.9)	48.3 (7.9)	23.1 (3.3)	11; 0; 5; 32
	All	209	151.4 (7.1)	51.6 (8.4)	22.5 (3.3)	53; 11; 59; 86

Notes: Values represent the mean (standard deviation). Primary industry jobs included agriculture and forestry. Secondary industry jobs involved manufacturing and construction. Tertiary industry jobs included food service and education. Abbreviations: BMI, body mass index; Pri, primary industry; Sec, secondary industry; Ter, tertiary industry.

Table 2. Tabulation results of spine parameters and SF8[TM] summary scores.

Age (Years)	Number	CSVA (mm)	CL (deg.)	T1S (deg.)	SVA (mm)	Presence of Spondylosis	PCS (Points)	MCS (Points)
Male								
50s	50	23.1 (13.9)	10.5 (10.3)	25.3 (5.9)	5.8 (25.8)	66.0%	50.2 (6.4)	49.0 (6.0)
60s	53	28.4 (15.0)	9.1 (11.1)	27.3 (8.4)	9.1 (37.9)	69.8%	50.1 (7.0)	49.5 (5.3)
70s	54	29.1 (12.1)	13.3 (12.1)	28.4 (8.5)	21.7 (30.5)	88.9%	46.8 (7.0)	50.5 (5.3)
80s	45	30.8 (17.0)	13.6 (15.1)	31.2 (9.9)	56.7 (48.6)	100.0%	43.6 (8.7)	52.0 (6.8)
All	202	27.8 (14.7)	11.6 (12.2)	28.0 (8.4)	22.2 (40.9)	80.7%	47.8 (7.7)	50.2 (5.9)
Female								
50s	47	17.8 (10.9)	8.6 (10.4)	22.8 (6.9)	−5.4 (26.3)	46.8%	50.7 (5.6)	46.6 (7.1)
60s	61	15.6 (7.7)	8.7 (9.1)	22.1 (7.2)	4.7 (29.5)	67.2%	50.1 (5.8)	50.1 (4.8)
70s	53	17.4 (10.1)	13.3 (11.0)	25.1 (10.3)	31.2 (36.3)	75.5%	46.5 (7.5)	49.9 (6.1)
80s	48	18.6 (15.6)	19.2 (12.2)	30.1 (13.6)	60.9 (59.7)	89.6%	42.0 (8.7)	50.7 (6.8)
All	209	17.2 (11.2)	12.3 (11.4)	24.8 (10.2)	22.1 (46.6)	69.9%	47.5 (7.7)	49.4 (6.3)

Note: Values represent the mean (standard deviation). Abbreviations: CSVA, C2-C7 sagittal vertical axis; CL, C2-C7 cervical lordosis; T1S, T1 slope; SVA, sagittal vertical axis; PCS, SF-8[TM] physical component summary score; MCS, SF-8[TM] mental component summary score.

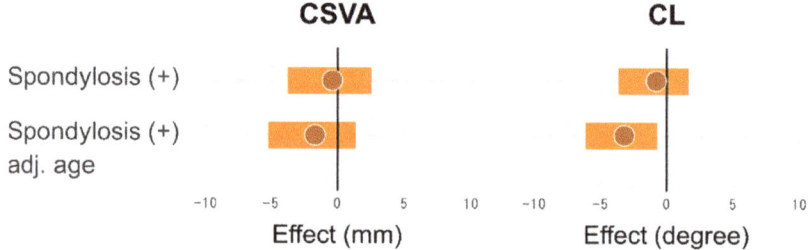

Figure 1. Impact of cervical spondylosis on cervical alignment parameters. Note: Bands represent 95% confidence interval. Abbreviations: CSVA, cervical sagittal vertical axis; CL, cervical lordosis; adj. age, multivariate analysis adjusted by age.

T1S minus CL displayed a significant moderate positive correlation with CSVA in both genders (Pearson correlation coefficient: 0.49 for males and 0.48 for females, both $p < 0.01$) (Figure 2). Only in males, however, did both CSVA and CL show mild positive correlations with SVA independently of age (Figure 3 and Table 3).

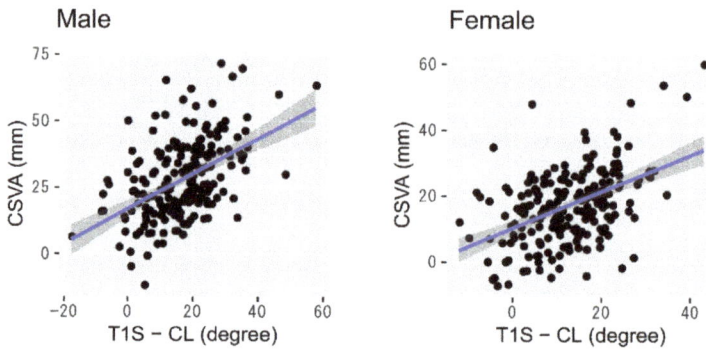

Figure 2. Relationship between cervical anteriorization and T1S minus CL. Abbreviations: CSVA, cervical sagittal vertical axis; T1S, T1 slope; CL, cervical lordosis.

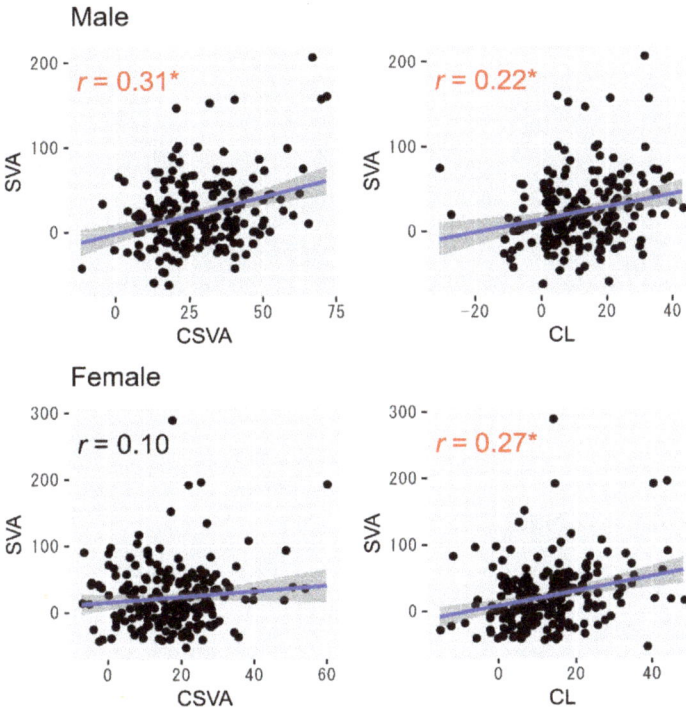

Figure 3. Relationship between subcervical alignment and cervical alignment parameters. Note: * denotes a significant association ($p < 0.05$). Abbreviations: SVA, sagittal vertical axis; CSVA, cervical sagittal vertical axis; CL, cervical lordosis.

Table 3. Relationship between subcervical alignment and cervical alignment parameters with and without age adjustment.

	Crude		Age-Adjusted	
	Correlation Coefficient	p-Value	Correlation Coefficient	p-Value
Male				
SVA and CSVA	0.31	<0.01 *	0.25	<0.01 *
SVA and CL	0.22	<0.01 *	0.20	<0.01 *
Female				
SVA and CSVA	0.10	0.15	0.07	0.31
SVA and CL	0.27	<0.01 *	0.09	0.19

Note: * denotes a significant difference ($p < 0.05$). Abbreviations: SVA, sagittal vertical axis; CSVA, cervical sagittal vertical axis; CL, cervical lordosis.

Tables 4 and 5 summarize how cervical and subcervical spinal alignment impacted HRQOL. Specifically, larger SVA was significantly associated with a lower PCS score in both genders independently of age. CSVA associated significantly with PCS score in females only, which was independent of age. Larger T1S minus CL was also significantly related to lower PCS scores after adjustment for age in women, with no clear association between cervical spinal alignment and HRQOL in men (Table 4). No remarkable associations were observed for cervical or subcervical spinal alignment among MCS scores (Table 5).

Table 4. Effects of cervical alignment parameters on SF-8™ physical component summary scores.

	Crude		Age-Adjusted	
	Effect	p-Value	Effect	p-Value
Male				
CSVA (+10 mm)	0.0 ± 0.4	0.98	0.3 ± 0.4	0.43
T1S-CL (+10 degrees)	−0.9 ± 0.5	0.08	−0.8 ± 0.5	0.08
SVA (+10 mm)	−0.5 ± 0.1	<0.01 *	−0.3 ± 0.1	0.04 *
Female				
CSVA (+10 mm)	−1.4 ± 0.5	<0.01 *	−1.2 ± 0.4	<0.01 *
T1S-CL (+10 degrees)	−0.5 ± 0.6	0.33	−1.0 ± 0.5	0.04 *
SVA (+10 mm)	−0.7 ± 0.1	<0.01 *	−0.4 ± 0.1	<0.01 *

Notes: Effect values represent the mean ± standard error. * Denotes a significant difference ($p < 0.05$). Abbreviations: CSVA, C2–C7 sagittal vertical axis; T1S-CL, T1 slope minus C2–C7 cervical lordosis; SVA, sagittal vertical axis.

Table 5. Effects of cervical alignment parameters on SF-8™ mental component summary scores.

	Crude		Age-Adjusted	
	Effect	p-Value	Effect	p-Value
Male				
CSVA (+10 mm)	0.0 ± 0.3	0.90	−0.1 ± 0.3	0.74
T1S-CL (+10 degrees)	−0.2 ± 0.4	0.62	−0.2 ± 0.4	0.53
SVA (+10 mm)	0.2 ± 0.1	0.06	0.1 ± 0.1	0.48
Female				
CSVA (+10 mm)	−0.5 ± 0.4	0.21	−0.5 ± 0.4	0.22
T1S-CL (+10 degrees)	−0.7 ± 0.5	0.12	−0.6 ± 0.5	0.21
SVA (+10 mm)	0.1 ± 0.1	0.33	0.0 ± 0.1	0.68

Note: Effect values represent the mean ± standard error. Abbreviations: CSVA, C2–C7 sagittal vertical axis; T1S-CL, T1 slope minus C2–C7 cervical lordosis; SVA, sagittal vertical axis.

4. Discussion

This study revealed that male community-dwelling elderly residents more frequently exhibited cervical spondylotic changes than female residents did, but without subaxial lordosis compensating for the anterior tilting of the subcervical spine. This non-compensation resulted in axis anteriorization accompanying deteriorated subcervical alignment. Thus, cervical sagittal spinal alignment deteriorations with cervical spondylosis may manifest as a compensatory function for diminished whole-spine balance rather than solely as a consequence of spinal degeneration.

The following is a possible pathomechanism of cervical decompensation, especially in males. First, SVA and T1S increase with aging [4]. However, there is insufficient lordotic compensation due to a range of motion decrease along with a higher prevalence of cervical spondylosis [6]. This leads to decompensated axis anteriorization. The cervical spine has variable normal morphology [8]. One author reported that SVA and T1S were important in determining cervical alignment [9]. A large T1S requires a correspondingly higher CL to preserve sagittal balance. Even in cervical laminoplasty patients, T1S is one of the most important factors determining postoperative cervical spinal alignment [10–12]. Figure 4 contrasts representative cervical spine alignment conditions. Cases A and B had virtually identical T1S. In Case A (female), CL suitable for T1S was formed such that the position of the center of gravity of the head was optimized and the front gaze posture was preserved. On the other hand, Case B (male) had obvious cervical spondylotic change and was unable to achieve CL suitable for T1S. As a result, the head has shifted anteriorly. Based on the results of this study, the A-type cervical spine may be less susceptible to changes in subcervical alignment, while the B-type spine may tend to situate more anteriorly due to its susceptibility to subcervical alignment.

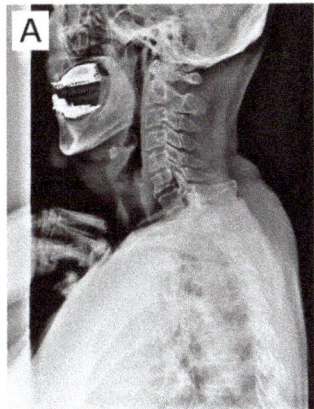 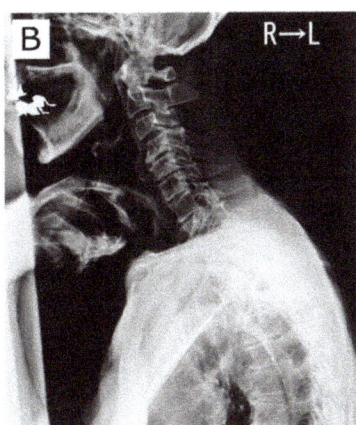

Figure 4. Effect of cervical spondylotic changes on cervical spine alignment. Notes: Case (**A**) (female) has a compensated cervical spine. Case (**B**) (male) has a decompensated cervical spine.

Larger values of either T1S minus CL or CSVA have been associated with low HRQOL condition in adult spinal deformity patients [13,14]. These cervical spine alignment parameters were also associated with the Neck Disability Index in cervical operation patients [15–17]. The subjects in our study were residents and not spinal deformity or cervical operation patients. Nevertheless, as with subcervical alignment, T1S minus CL and CSVA were significantly associated with HRQOL. It was noteworthy that these relationships between alignment parameters and HRQOL in cervical spine surgery patients were present even in pre-disease populations. However, such associations were significant only in females in our cohort. The reason for this gender difference is unclear and requires further examination. The effect size is small and may be irrelevant given the size of the effect.

Another study of 50–89-year-old Japanese residents (the TOEI study) showed that cervical deformity (i.e., CSVA $\geq$ 40 mm) residents had significantly lower HRQOL index scores [18]. Although the results in females agreed with our own, those for males did not. This could have been due to differences in the prevalence of cervical deformity in the target population; the TOEI study had cervical deformity prevalences of 31% for male and 9% for female, which were 19% and 2% respectively in this study and significantly lower ($p < 0.01$, Fisher's exact test). Our earlier studies revealed that the change in spinal alignment with aging in males first appears in the cervical spine and that an age-related increase in CSVA was not noticeable in females [4]. On the other hand, larger CSVA was associated with physical performance deterioration [19]. Insufficient physical performance affects HRQOL, even in healthy local residents [20]. Cervical spine anteriorization in females may occur in a low physical tolerance condition as compared to males.

Lastly, it is difficult to ascertain a direct causal relationship between mental health and spinal posture, and their precise association remains unclear. Although this study found no significant relationship between the factors, there have been reports of a link of recurring depressive episodes to poor spinal posture [21]. Health status is holistic, and clinically useful associations may be identified in the future for mental health and spinal posture.

The limitations of the current investigation include the possibility of inter-observer bias. The high concordance rate was proof that the evaluation was legitimate, but the possibility of bias risk could be further reduced by adding the evaluations of radiologists from a different specialty. As this research was cross-sectional, the direction of the causal relationship between spinal alignments could not be specified. Longitudinal surveys are needed to obtain a definitive conclusion on aging-dependent changes. In this non-compulsory survey, the proportion of people randomly sampled who were ultimately enrolled was less than one third, with 882 people refusing to participate, implying incomplete selection bias and participation bias elimination. Furthermore, no a priori calculations were made regarding a sample size that would ensure sufficient clinical variation to support conclusions that could be generalized; thus, the findings could have been influenced by the composition and prevalence of spondylosis and spinal deformity of the patients who agreed to participate. Regional characteristics were also a limitation of this study in that we sampled subjects from a relatively small town. Although the benefits of recruiting in such regions are lower resident displacement and greater ease in performing an epidemiological survey, the results may differ from those of urban-dwelling residents. Moreover, we could not prove the absence of selection bias by presenting the results of a cohort in one town. Previous papers [4] have shown that the spinal alignment status of Obuse residents was comparable to that from other parts of Japan, implying no particular physical characteristics in our test group, at least among the Japanese. On the other hand, it is very likely that other ethnic groups have different physical characteristics, and so further study is needed in other populations. This study analyzed the relationship among age, gender, and spinal alignment. Spinal alignment can also be affected by a variety of other factors, including activity level and profession. These will be addressed in future studies to deepen our findings. The mechanism of female alignment change could also not be ascertained in this report. Cervical spinal alignment change is more likely to occur in males, but the effects of changes in the cervical spine on HRQOL are more apparent in females. We suspect that cervical alignment is not linearly related to HRQOL, and that females with poor alignment may be subject to lower HRQOL than males with similar findings. Longitudinal studies on this point are needed.

5. Conclusions

In conclusion, cervical sagittal spinal alignment changes accompanying spondylosis in the general elderly population manifested as hypofunction to compensate for whole-spine imbalance. Men have a higher prevalence of cervical spondylosis, and their inflexible cervical spine has difficulty compensating for subcervical alignment deterioration. This is likely why males are more prone to large CSVA as a sagittal spinal misalignment. In contrast, cervical spinal misalignment was more clearly associated with low HRQOL in females.

Author Contributions: S.I. designed the study, performed the data analysis, and wrote the manuscript. M.U., R.T., H.N., N.S. and H.H. provided clinical experience and wrote the manuscript. H.K. and J.T. supervised the whole study. All authors read and approved the final manuscript.

Funding: This work was supported by a grant from the Japan Orthopaedics and Traumatology Research Foundation, Inc. (number: 339) as well as research funds from the Promotion Project of Education, Research, and Medical Care from Shinshu University Hospital, the Japanese Orthopaedic Association, the Japanese Society for Musculoskeletal Medicine, the Shinshu Public Utility Foundation for Promotion of Medical Sciences, and the Nakatomi Foundation.

Institutional Review Board Statement: This study was approved by the investigational review board of our hospital (approval number: 2792). Written consent was obtained from all participants. All research was conducted in accordance with the STROBE guidelines for observational research.

Informed Consent Statement: Informed consent was obtained from all subjects involved in the study.

Data Availability Statement: The complete database of the cohort can be accessed at the Zenodo repository (doi.org/10.5281/zenodo.5723125).

Acknowledgments: We thank Hironobu Sato of the Obuse Town Institute for Community Health Promotion, Takashi Igarashi of the Center for Clinical Research at Shinshu University Hospital, and the Obuse town office for sample selection in this study.

Conflicts of Interest: The authors declared no potential conflict of interest with respect to the research, authorship, and/or publication of this article.

References

1. Glassman, S.D.; Bridwell, K.H.; Dimar, J.R.; Horton, W.; Berven, S.; Schwab, F. The impact of positive sagittal balance in adult spinal deformity. *Spine* **2005**, *30*, 2024–2029. [CrossRef] [PubMed]
2. Oe, S.; Togawa, D.; Nakai, K.; Yamada, T.; Arima, H.; Banno, T.; Yasuda, T.; Kobayasi, S.; Yamato, Y.; Hasegawa, T.; et al. The influence of age and sex on cervical spinal alignment among volunteers aged over 50. *Spine* **2015**, *40*, 1487–1494. [CrossRef] [PubMed]
3. Asai, Y.; Tsutsui, S.; Oka, H.; Yoshimura, N.; Hashizume, H.; Yamada, H.; Akune, T.; Muraki, S.; Matsudaira, K.; Kawaguchi, H.; et al. Sagittal spino-pelvic alignment in adults: The Wakayama Spine Study. *PLoS ONE* **2017**, *12*, e0178697. [CrossRef] [PubMed]
4. Uehara, M.; Takahashi, J.; Ikegami, S.; Tokida, R.; Nishimura, H.; Sakai, N.; Kato, H. Sagittal spinal alignment deviation in the general elderly population: A Japanese cohort survey randomly sampled from a basic resident registry. *Spine J.* **2019**, *19*, 349–356. [CrossRef] [PubMed]
5. Cohen, L.; Pappas, E.; Refshauge, K.; Dennis, S.; Simic, M. Associations between potentially modifiable clinical factors and sagittal balance of the spine in older adults from the general population. *Spine Deform.* **2021**, in press. [CrossRef]
6. Ferrara, L.A. The biomechanics of cervical spondylosis. *Adv. Orthop.* **2012**, *2012*, 493605. [CrossRef] [PubMed]
7. Staub, B.N.; Lafage, R.; Kim, H.J.; Shaffrey, C.I.; Mundis, G.M.; Hostin, R.; Burton, D.; Lenke, L.; Gupta, M.C.; Ames, C.; et al. Cervical mismatch: The normative value of T1 slope minus cervical lordosis and its ability to predict ideal cervical lordosis. *J. Neurosurg. Spine* **2018**, *30*, 31–37. [CrossRef] [PubMed]
8. Hey, H.W.D.; Lau, E.T.; Wong, G.C.; Tan, K.A.; Liu, G.K.; Wong, H.K. Cervical Alignment Variations in Different Postures and Predictors of Normal Cervical Kyphosis: A New Understanding. *Spine* **2017**, *42*, 1614–1621. [CrossRef]
9. Lee, S.H.; Son, E.S.; Seo, E.M.; Suk, K.S.; Kim, K.T. Factors determining cervical spine sagittal balance in asymptomatic adults: Correlation with spinopelvic balance and thoracic inlet alignment. *Spine J.* **2015**, *15*, 705–712. [CrossRef] [PubMed]
10. Lin, B.J.; Hong, K.T.; Lin, C.; Chung, T.T.; Tang, C.T.; Hueng, D.Y.; Hsia, C.C.; Ju, D.T.; Ma, H.I.; Liu, M.Y.; et al. Impact of global spine balance and cervical regional alignment on determination of postoperative cervical alignment after laminoplasty. *Medicine* **2018**, *97*, e13111. [CrossRef]
11. Sharma, R.; Borkar, S.A.; Goda, R.; Kale, S.S. Which factors predict the loss of cervical lordosis following cervical laminoplasty? A review of various indices and their clinical implications. *Surg. Neurol. Int.* **2019**, *10*, 147. [CrossRef] [PubMed]
12. Kim, B.; Yoon, D.H.; Ha, Y.; Yi, S.; Shin, D.A.; Lee, C.K.; Lee, N.; Kim, K.N. Relationship between T1 slope and loss of lordosis after laminoplasty in patients with cervical ossification of the posterior longitudinal ligament. *Spine J.* **2016**, *16*, 219–225. [CrossRef] [PubMed]
13. Iyer, S.; Nemani, V.M.; Nguyen, J.; Elysee, J.; Burapachaisri, A.; Ames, C.P.; Kim, H.J. Impact of Cervical Sagittal Alignment Parameters on Neck Disability. *Spine* **2016**, *41*, 371–377. [CrossRef] [PubMed]
14. Protopsaltis, T.S.; Scheer, J.K.; Terran, J.S.; Smith, J.S.; Hamilton, D.K.; Kim, H.J.; Mundis, G.M., Jr.; Hart, R.A.; McCarthy, I.M.; Klineberg, E.; et al. How the neck affects the back: Changes in regional cervical sagittal alignment correlate to HRQOL improvement in adult thoracolumbar deformity patients at 2-year follow-up. *J. Neurosurg. Spine* **2015**, *23*, 153–158. [CrossRef]
15. Hyun, S.J.; Kim, K.J.; Jahng, T.A.; Kim, H.J. Relationship Between T1 Slope and Cervical Alignment Following Multilevel Posterior Cervical Fusion Surgery: Impact of T1 Slope Minus Cervical Lordosis. *Spine* **2016**, *41*, E396–E402. [CrossRef]
16. Hyun, S.J.; Kim, K.J.; Jahng, T.A.; Kim, H.J. Clinical Impact of T1 Slope Minus Cervical Lordosis After Multilevel Posterior Cervical Fusion Surgery: A Minimum 2-Year Follow Up Data. *Spine* **2017**, *42*, 1859–1864. [CrossRef] [PubMed]
17. Lan, Z.; Huang, Y.; Xu, W. Relationship Between T1 Slope Minus C2-7 Lordosis and Cervical Alignment Parameters After Adjacent 2-Level Anterior Cervical Diskectomy and Fusion of Lower Cervical Spine. *World Neurosurg.* **2019**, *122*, e1195–e1201. [CrossRef] [PubMed]
18. Oe, S.; Togawa, D.; Yoshida, G.; Hasegawa, T.; Yamato, Y.; Kobayashi, S.; Yasuda, T.; Banno, T.; Mihara, Y.; Matsuyama, Y. Difference in Spinal Sagittal Alignment and Health-Related Quality of Life between Males and Females with Cervical Deformity. *Asian Spine J.* **2017**, *11*, 959–967. [CrossRef]
19. Tokida, R.; Uehara, M.; Ikegami, S.; Takahashi, J.; Nishimura, H.; Sakai, N.; Kato, H. Association Between Sagittal Spinal Alignment and Physical Function in the Japanese General Elderly Population: A Japanese Cohort Survey Randomly Sampled from a Basic Resident Registry. *J. Bone Joint Surg. Am.* **2019**, *101*, 1698–1706. [CrossRef]
20. Ikegami, S.; Takahashi, J.; Uehara, M.; Tokida, R.; Nishimura, H.; Sakai, A.; Kato, H. Physical performance reflects cognitive function, fall risk, and quality of life in community-dwelling older people. *Sci. Rep.* **2019**, *9*, 12242. [CrossRef] [PubMed]
21. Canales, J.Z.; Fiquer, J.T.; Campos, R.N.; Soeiro-de-Souza, M.G.; Moreno, R.A. Investigation of associations between recurrence of major depressive disorder and spinal posture alignment: A quantitative cross-sectional study. *Gait Posture* **2017**, *52*, 258–264. [CrossRef] [PubMed]

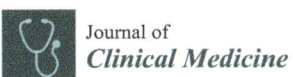

Article

Time Course of Acute Vertebral Fractures: A Prospective Multicenter Cohort Study

Hiroyuki Inose [1,*], Tsuyoshi Kato [2], Shinichi Shirasawa [3], Shinji Takahashi [4], Masatoshi Hoshino [5], Yu Yamato [6], Yu Matsukura [7], Takashi Hirai [7], Toshitaka Yoshii [7] and Atsushi Okawa [7]

1. Department of Orthopedic and Trauma Research, Graduate School, Tokyo Medical and Dental University, Tokyo 108-0075, Japan
2. Department of Orthopaedics, Ome Municipal General Hospital, Tokyo 198-0042, Japan; katoorth@gmail.com
3. Department of Orthopaedics, Suwa Central Hospital, Nagano 391-8503, Japan; sshirasawa@aol.com
4. Department of Orthopedic Surgery, Graduate School of Medicine, Osaka City University, Osaka 545-8585, Japan; shinji@med.osaka-cu.ac.jp
5. Department of Orthopedic Surgery, Osaka City General Hospital, Osaka 534-0021, Japan; hoshino717@gmail.com
6. Division of Geriatric Musculoskeletal Health, Hamamatsu University School of Medicine, Shizuoka 431-3192, Japan; yamato@hama-med.ac.jp
7. Department of Orthopaedics, Graduate School, Tokyo Medical and Dental University, Tokyo 108-0075, Japan; matsukura.orth@tmd.ac.jp (Y.M.); hirai.orth@tmd.ac.jp (T.H.); yoshii.orth@tmd.ac.jp (T.Y.); okawa.orth@tmd.ac.jp (A.O.)
* Correspondence: inose.orth@tmd.ac.jp; Tel.: +81-3-5803-5279

Abstract: To date, it is still unclear how fresh osteoporotic vertebral fractures (OVFs) affect the patient's quality of life and low back pain during a follow-up period of more than 1 year. In the previous trial, women with fresh OVF were randomized to rigid or soft brace for 12 weeks, then both groups were followed for the subsequent 48 weeks. In women completing this trial at our affiliated hospitals, we conducted a follow-up study to investigate the long-term course of an acute vertebral fracture in terms of pain and quality of life. When comparing visual analog scale scores for low back pain and European Quality of Life-5 Dimensions Questionnaire scores between consecutive time points, a significant difference was found between 0 and 12 weeks, but not between 12 and 48 weeks or between 48 weeks and final follow-up. A total 25% had residual low back pain at the final follow-up. A stepwise logistic regression analysis identified age and previous vertebral fracture as predictors of residual low back pain at the final follow-up. Therefore, the degree of low back pain and impairment of the quality of life improved by 12 weeks after injury and did not change thereafter until a mean follow-up of 5.3 years.

Keywords: osteoporotic vertebral fracture; residual pain; visual analog scale; quality of life

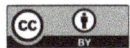

1. Introduction

Vertebral fractures are the most common osteoporotic fracture [1]. When osteoporotic vertebral body fractures occur, the symptoms improve approximately 3 months after the injury in most cases [2]. However, in some cases, the symptoms persist chronically. A study found that patients with new vertebral fractures had significantly more back pain and poorer physical function at all time points up to 12 months after fracture than those without fractures [2]. In addition, if there is a history of vertebral fractures, recovery after a new vertebral fracture is even worse. In a study comparing the post-vertebral fracture course, patients with a history of vertebral fracture had significantly lower physical motor function, activities of daily living, and quality of life (QOL) up to 12 months after injury than patients without a history of vertebral fracture [3]. However, it is still unclear how fresh vertebral fractures affect the patient's QOL and low back pain during a follow-up period of more than 1 year. Thus, this study aimed to describe the course of acute vertebral fractures in terms of pain and QOL and to characterize patients with residual low back pain long after a vertebral fracture.

2. Materials and Methods

This study was a follow-up study of women involved in the previous prospective randomized study (UMIN000014876) that compared the effectiveness of rigid and soft braces for acute thoracolumbar OVFs [4]. Briefly, the original trial enrolled 284 patients aged between 65 and 85 years who were diagnosed with one fresh OVF between T10 and L2 within four weeks of injury; 141 of these patients were randomly assigned to wear rigid braces and 143 were assigned to wear soft braces. Patients wore ready-made braces until a custom-made thoracolumbar sacral rigid or soft brace was applied. Patients in the rigid-brace group received a rigid thoracolumbosacral orthosis. Patients in the soft-brace group received a soft thoracolumbosacral orthosis. In both the rigid and flexible bracing groups, the patients were instructed to always wear the braces, when possible. All the participants were instructed to wear the brace for a total of 12 weeks. Detailed inclusion and exclusion criteria of the study have been described previously [4].

Among the patients who completed the previous brace trial, patients from hospitals that agreed to participate in this study were included in this study. Accordingly, a total of 73 patients were enrolled. Of the 73, 3 died, 2 refused to cooperate, and 28 could not be contacted. Finally, 40 patients with mean 5.3 years of follow-up were included in this study. With regard to the use of anti-osteoporosis treatments during the 48-week brace treatment prospective randomized study, the patients were allowed to use only the medications that were used prior to the injury or newly prescribed active vitamin D [4]. During the subsequent follow-up period, prescription of any anti-osteoporosis medication was allowed.

This study was approved by each hospital's institutional review board, and informed consent was obtained from all the participants included in the study.

2.1. Patient-Reported Outcome Measures

Regarding the patient-reported outcome measures (PROMs), scores on the European Quality of Life-5 Dimensions (EQ-5D; range, −0.111 to 1, with higher scores indicating a better QOL) [5] and the visual analog scale (VAS) for low back pain (range, 0–10, with higher scores indicating more severe pain) [6] were used. These questionnaires were provided at a regular hospital visit (0, 12, and 48 weeks after brace application) but were completed without assistance from the surgeon or any other person involved in this study. After 48 weeks, since regular visits to the hospital were not mandatory, outcome assessment at the last follow-up was completed by mailing a questionnaire. To maximize participant retention, we decided to mail the questionnaires. This is because, according to previous research, comparing three different methods of administering a brief screening questionnaire to the elderly, response rates were higher for the postal questionnaire than the interview method [7].

2.2. Radiographic Assessment

Lateral radiography was performed at 0, 12, and 48 weeks. MRI was performed at enrollment. In the radiographic analysis, the anterior vertebral body compression percentage [4,8], which is defined as the ratio between the vertical height of the compressed anterior section of the injured vertebral body and the posterior vertebral body height at the same level, was measured independently at 0, 12, and 48 weeks after brace application by two radiologists. The mean values of the two evaluators were used. In this study, a previous vertebral fracture was defined as a decrease of at least 20% in the height of any vertebral body at Week 0 [9]. To investigate the presence of degenerative spinal diseases that can cause low back pain, we investigated lumbar spinal canal stenosis and lumbar disc herniation by MRI at enrollment. Lumbar spinal canal stenosis was diagnosed as C or higher in Schizas' classification [10].

2.3. Data Analysis

All data were collected by a clinical research assistant. An analysis of variance with repeated measures was used to analyze the data over time. When there was a significant main effect of time, Tukey's HSD analysis was performed to identify the differences among time points.

In this study, "residual low back pain" was defined as VAS for low back pain ≥3.5 at the final follow-up; VAS score <3.5 is used to describe mild pain, and VAS score ≥ 3.5 is used to describe moderate or severe pain [11]. We performed outcome and risk factor analyses by comparing patients with VAS scores <3.5 and ≥3.5 for low back pain. We analyzed the differences between the two groups using the Mann–Whitney U test for continuous variables and Fisher's exact test or chi-squared test for nominal variables. To identify the most significant risk factors for residual low back pain at the final follow-up, we performed risk factor analysis using multivariable logistic regression analysis with a forward-backward stepwise procedure ($p < 0.1$ for entry). We then calculated the odds ratios (ORs) and their approximate 95% confidence intervals (CIs) for residual low back pain. For continuous variables, the OR reflects the incremental risk associated with a one-unit change in that variable. JMP version 12 (SAS Institute, Cary, NC, USA) was used for all statistical analyses. All tests were two-sided, and p-values < 0.05 were considered significant.

3. Results

3.1. Demographics

A total of 40 patients with a mean follow-up of 5.3 years were included in this study. The mean age was 73.9 years. Figure 1 shows the time course of VAS for low back pain and EQ-5D after OVF. Time had a significant main effect on VAS for low back pain and EQ-5D ($p < 0.001$ and $p < 0.001$, respectively). Comparison of VAS scores for low back pain between consecutive time points showed a significant difference between 0 and 12 weeks ($p < 0.001$), but not between 12 and 48 weeks ($p = 0.97$), or between 48 weeks and final follow-up ($p = 0.99$) (Figure 1). Comparison of EQ-5D scores between consecutive time points showed a significant difference between 0 and 12 weeks ($p < 0.001$), but not between 12 and 48 weeks ($p = 0.82$), or between 48 weeks and final follow-up ($p = 0.99$) (Figure 1).

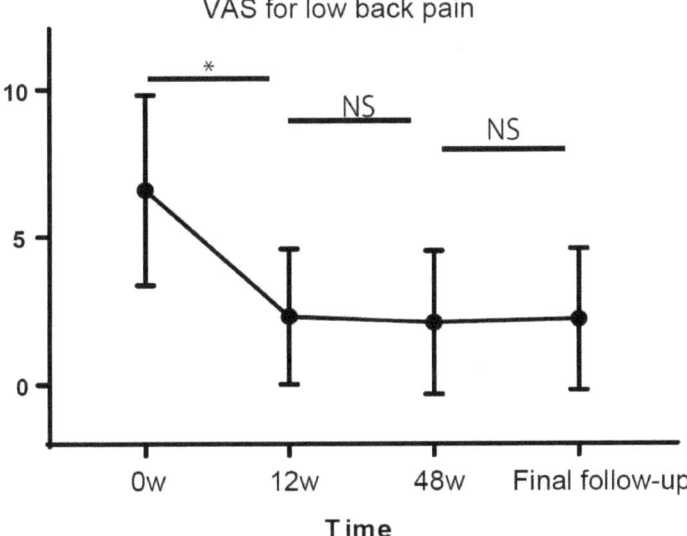

Figure 1. Cont.

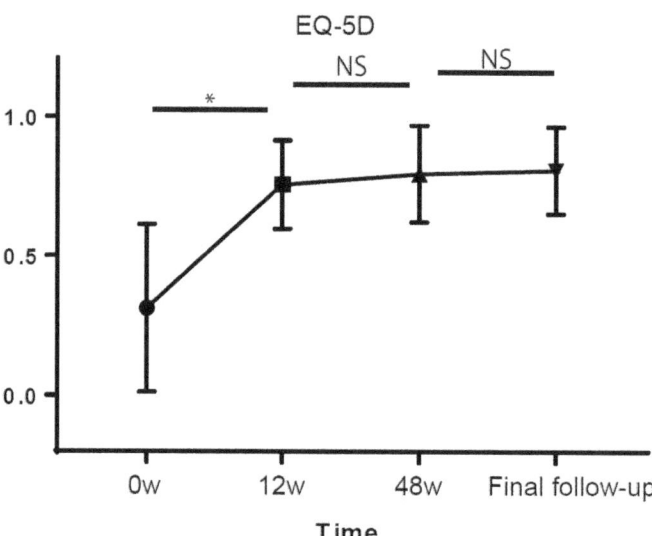

Figure 1. Temporal trends in outcome measures. The visual analog scale (VAS) for low back pain (0–10, with higher scores indicating severe pain) and the European Quality of Life-5 Dimensions Questionnaire (EQ-5D, −0.111 to 1, with higher scores indicating better quality of life). Means with standard deviations at baseline and each follow-up are shown. * $p < 0.05$, NS not significant.

3.2. Characteristics of Patients with Residual Low Back Pain at 5 Years after OVF

We then divided the patients into two groups according to their VAS score at the last follow-up: the residual low back pain group and the no low back pain group. Of the 40 patients analyzed in this study, 10 (25.0%) reported residual low back pain at a mean 5.3 years after OVFs. The baseline characteristics of the patients are shown in Table 1. In the residual low back pain group, the patients were older, and the percentage of patients with a history of pre-existing vertebral fracture was higher. No significant differences were observed in the other background variables between the two groups.

Table 1. Baseline characteristics of the patients.

Characteristics	VAS < 3.5 (n = 30)	VAS ≥ 3.5 (n = 10)	p Value
Age (years)	72.8 ± 5.5	77.1 ± 4.8	0.03 *
Receiving osteoporosis therapy at enrollment	5 (17)	3 (30)	0.38
Any previous vertebral fracture	6 (20)	6 (60)	0.04 *
Spinal disorders	9 (30)	1 (10)	0.40
Lumbar canal stenosis	8 (27)	0 (0)	
Lumbar disc hernia	1 (3)	1 (10)	
Level			0.70
T10	1 (3)	0 (0)	
T11	2 (7)	0 (0)	
T12	7 (23)	3 (30)	
L1	11 (37)	3 (30)	
L2	9 (30)	4 (40)	
Type of brace			
Rigid	15 (50)	4 (40)	0.58
Soft	15 (50)	6 (60)	
Follow-up period, days	1922 ± 255	1898 ± 213	0.75
Receiving osteoporosis therapy at final follow-up	13 (43)	4 (40)	0.85

Data are presented as mean ± standard deviation or n (%). * $p < 0.05$. VAS, visual analog scale.

Table 2 shows the differences in PROMs between the groups with VAS scores < 3.5 and ≥3.5 at the final follow-up. VAS scores for low back pain did differ not significantly between the two groups at 0 and 12 weeks, but were significantly worse in the residual low back pain group at 48 weeks and final follow-up ($p < 0.001$ and <0.001, respectively). The EQ-5D score was not significantly different between the two groups at 0 and 12 weeks, but was significantly worse in the residual low back pain group at 48 weeks and final follow-up ($p < 0.001$ and $p = 0.001$, respectively). We then examined the trends in the VAS score for low back pain in the residual low back pain group and no low back pain group. In the no low back pain group, a significant difference was found between VAS scores at 0 and 12 weeks ($p < 0.001$), but no significant difference was noted in the VAS scores between 12 and 48 weeks or between 12 weeks and final follow-up ($p = 0.41$ and 0.30, respectively). In the residual low back pain group, no significant difference was found in the VAS scores between 12 and 48 weeks ($p = 0.08$), but a significant difference was noted in the VAS scores between 0 and 12 weeks and between 12 weeks and final follow-up ($p < 0.001$ and $p = 0.02$, respectively).

Table 2. Patient-reported outcome measures.

Characteristic	VAS < 3.5 (n = 30)	VAS ≥ 3.5 (n = 10)	p
EQ-5D			
Week 0	0.31 ± 0.33	0.31 ± 0.23	0.78
12 weeks	0.78 ± 0.16	0.68 ± 0.14	0.09
48 weeks	0.85 ± 0.15	0.61 ± 0.08	<0.001 *
Final follow-up	0.85 ± 0.14	0.65 ± 0.07	0.001 *
VAS low back pain			
Week 0	6.1 ± 3.4	8.0 ± 2.5	0.08
12 weeks	2.1 ± 2.4	2.7 ± 2.1	0.30
48 weeks	1.2 ± 1.6	5.1 ± 2.3	<0.001 *
Final follow-up	1.1 ± 1.3	5.7 ± 1.5	<0.001 *

* $p < 0.05$. VAS, visual analog scale; EQ-5D, European Quality of Life-5 Dimensions.

Table 3 shows the differences in the radiographic assessment between the groups with VAS scores of <3.5 and ≥3.5. No significant difference was observed in the anterior vertebral body compression percentage between the two groups, although there was a trend toward lower anterior vertebral body compression percentage in the residual low back pain group throughout the period from 0 to 48 weeks ($p = 0.17$, 0.11, and 0.09, respectively).

Table 3. Radiographic assessment.

Characteristic	VAS < 3.5 (n = 30)	VAS ≥ 3.5 (n = 10)	p Value
Anterior Vertebral Body Compression Percentage			
0 week	74.6 ± 12.6	65.4 ± 20.3	0.17
12 weeks	62.4 ± 15.6	51.5 ± 15.1	0.11
48 weeks	61.9 ± 16.2	50.5 ± 18.0	0.09

Data are presented as mean ± standard deviation or n (%). $p < 0.05$. VAS, visual analog scale.

Lastly, the predictors at 12 weeks after OVFs for residual low back pain at the final follow-up were evaluated using a stepwise multiple logistic regression analysis (Table 4). Based on the univariate analysis, the dependent variable was defined as the presence of residual low back pain at the final follow-up, and the independent variables were age, previous vertebral fracture, and EQ-5D score at 12 weeks after OVF. As a result, the independent risk factors at 12 weeks were identified as age (OR = 1.19; 95% CI, 1.01–1.46; $p = 0.04$) and previous vertebral fracture (OR = 6.28; 95% CI, 1.24–39.83; $p = 0.03$).

Table 4. Multiple logistic regression analysis: independent risk factors of residual low back pain (VAS ≥ 3.5 at final follow-up).

Variable	Odds Ratio	95% Confidence Interval	p
12 weeks			
History of vertebral fracture	6.28	1.24–39.83	0.03 *
Age	1.19	1.01–1.46	0.04 *

* $p < 0.05$. VAS, visual analog scale.

4. Discussion

This study investigated the course of acute vertebral fracture in terms of pain and QOL. When comparing VAS for low back pain and EQ-5D scores between consecutive time points, a significant difference was observed between 0 and 12 weeks, but not between 12 and 48 weeks or between 48 weeks and final follow-up. Twenty-five percent of patients had residual low back pain at the final follow-up. The patients with residual low back pain after OVF had a higher percentage of pre-existing vertebral fractures and were older than those who did not have residual low back pain. A stepwise logistic regression analysis identified age and previous vertebral fracture as predictors of residual low back pain at the final follow-up.

This study showed that when comparing VAS scores for low back pain and EQ-5D scores between consecutive time points, a significant difference was found between 0 and 12 weeks, but not between 12 and 48 weeks or between 48 weeks and final follow-up. This result is consistent with previous reports that pain improved by 3 months after the fracture and did not change significantly until 12 months thereafter [12]. Collectively, these results suggest that if severe pain remains after the acute phase, it might be unlikely that the pain will improve spontaneously.

Among patients with acute vertebral fractures, 25% had mild or severe low back pain for an average of 5.3 years after injury based on VAS for low back pain. Patients with mild or severe low back pain were older and had a higher percentage of patients with pre-existing vertebral fractures than those with moderate or no pain. The results were partially consistent with a previous report stating that chronic pain after acute spine fractures was only maintained in patients with multiple compression fractures, reduced height, and low bone density [13].

In this study, the VAS score for low back pain was not significantly different between the residual low back pain group and no low back pain group at 0 and 12 weeks, but was significantly worse in the residual low back pain group at 48 weeks and final follow-up. Regarding the transition of pain within the group, although not significant, the low back pain tended to improve after 12 weeks in the no low back pain group. By contrast, back pain deteriorated after 12 weeks in the residual low back pain group. In a randomized controlled trial comparing vertebroplasty and conservative treatment for patients with vertebral fractures who reported severe pain for more than 3 months, vertebroplasty was associated with better pain relief and improved functional outcomes at 1 year compared with conservative treatment [14]. Therefore, taking into account the improvement of pain in patients who report severe low back pain 3 months after a vertebral fracture, vertebroplasty should be considered rather than conservative treatment. This treatment strategy should be tested in the future.

Since OVF-induced pain significantly improves by 12 weeks, we decided to investigate predictors for residual low back pain at 12 weeks after OVF. A stepwise logistic regression analysis identified age and previous vertebral fracture as predictors for residual low back pain at a mean of 5.3 years after OVFs. Therefore, when a new vertebral fracture occurs in an older patient with a pre-existing vertebral fracture, the patient is likely to have residual low back pain in the future. Furthermore, risk factors for OVFs include older age, low bone mineral density, and pre-existing vertebral fractures [15]. Therefore, elderly patients with new OVF and pre-existing vertebral fractures are at risk of further subsequent fractures. In this study, we do not know whether subsequent vertebral fractures occurred in this group of patients after 48 weeks, because imaging evaluation was not performed in the final follow-up. According to a post-hoc analysis of the original prospective study, patients with subsequent vertebral fractures at Week 48 had significantly more severe low back pain than those without subsequent fractures at Week 48 [16]. Therefore, in this study, it cannot be ruled out that the presence of subsequent vertebral fractures at the time of the final follow-up may be associated with residual low back pain. However, if a new OVF occurs in an older patient with a pre-existing vertebral fracture, it may be desirable to provide intensive osteoporosis treatment to prevent subsequent fractures. Further research is needed to determine which osteoporosis drugs are the most effective in reducing subsequent fractures in elderly patients with pre-existing vertebral fractures.

This study had some limitations. First, several patients were excluded after enrollment which might have led to a slight decrease in the sample size. Accordingly, attrition bias may limit the internal validity of this study. Second, we did not investigate the bone mineral density in this study. Although it is undeniable that the severity of osteoporosis may affect back pain, a decrease in bone mineral density does not necessarily lead to an increase in low back pain. In fact, the authors of several studies concluded that there is no evidence supporting a relationship between low back pain and bone mineral density [17,18]. Third, given the small percentage of patients who continued to attend the hospital, no radiographic evaluation was performed at the last follow-up. This prevented us from assessing the relationship between residual low back pain and non-union, subsequent fractures, and spinal alignment at the final follow-up. Lastly, the results of the multiple logistic regression analysis showed that there were two independent variables. Accordingly, the event per variable (EPV) was five in this model. However, the rule of thumb of 10 or more EPV in logistic models is not a well-defined bright line [19]. A simulation study showed that statistical problems are uncommon with 5–9 EPV, and still observed with 10–16 EPV [19]. Further studies are required to address these limitations and to validate our findings.

5. Conclusions

This study demonstrated that the degree of pain and impairment of QOL after OVF improved by 12 weeks after injury and did not change thereafter, until a mean follow-up period of 5.3 years. In addition, patients with residual low back pain after OVF had a higher percentage of pre-existing vertebral fractures and were older than those who did not have residual low back pain.

Author Contributions: Conceptualization, H.I.; formal analysis, H.I.; investigation, H.I, T.K., S.S., S.T., M.H., Y.Y., Y.M., T.H. and T.Y.; data curation, H.I.; writing—original draft preparation, H.I.; writing—review and editing, H.I. and T.K.; visualization, H.I.; supervision, A.O.; project administration, H.I.; All authors have read and agreed to the published version of the manuscript.

Funding: This research received no external funding.

Institutional Review Board Statement: The study was conducted according to the guidelines of the Declaration of Helsinki, and approved by the Institutional Review Board of the Tokyo Medical and Dental University (M2019-254).

Informed Consent Statement: Informed consent was obtained from all subjects involved in the study.

Data Availability Statement: Not available.

Acknowledgments: We acknowledge the following contributions: Nobuko Nakajima was the patient-reported outcomes manager. The authors wish to thank all the participants and doctors involved in this study.

Conflicts of Interest: The authors declare no conflict of interest.

References

1. Cauley, J.A.; Hochberg, M.C.; Lui, L.Y.; Palermo, L.; Ensrud, K.E.; Hillier, T.A.; Nevitt, M.C.; Cummings, S.R. Long-term risk of incident vertebral fractures. *Jama* **2007**, *298*, 2761–2767. [CrossRef] [PubMed]
2. Silverman, S.; Viswanathan, H.N.; Yang, Y.C.; Wang, A.; Boonen, S.; Ragi-Eis, S.; Fardellone, P.; Gilchrist, N.; Lips, P.; Nevitt, M.; et al. Impact of clinical fractures on health-related quality of life is dependent on time of assessment since fracture: Results from the FREEDOM trial. *Osteoporos. Int.* **2012**, *23*, 1361–1369. [CrossRef] [PubMed]
3. Suzuki, N.; Ogikubo, O.; Hansson, T. Previous vertebral compression fractures add to the deterioration of the disability and quality of life after an acute compression fracture. *Eur. Spine J.* **2010**, *19*, 567–574. [CrossRef] [PubMed]
4. Kato, T.; Inose, H.; Ichimura, S.; Tokuhashi, Y.; Nakamura, H.; Hoshino, M.; Togawa, D.; Hirano, T.; Haro, H.; Ohba, T.; et al. Comparison of Rigid and Soft-Brace Treatments for Acute Osteoporotic Vertebral Compression Fracture: A Prospective, Randomized, Multicenter Study. *J. Clin. Med.* **2019**, *8*, 198. [CrossRef] [PubMed]
5. Szende, A.; Oppe, M.; Devlin, N. *EQ-5D Value Sets: Inventory, Comparative Review and User Guide*; Springer: Rotterdam, The Netherlands, 2007.
6. McCormack, H.M.; Horne, D.J.; Sheather, S. Clinical applications of visual analogue scales: A critical review. *Psychol. Med.* **1988**, *18*, 1007–1019. [CrossRef] [PubMed]
7. Smeeth, L.; Fletcher, A.E.; Stirling, S.; Nunes, M.; Breeze, E.; Ng, E.; Bulpitt, C.J.; Jones, D. Randomised comparison of three methods of administering a screening questionnaire to elderly people: Findings from the MRC trial of the assessment and management of older people in the community. *BMJ* **2001**, *323*, 1403–1407. [CrossRef] [PubMed]
8. Keynan, O.; Fisher, C.G.; Vaccaro, A.; Fehlings, M.G.; Oner, F.C.; Dietz, J.; Kwon, B.; Rampersaud, R.; Bono, C.; France, J.; et al. Radiographic measurement parameters in thoracolumbar fractures: A systematic review and consensus statement of the spine trauma study group. *Spine* **2006**, *31*, E156–E165. [CrossRef] [PubMed]
9. Fujiwara, S.; Kasagi, F.; Masunari, N.; Naito, K.; Suzuki, G.; Fukunaga, M. Fracture prediction from bone mineral density in Japanese men and women. *J. Bone Miner. Res.* **2003**, *18*, 1547–1553. [CrossRef] [PubMed]
10. Schizas, C.; Theumann, N.; Burn, A.; Tansey, R.; Wardlaw, D.; Smith, F.W.; Kulik, G. Qualitative grading of severity of lumbar spinal stenosis based on the morphology of the dural sac on magnetic resonance images. *Spine* **2010**, *35*, 1919–1924. [CrossRef] [PubMed]
11. Boonstra, A.M.; Schiphorst Preuper, H.R.; Balk, G.A.; Stewart, R.E. Cut-off points for mild, moderate, and severe pain on the visual analogue scale for pain in patients with chronic musculoskeletal pain. *Pain* **2014**, *155*, 2545–2550. [CrossRef] [PubMed]
12. Suzuki, N.; Ogikubo, O.; Hansson, T. The course of the acute vertebral body fragility fracture: Its effect on pain, disability and quality of life during 12 months. *Eur. Spine J.* **2008**, *17*, 1380–1390. [CrossRef] [PubMed]
13. Silverman, S.L. The clinical consequences of vertebral compression fracture. *Bone* **1992**, *13* (Suppl. 2), S27–S31. [CrossRef]
14. Chen, D.; An, Z.Q.; Song, S.; Tang, J.F.; Qin, H. Percutaneous vertebroplasty compared with conservative treatment in patients with chronic painful osteoporotic spinal fractures. *J. Clin. Neurosci.* **2014**, *21*, 473–477. [CrossRef] [PubMed]
15. Chen, P.; Krege, J.H.; Adachi, J.D.; Prior, J.C.; Tenenhouse, A.; Brown, J.P.; Papadimitropoulos, E.; Kreiger, N.; Olszynski, W.P.; Josse, R.G.; et al. Vertebral fracture status and the World Health Organization risk factors for predicting osteoporotic fracture risk. *J. Bone Miner Res.* **2009**, *24*, 495–502. [CrossRef] [PubMed]
16. Inose, H.; Kato, T.; Ichimura, S.; Nakamura, H.; Hoshino, M.; Togawa, D.; Hirano, T.; Tokuhashi, Y.; Ohba, T.; Haro, H.; et al. Risk factors for subsequent vertebral fracture after acute osteoporotic vertebral fractures. *Eur. Spine J.* **2021**, *30*, 2698–2707. [CrossRef] [PubMed]
17. Zetterberg, C.; Mannius, S.; Mellstrom, D.; Rundgren, A.; Astrand, K. Osteoporosis and back pain in the elderly. A controlled epidemiologic and radiographic study. *Spine* **1990**, *15*, 783–786. [CrossRef] [PubMed]
18. Ahn, S.; Song, R. Bone mineral density and perceived menopausal symptoms: Factors influencing low back pain in post-menopausal women. *J. Adv. Nurs.* **2009**, *65*, 1228–1236. [CrossRef] [PubMed]
19. Vittinghoff, E.; McCulloch, C.E. Relaxing the rule of ten events per variable in logistic and Cox regression. *Am. J. Epidemiol.* **2007**, *165*, 710–718. [CrossRef] [PubMed]

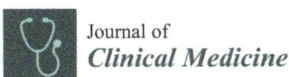

Article

Perioperative Predictive Factors for Positive Outcomes in Spine Fusion for Adult Deformity Correction

Alice Baroncini [1,2,3,*], Filippo Migliorini [2], Francesco Langella [1], Paolo Barletta [1], Per Trobisch [3], Riccardo Cecchinato [1], Marco Damilano [1], Emanuele Quarto [1], Claudio Lamartina [1] and Pedro Berjano [1]

[1] IRCCS Istituto Ortopedico Galeazzi, Via Riccardo Galeazzi, 4, 20161 Milan, Italy; francesco.langella.md@gmail.com (F.L.); paolo.barletta@grupposandonato.it (P.B.); dott.cecchinato@gmail.com (R.C.); marco.damilano@gmail.com (M.D.); emanuelequarto88@gmail.com (E.Q.); c.lamartina@chirurgiavertebrale.net (C.L.); pberjano@gmail.com (P.B.)
[2] Department of Orthopaedic Surgery, RWTH Uniklinik Aachen, 52074 Aachen, Germany; fmigliorini@ukaachen.de
[3] Department of Spine Surgery, Eifelklinik St. Brigida, 52152 Simmerath, Germany; per.trobisch@artemed.de
* Correspondence: alice.baroncini@artemed.de; Tel.: +39-0266-2141

Abstract: Purpose: Identifying perioperative factors that may influence the outcomes of long spine fusion for the treatment of adult deformity is key for tailored surgical planning and targeted informed consent. The aim of this study was to analyze the association between demographic or perioperative factors and clinical outcomes 2 years after long spine fusion for the treatment of adult deformity. Methods: This study is a multivariate analysis of retrospectively collected data. All patients who underwent long fusion of the lumbar spine for adult spinal deformity (January 2016–June 2019) were included. The outcomes of interest were the Oswestry disability index (ODI), visual analogic scale (VAS) preoperatively and at 1 and 2 years' follow up, age, body mass index, American Society of Anaesthesiologists (ASA) score, upper and lowest instrumented vertebrae (UIV and LIV, respectively), length of surgery, estimated blood loss, and length of hospital stay. Results: Data from 192 patients were available. The ODI at 2 years correlated weakly to moderately with age ($r = 0.4$), BMI ($r = 0.2$), ASA ($r = 0.3$), and LIV ($r = 0.2$), and strongly with preoperative ODI ($r = 0.6$). The leg VAS at 2 years moderately correlated with age ($r = 0.3$) and BMI ($r = 0.3$). Conclusion: ODI and VAS at 2 years' follow-up had no to little association to preoperative age, health status, LIV, or other perioperative data, but showed a strong correlation with preoperative ODI and pain level.

Keywords: adult spine deformity; adult spine fusion; deformity correction; perioperative parameters; ODI; VAS; disability

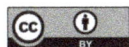

1. Introduction

The social burden caused by low back pain (LBP) is relevant, having a first-ever episode incidence of 15% and an 80% recurrence rate within a year [1]. This percentage increases in patients affected by adult spine deformity [2] and various studies showed that this condition has a negative impact on the patients' quality of life [3,4]. Surgical deformity correction involves complex procedures; given the advances in surgical and anesthesiological techniques, it is now possible to perform surgery in patients at an older age and with more comorbidities [5–8]. So, disability and pain levels play a decisive role in the assessment of a patient and in the decision-making process [9]. However, the postoperative motion restriction following fusion of the lumbar spine should be considered when indicating surgical management to ensure that the benefits of the surgery outweigh the limitations [10].

Patient-reported outcome measures (PROMs) are used to obtain a more complete overview of a patient's status, as they allow to match objective informations such as radiographic findings with subjective data regarding different aspects of the patient's quality of life [11]. In particular, the Oswestry disability index (ODI) and the visual analogic scale (VAS) are two parameters widely used for pre- and postoperative assessment of patients undergoing spine surgery [12,13].

The effects of the correction of sagittal and coronal parameters on disability and pain levels have been evaluated in multiple studies [14–17]. However, the effects of demographic and perioperative data on the postoperative outcome has not yet been thoroughly investigated, and patients with a low risk of a poor clinical outcome have not yet been characterized [18]. Thus, the aim of this study was to analyze the demographic and perioperative data of adult spine deformity patients undergoing long fusion involving the lumbar spine, in order to seek possible associations between these parameters and levels of disability (ODI) and pain (VAS back and leg) at the one- and two-year follow-up.

2. Materials and Methods

2.1. Patient Recruitment

The present retrospective study was conducted according to the Strengthening the Reporting of Observational Studies in Epidemiology: the STROBE Statement [19].

All patients who underwent spine fusion at IRCCS Istituto Ortopedico Galeazzi (Milano, Italy) between January 2016 and June 2019 were retrospectively screened for inclusion on the local spine registry using the ICD (International Classification of Diseases) diagnosis and procedure codes listed in Table 1. The use of ICD codes for diagnosis and procedure allows to retrieve data from the registry, but also offers an internationally acknowledged key to replicate data extraction, if necessary. Inclusion criteria for the current study were age ≥ 18, diagnosis of adult spine deformity, and fusion of at least four segments—at least three of which in the lumbar spine. Patients who did not have an ODI and/or VAS preoperatively and at the one- or two-year follow-up were not eligible for the study.

Table 1. List of all ICD diagnosis and procedure codes used for data extraction from the local spine registry.

ICD Diagnosis Codes	
737.30, 737.31, 737.32, 737.34, 737.0, 737.10, 737.12, 737.22, 737.40, 737.41, 737.43, 737.19, 738.5, 737.39	
ICD Procedure Codes	
Primary surgery	81.05, 81.06, 81.08, 81.63, 81.64
Revision surgery	996.49, V45.4, 996.78, 998.89

ICD, International Classification of Diseases.

2.2. Outcomes of Interest

We analyzed the effects of demographic and perioperative parameters on ODI and VAS over time, as well as the mutual association between ODI and VAS at different follow-ups. Furthermore, question n. 11 of the COME back questionnaire (CB11) [20] was used to identify whether patients felt overall that surgery had helped or not (0 = helped a lot, 4 = made things worse). Demographic parameters included age, sex, body mass index (BMI), and American Society of Anaesthesiologists (ASA) score. The level of the upper and lowest instrumented vertebra (UIV and LIV, respectively) was analyzed. Length of surgery, estimated blood loss (EBL), and length of hospital stay were also considered.

2.3. Statistical Analysis

For the statistical analysis, STATA software (StataCorp, College Station, TX, USA) was used. Continuous variables are expressed as mean $\pm$ standard deviation. Comparisons between continuous variables across the follow-ups were assessed through the mean difference and t-test, with values of $p < 0.05$ considered statistically significant. A multivariate diagnostic through the Pearson product-moment correlation coefficient (r) was performed to investigate potential correlations between continuous variables. According to the Cauchy–Schwarz equation of inequality, the final effect can score between +1 (positive linear correlation) and −1 (negative linear correlation). Values of $0.1 > |r| < 0.3$, $0.3 < |r| < 0.5$, and $|r| > 0.5$ indicate weak, moderate, and strong association, respectively. The test of overall significance was performed through the $\chi 2$ test, with values of $p > 0.05$ considered statistically significant.

3. Results

3.1. Patient Recruitment and Demographics

After cross-referencing the ICD diagnosis and procedure codes, 821 eligible patients were identified on the local spine registry. Of them, 128 were excluded because they were <18 years old. A further 210 were excluded because their level or extent of instrumentation did not match the requirements of this study. A further 291 patients were excluded due to the lack of a sufficient follow-up, leaving 192 patients available for the analysis. The flowchart of the patients' recruitment is presented in Figure 1.

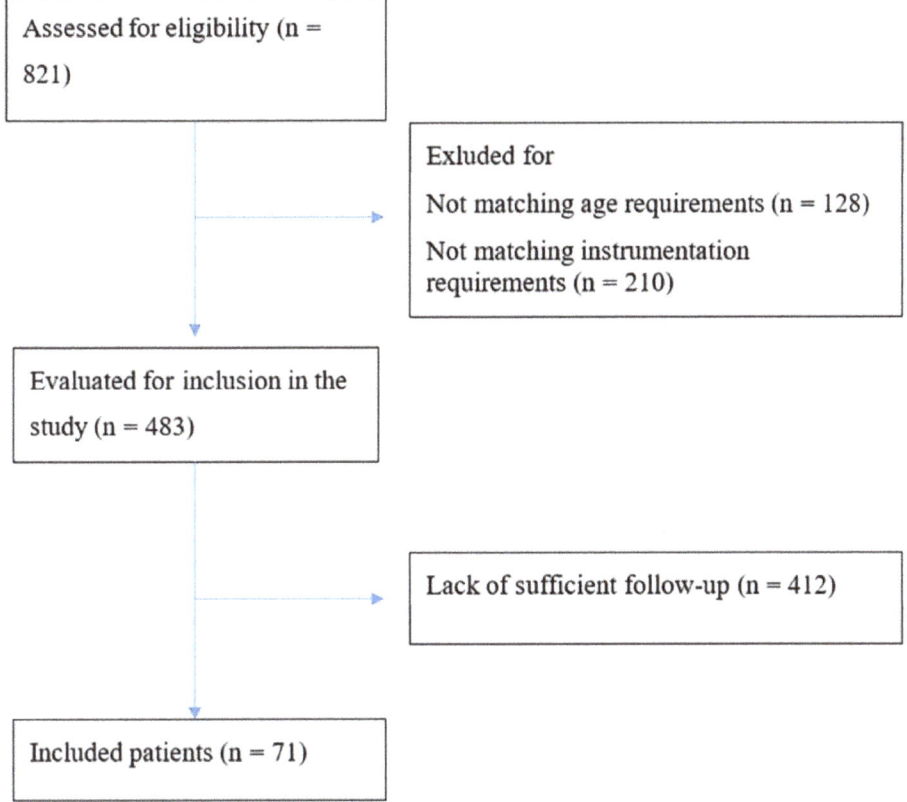

Figure 1. STROBE flow diagram of patient selection.

Summaries of the patients' demographics and the considered intraoperative data are shown in Tables 2 and 3, respectively. An overview of ODI, VAS, and CB11 in the different follow-ups is presented in Table 4.

Table 2. Overview of the patients' demographics.

Demographic Data	
Age (years)	53.4 ± 16.7
Sex	149 women (78%), 43 men (22%)
BMI (kg/cm^2)	24.2 ± 3.9

BMI, body mass index.

Table 3. Summary of perioperative data.

Perioperative Data	
UIV	C7: 1; T1: 5; T2: 7; T3: 28; T4: 29; T5: 15; T6: 4; T7: 3; T8: 11; T9: 16; T10: 44; T11: 5; T12: 3; L1: 5; L2: 13; L3: 3
LIV	L3: 11; L4: 35; L5: 24; S1: 62; Ilium: 60
Access	Posterior only: 192; postero-anterior: 21; postero-lateral: 38
Curve correction method	SPO: 21; PSO: 13; ALIF: 21; LLIF 38
Length of surgery (min)	430 ± 150
% EBL	18 ± 15.3
EBL (mL)	1264 ± 1073
Length of hospital stay (days)	8.5 ± 4.5

UIV, upper instrumented vertebra; LIV, lowest instrumented vertebra; SPO, Smith Petersen osteotomy; PSO, pedicle substraction osteotomy; ALIF, anterior lumbar interbody fusion; LLIF, latera lumbar interbody fusion; EBL, estimated blood loss.

Table 4. Overview of ODI, back and leg VAS, and CB11 values over time.

ODI, VAS and CB11 Overview				
	Preop	1-year FU	2-years FU	p (Preop vs. 2-year FU)
ODI	42.5 ± 20.3	26.7 ± 21.4	26.8 ± 20.7	<0.0001
VAS back	6.8 ± 2.7	3.8 ± 3	4 ± 3.1	<0.0001
VAS leg	4.8 ± 3.7	3.4 ± 3.1	3.6 ± 3.5	0.01
CB11	-	0.9 ± 1.1	0.9 ± 1.2	-

ODI, Oswestry disability index; VAS, visual analogic scale; CB11, question n. 11 of the COME back questionnaire; FU, follow-up.

3.2. Multivariate Analysis

Age and BMI showed a significant, weak-to-moderate correlation with most of the considered PROMs (ODI and leg VAS before and after surgery, and back VAS preoperatively and at 12 months, CB11). The ASA class correlated moderately with the ODI at all follow-ups and with the VAS leg before surgery and at 1 year, and with the CB11 at both follow-ups. Length of surgery, EBL, and length of hospital stay had a little correlation to ODI, VAS, and CB11 at different follow-ups. While UIV showed no significant correlation with postoperative outcomes, LIV had a weak-to-moderate correlation with postoperative ODI, leg VAS, and CB11. Numerous, mostly medium-to-strong correlations were observed among ODI, leg and back VAS, and CB11.

Other moderate correlations of interest were observed between age and BMI (r = 0.52, p < 0.001), ASA (r = 0.51, p < 0.001), and LIV (r = 0.54, p < 0.001); and between LIV and BMI (r = 0.35, p < 0.001), ASA (r = 0.38, p < 0.001), and length of hospital stay (r = 0.31, p < 0.001). Length of surgery correlated with EBL (r = 0.46, p < 0.001) and length of hospital stay (r = 0.33, p < 0.001). The details of the correlations are shown in Figure 2.

		Age	BMI	ASA	Length of surgery	Estimated blood loss	Length of hospital stay	UIV	LIV	ODI preoperative	ODI 1 year	ODI 2 years	VAS back preoperative	VAS leg preoperative	VAS back 1 year	VAS leg 1 year	VAS back 2 years	VAS leg 2 years	CB11 1 year	CB11 2 years
Age	r	1.00																		
	p	0.0000																		
BMI	r	0.53	1.00																	
	p	0.0000	0.0000																	
ASA	r	0.52	0.29	1.00																
	p	0.0000	0.0001	0.0000																
Length of surgery	r	0.22	0.13	0.24	1.00															
	p	0.0025	0.0784	0.0008	0.0000															
Estimated blood loss	r	0.19	0.07	0.20	0.46	1.00														
	p	0.0114	0.3310	0.0076	0.0000	0.0000														
Length of hospital stay	r	0.24	0.18	0.28	0.36	0.28	1.00													
	p	0.0007	0.0136	0.0001	0.0000	0.0001	0.0000													
UIV	r	0.18	0.13	0.00	-0.17	-0.20	-0.15	1.00												
	p	0.0126	0.0766	0.9934	0.0205	0.0068	0.0402	0.0000												
LIV	r	0.55	0.36	0.38	0.25	0.27	0.31	0.22	1.00											
	p	0.0000	0.0000	0.0000	0.0006	0.0002	0.0000	0.0019	0.0000											
ODI preoperative	r	0.47	0.34	0.41	0.11	0.08	0.23	0.11	0.35	1.00										
	p	0.0000	0.0000	0.0000	0.1412	0.2582	0.0016	0.1182	0.0000	0.0000										
ODI 1 year	r	0.58	0.40	0.54	0.16	0.18	0.21	0.03	0.40	0.64	1.00									
	p	0.0000	0.0000	0.0000	0.1115	0.0673	0.0258	0.7712	0.0000	0.0000	0.0000									
ODI 2 years	r	0.40	0.27	0.30	-0.18	-0.03	-0.16	0.17	0.25	0.69	0.85	1.00								
	p	0.0006	0.0232	0.0099	0.1373	0.8298	0.1829	0.1605	0.0348	0.0000	0.0000	0.0000								
VAS back preoperative	r	0.17	0.14	0.05	0.02	0.09	0.12	0.03	0.07	0.54	0.18	0.26	1.00							
	p	0.0194	0.0615	0.4734	0.7721	0.2115	0.0942	0.6710	0.3048	0.0000	0.0604	0.0284	0.0000							
VAS leg preoperative	r	0.35	0.27	0.33	0.09	0.15	0.20	0.17	0.32	0.52	0.45	0.40	0.38	1.00						
	p	0.0000	0.0001	0.0000	0.2406	0.0410	0.0043	0.0154	0.0000	0.0000	0.0000	0.0005	0.0000	0.0000						
VAS back 1 year	r	0.20	0.21	0.12	0.01	0.00	-0.04	-0.08	0.05	0.29	0.62	0.48	0.28	0.30	1.00					
	p	0.0373	0.0301	0.2004	0.9104	0.9718	0.6591	0.4091	0.6061	0.0027	0.0000	0.0016	0.0041	0.0016	0.0000					
VAS leg 1 year	r	0.40	0.31	0.36	0.17	0.20	0.02	0.00	0.34	0.42	0.70	0.63	0.07	0.40	0.55	1.00				
	p	0.0000	0.0010	0.0002	0.0897	0.0415	0.8154	0.9749	0.0004	0.0000	0.0000	0.0000	0.4681	0.0000	0.0000	0.0000				
VAS back 2 years	r	0.05	0.08	0.00	-0.25	-0.20	-0.31	0.11	-0.13	0.32	0.47	0.58	0.29	0.30	0.77	0.49	1.00			
	p	0.6803	0.5214	0.9706	0.0455	0.1247	0.0101	0.3673	0.2895	0.0089	0.0031	0.0000	0.0158	0.0133	0.0000	0.0020	0.0000			
VAS leg 2 years	r	0.34	0.31	0.21	0.07	0.06	-0.11	0.08	0.10	0.41	0.59	0.57	0.12	0.31	0.53	0.74	0.55	1.00		
	p	0.0043	0.0110	0.0879	0.5887	0.6297	0.3585	0.5445	0.4024	0.0006	0.0001	0.0000	0.3396	0.0097	0.0007	0.0000	0.0000	0.0000		
CB11 1 year	r	0.35	0.23	0.32	-0.06	-0.01	-0.06	-0.03	0.20	0.25	0.70	0.65	0.05	0.28	0.52	0.50	0.43	0.40	1.00	
	p	0.0002	0.0130	0.0005	0.5119	0.9139	0.5507	0.7287	0.0340	0.0081	0.0000	0.0000	0.6136	0.0026	0.0000	0.0000	0.0066	0.0122	0.0000	
CB11 2 years	r	0.30	0.02	0.32	-0.03	0.09	0.03	0.01	0.11	0.33	0.62	0.66	0.07	0.14	0.35	0.47	0.39	0.36	0.78	1.00
	p	0.0115	0.8459	0.0059	0.8256	0.4692	0.8335	0.9421	0.3429	0.0048	0.0000	0.0000	0.5728	0.2319	0.0286	0.0024	0.0011	0.0032	0.0000	0.0000

Figure 2. Overview of all the observed correlations among the considered parameters. Red, orange and yellow color indicate significant weak, moderate and strong correlations, respectively.

4. Discussion

Overall, we observed a significant improvement in ODI and leg and back VAS at the last follow-up. CB11 analysis highlighted a high level of satisfaction after surgery, confirming the results of previous studies, which reported positive outcomes after surgical therapy for adult spine deformity [21,22].

The correlation between ODI and age, BMI, or ASA was moderate at the one-year follow-up, but the strength of these correlations was reduced at the two-year follow-up. The correlation between leg and back VAS and age, BMI, and ASA showed similar trends to those observed for the ODI: back pain weakly correlated with age and BMI before surgery and at the 1 year follow-up, but no significant correlation was observed at 2 years, or with ASA at any follow-up. Leg pain showed a weak-to-moderate correlation with all parameters and at all follow-up, except with ASA at the last follow-up. Similar trends were also observed for CB11. These data confirmed that older age and poorer overall health condition may have a moderate negative impact on the level of complications and disability or pain after surgery [23–25], but this negative influence dissipates over time. Thus, these patients can also expect positive outcomes after long spine fusion [26–29], but have to be adequately informed that a poorer preoperative health status correlates with longer recovery time. Surgeons, however, need to consider that obesity and age or comorbidities have a relevant impact on intraoperative blood loss, length of surgery, and complication rate; thus, preoperative BMI and ASA should still be considered when planning long spine fusion [30–32].

Length of surgery, estimated blood loss, and length of hospital stay showed no or only weak correlation with ODI, VAS, and CB11. This aspect is also key for the informed consent of the patients and their attitude toward the recovery process, as a prolonged hospital stay does not have a negative impact on the long-term outcomes of surgery.

Analyzing the correlation of ODI, VAS, or CB with the extent of the instrumentation, we found that the level of the UIV did not affect any of the outcomes of interest. Given the relative limited mobility of the thoracic spine [33], these data are not surprising. It is however striking that the moderate correlation between ODI and LIV at the one-year follow-up was further reduced at the two-year follow-up. Similar results were obtained in other studies observing different PROMs and the ability of patients to perform determined activities after spinal fusion: over time, a gradual ODI improvement could be observed even in patients with fusion to the pelvis [10,34]. The explanation for this finding may lie in the postoperative movement restrictions required by many surgeons after fusion (e.g., avoiding forward bending or heavy lifting), which then ease over time, or in the fact that patients adapt to the movement restrictions imposed by the instrumentation and develop strategies to overcome them. This topic requires further investigation: if the developing of these strategies is the key in reducing postoperative disability after spine fusion, specific pre- or postoperative physiotherapy programs may be implemented to support patients and improve their quality of life after surgery.

Overall, the ODI, VAS, and CB parameters showed multiple moderate and strong correlations amongst each other, confirming how different aspects of a patient's health, quality of life, and satisfaction regarding treatment are interconnected [35]. Regarding the ODI, a strong correlation was observed between pre- and postoperative disability levels; this suggests that patients starting with high ODI values have lower chances of achieving a low ODI postoperatively. This represents a key factor in planning the timing of surgery. Different to what was observed for the ODI, the preoperative VAS only weakly to moderately associated with levels of back and pain level at the two-year follow-up. Thus, even patients with a high preoperative pain level can expect an improvement with respect to the painful symptoms two years after surgery. Unsurprisingly, the level of satisfaction with the treatment (CB11) correlated with ODI and VAS both at the one- and two-year follow-ups. However, while the correlation with pain level was of moderate intensity and declined at the two-year follow-up, the correlation to disability was strong at both follow-ups. A similar correlation between patients' satisfaction and PROMs was also observed by another study group [35].

This study is not without limitations, the main one being its retrospective nature. The relationship between ODI, pain, and satisfaction with treatment and pre- and perioperative data proved to be a complex, and further research on a wider patient cohort will be required to investigate it. Furthermore, the patients in our cohort presented different types of instrumentations (e.g., different types or levels of interbody implants) and deformity correction techniques. While it was not possible to investigate the effect of different surgical techniques on the outcome of interest due to the limited number of observations, this topic deserves further analysis in the future.

5. Conclusions

The main finding of this work was that preoperative ODI showed the strongest association with the postoperative clinical outcomes after spine fusion for adult deformity correction. Other parameters such as age, health status, or LIV presented only a weak association with the long-term ODI or VAS values. Thus, surgery should be performed in a timely manner to avoid patients reaching high preoperative ODI values.

Author Contributions: A.B., conception, data interpretation, draft and revision, final approval of the work; F.M., statistical analysis, draft and revision, final approval of the work; P.B. (Paolo Barletta), data acquisition, draft and revision, final approval of the work; F.L., C.L., P.B. (Pedro Berjano), P.T., E.Q., R.C. and M.D., data interpretation, draft and revision, final approval of the work, logistic support. All authors have read and agreed to the published version of the manuscript.

Funding: Funding for this study was provided by the Italian Ministry of Health (CO-2016-02364645).

Institutional Review Board Statement: Ethical approval for this study was asked for and waived by the local Medical Research Ethics Committee (Fourth Amendment to the SPINEREG Protocol,

Issued on 10 October 2019). The study fell outside the remit of the law for Medical Research Involving Human Subjects Act and was approved by the local ethical committee.

Informed Consent Statement: Waived as not required by local law for retrospective studies.

Data Availability Statement: The dataset used and/or analyzed in the present study is available from the corresponding author upon reasonable request.

Conflicts of Interest: Berjano, P. and Lamartina, C. disclose grants and personal fees from Nuvasive, personal fees from Depuy Sinthes, personal fees from Medacta, personal fees from Zimmer, personal fees from K2M, personal fees from Medtronic, grants from Stoeckli Medical, outside the submitted work. Trobisch, P. is a consultant for Globus Medical and Zimmer Biomet. Cecchinato, R. and Damilano, M. disclose personal fees from Nuvasive and Medacta. Baroncini, A., Migliorini, F., Langella, F., Barletta, P., and Quarto, E. have no conflict of interest to disclose.

References

1. Hoy, D.; Brooks, P.; Blyth, F.; Buchbinder, R. The Epidemiology of low back pain. *Best Pract. Res. Clin. Rheumatol.* **2010**, *24*, 769–781. [CrossRef] [PubMed]
2. Kostuik, J.P.; Bentivoglio, J. The incidence of low-back pain in adult scoliosis. *Spine* **1981**, *6*, 268–273. [CrossRef]
3. Berven, S.; Deviren, V.; Demir-Deviren, S.; Hu, S.S.; Bradford, D.S. Studies in the modified Scoliosis Research Society Outcomes Instrument in adults: Validation, reliability, and discriminatory capacity. *Spine* **2003**, *28*, 2164–2169. [CrossRef] [PubMed]
4. Ogura, Y.; Shinozaki, Y.; Kobayashi, Y.; Kitagawa, T.; Yonezawa, Y.; Takahashi, Y.; Yoshida, K.; Yasuda, A.; Ogawa, J. Impact of sagittal spinopelvic alignment on clinical outcomes and health-related quality of life after decompression surgery without fusion for lumbar spinal stenosis. *J. Neurosurg. Spine* **2019**, 1–6. [CrossRef]
5. Daniels, A.H.; Reid, D.B.; Tran, S.N.; Hart, R.A.; Klineberg, E.O.; Bess, S.; Burton, D.; Smith, J.S.; Shaffrey, C.; Gupta, M.; et al. Evolution in Surgical Approach, Complications, and Outcomes in an Adult Spinal Deformity Surgery Multicenter Study Group Patient Population. *Spine Deform.* **2019**, *7*, 481–488. [CrossRef]
6. Berjano, P.; Langella, F.; Ismael, M.-F.; Damilano, M.; Scopetta, S.; Lamartina, C. Successful correction of sagittal imbalance can be calculated on the basis of pelvic incidence and age. *Eur. Spine J.* **2014**, *23*, 587–596. [CrossRef] [PubMed]
7. Campagner, A.; Berjano, P.; Lamartina, C.; Langella, F.; Lombardi, G.; Cabitza, F. Assessment and prediction of spine surgery invasiveness with machine learning techniques. *Comput. Biol. Med.* **2020**, *121*, 103796. [CrossRef]
8. Langella, F.; Villafañe, J.H.; Damilano, M.; Cecchinato, R.; Pejrona, M.; Ismael, M.; Berjano, P. Predictive Accuracy of Surgimap Surgical Planning for Sagittal Imbalance: A Cohort Study. *Spine* **2017**, *42*, E1297–E1304. [CrossRef]
9. Bess, S.; Boachie-Adjei, O.; Burton, D.; Cunningham, M.; Shaffrey, C.; Shelokov, A.; Hostin, R.; Schwab, F.; Wood, K.; Akbarnia, B. Pain and disability determine treatment modality for older patients with adult scoliosis, while deformity guides treatment for younger patients. *Spine* **2009**, *34*, 2186–2190. [CrossRef]
10. Togawa, D.; Hasegawa, T.; Yamato, Y.; Yoshida, G.; Kobayashi, S.; Yasuda, T.; Oe, S.; Banno, T.; Arima, H.; Mihara, Y.; et al. Postoperative Disability After Long Corrective Fusion to the Pelvis in Elderly Patients with Spinal Deformity. *Spine* **2018**, *43*, E804–E812. [CrossRef]
11. Finkelstein, J.A.; Schwartz, C.E. Patient-reported outcomes in spine surgery: Past, current, and future directions. *J. Neurosurg. Spine* **2019**, *31*, 155–164. [CrossRef] [PubMed]
12. Gum, J.L.; Carreon, L.Y.; Glassman, S.D. State-of-the-art: Outcome assessment in adult spinal deformity. *Spine Deform.* **2020**, *9*, 1–11. [CrossRef] [PubMed]
13. Langella, F.; Barletta, P.; Baroncini, A.; Agarossi, M.; Scaramuzzo, L.; Luca, A.; Bassani, R.; Peretti, G.M.; Lamartina, C.; Villafañe, J.H.; et al. The use of electronic PROMs provides same outcomes as paper version in a spine surgery registry. Results from a prospective cohort study. *Eur. Spine J.* **2021**, *30*, 2645–2653. [CrossRef]
14. Diebo, B.G.; Varghese, J.J.; Lafage, R.; Schwab, F.J.; Lafage, V. Sagittal alignment of the spine: What do you need to know? *Clin. Neurol. Neurosurg.* **2015**, *139*, 295–301. [CrossRef]
15. Garbossa, D.; Pejrona, M.; Damilano, M.; Sansone, V.; Ducati, A.; Berjano, P. Pelvic parameters and global spine balance for spine degenerative disease: The importance of containing for the well being of content. *Eur. Spine J.* **2014**, *23* (Suppl. 6), 616–627. [CrossRef] [PubMed]
16. Johnson, R.; Valore, A.; Villaminar, A.; Comisso, M.; Balsano, M. Sagittal balance and pelvic parameters–a paradigm shift in spinal surgery. *J. Clin. Neurosci.* **2013**, *20*, 191–196. [CrossRef] [PubMed]
17. Yamato, Y.; Hasegawa, T.; Togawa, D.; Yoshida, G.; Banno, T.; Arima, H.; Oe, S.; Mihara, Y.; Ushirozako, H.; Kobayashi, S.; et al. Rigorous Correction of Sagittal Vertical Axis Is Correlated with Better ODI Outcomes After Extensive Corrective Fusion in Elderly or Extremely Elderly Patients with Spinal Deformity. *Spine Deform.* **2019**, *7*, 610–618. [CrossRef]
18. Yagi, M.; Michikawa, T.; Suzuki, S.; Okada, E.; Nori, S.; Tsuji, O.; Nagoshi, N.; Asazuma, T.; Hosogane, N.; Fujita, N.; et al. Characterization of Patients with Poor Risk for Clinical Outcomes in Adult Symptomatic Lumbar Deformity Surgery. *Spine* **2021**, *46*, 813–821. [CrossRef] [PubMed]

19. Von Elm, E.; Altman, D.G.; Egger, M.; Pocock, S.J.; Gøtzsche, P.C.; Vandenbroucke, J.P. The Strengthening the Reporting of Observational Studies in Epidemiology (STROBE) Statement: Guidelines for reporting observational studies. *Int. J. Surg.* **2014**, *12*, 1495–1499. [CrossRef]
20. Mannion, A.F.; Porchet, F.; Kleinstück, F.S.; Lattig, F.; Jeszenszky, D.; Bartanusz, V.; Dvorak, J.; Grob, D. The quality of spine surgery from the patient's perspective: Part 2. Minimal clinically important difference for improvement and deterioration as measured with the Core Outcome Measures Index. *Eur. Spine J.* **2009**, *18* (Suppl. 3), 374–379. [CrossRef]
21. Ledonio, C.G.T.; Polly, D.W.; Crawford, C.H.; Duval, S.; Smith, J.S.; Buchowski, J.; Yson, S.C.; Larson, A.N.; Sembrano, J.N.; Santos, E.R.G. Adult Degenerative Scoliosis Surgical Outcomes: A Systematic Review and Meta-analysis. *Spine Deform.* **2013**, *1*, 248–258. [CrossRef]
22. Smith, J.S.; Kelly, M.P.; Yanik, E.L.; Baldus, C.R.; Buell, T.J.; Lurie, J.D.; Edwards, C.; Glassman, S.D.; Lenke, L.G.; Boachie-Adjei, O.; et al. Operative versus nonoperative treatment for adult symptomatic lumbar scoliosis at 5-year follow-up: Durability of outcomes and impact of treatment-related serious adverse events. *J. Neurosurg. Spine* **2021**, *35*, 1–13. [CrossRef] [PubMed]
23. Dinizo, M.; Dolgalev, I.; Passias, P.G.; Errico, T.J.; Raman, T. Complications after Adult Spinal Deformity Surgeries: All Are Not Created Equal. *Int. J. Spine Surg.* **2021**, *15*, 137–143. [CrossRef]
24. Alas, H.; Passias, P.G.; Brown, A.E.; Pierce, K.E.; Bortz, C.; Bess, S.; Lafage, R.; Lafage, V.; Ames, C.P.; Burton, D.C.; et al. Predictors of serious, preventable, and costly medical complications in a population of adult spinal deformity patients. *Spine J.* **2021**, *21*, 1559–1566. [CrossRef] [PubMed]
25. Brown, A.E.; Alas, H.; Pierce, K.E.; Bortz, C.A.; Hassanzadeh, H.; Labaran, L.A.; Puvanesarajah, V.; Vasquez-Montes, D.; Wang, E.; Raman, T.; et al. Obesity negatively affects cost efficiency and outcomes following adult spinal deformity surgery. *Spine J.* **2020**, *20*, 512–518. [CrossRef]
26. Hashimoto, Y.; Yoshii, T.; Sakai, K.; Hirai, T.; Yuasa, M.; Inose, H.; Kawabata, A.; Utagawa, K.; Matsukura, Y.; Tomori, M.; et al. Impact of body mass index on surgical outcomes and complications in adult spinal deformity. *J. Orthop. Sci.* **2021**, in press. [CrossRef]
27. Khan, J.M.; Basques, B.A.; Harada, G.K.; Louie, P.K.; Chen, I.; Vetter, C.; Kadakia, K.; Elboghdady, I.; Colman, M.; An, H.S. Does increasing age impact clinical and radiographic outcomes following lumbar spinal fusion? *Spine J.* **2020**, *20*, 563–571. [CrossRef]
28. Drazin, D.; Shirzadi, A.; Rosner, J.; Eboli, P.; Safee, M.; Baron, E.M.; Liu, J.C.; Acosta, F.L. Complications and outcomes after spinal deformity surgery in the elderly: Review of the existing literature and future directions. *Neurosurg. Focus* **2011**, *31*, E3. [CrossRef]
29. Lovato, Z.R.; Deckey, D.G.; Chung, A.S.; Crandall, D.G.; Revella, J.; Chang, M.S. Adult spine deformity surgery in elderly patients: Are outcomes worse in patients 75 years and older? *Spine Deform.* **2020**, *8*, 1353–1359. [CrossRef] [PubMed]
30. Lingutla, K.K.; Pollock, R.; Benomran, E.; Purushothaman, B.; Kasis, A.; Bhatia, C.K.; Krishna, M.; Friesem, T. Outcome of lumbar spinal fusion surgery in obese patients: A systematic review and meta-analysis. *Bone Jt. J.* **2015**, *97-B*, 1395–1404. [CrossRef]
31. Pierce, K.E.; Passias, P.G.; Alas, H.; Brown, A.E.; Bortz, C.A.; Lafage, R.; Lafage, V.; Ames, C.; Burton, D.C.; Hart, R.; et al. Does Patient Frailty Status Influence Recovery Following Spinal Fusion for Adult Spinal Deformity?: An Analysis of Patients With 3-Year Follow-up. *Spine* **2020**, *45*, E397–E405. [CrossRef] [PubMed]
32. Scheer, J.K.; Smith, J.S.; Schwab, F.; Lafage, V.; Shaffrey, C.I.; Bess, S.; Daniels, A.H.; Hart, R.A.; Protopsaltis, T.S.; Mundis, G.M.; et al. Development of a preoperative predictive model for major complications following adult spinal deformity surgery. *J. Neurosurg. Spine* **2017**, *26*, 736–743. [CrossRef] [PubMed]
33. Pan, F.; Firouzabadi, A.; Reitmaier, S.; Zander, T.; Schmidt, H. The shape and mobility of the thoracic spine in asymptomatic adults—A systematic review of in vivo studies. *J. Biomech.* **2018**, *78*, 21–35. [CrossRef] [PubMed]
34. Yoshida, G.; Boissiere, L.; Larrieu, D.; Bourghli, A.; Vital, J.M.; Gille, O.; Pointillart, V.; Challier, V.; Mariey, R.; Pellisé, F.; et al. Advantages and Disadvantages of Adult Spinal Deformity Surgery and Its Impact on Health-Related Quality of Life. *Spine* **2017**, *42*, 411–419. [CrossRef] [PubMed]
35. Kyrölä, K.; Kautiainen, H.; Pekkanen, L.; Mäkelä, P.; Kiviranta, I.; Häkkinen, A. Long-term clinical and radiographic outcomes and patient satisfaction after adult spinal deformity correction. *Scand. J. Surg. SJS* **2019**, *108*, 343–351. [CrossRef] [PubMed]

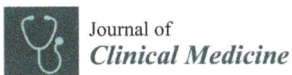

Article

Differences in Demographic and Radiographic Characteristics between Patients with Visible and Invisible T1 Slopes on Lateral Cervical Radiographic Images

Sadayuki Ito [1], Hiroaki Nakashima [1,*], Akiyuki Matsumoto [2], Kei Ando [1], Masaaki Machino [1], Naoki Segi [1], Hiroyuki Tomita [1], Hiroyuki Koshimizu [1] and Shiro Imagama [1]

1. Department of Orthopedic Surgery, Nagoya University Graduate School of Medicine, Nagoya 466-8560, Japan; sadaito@med.nagoya-u.ac.jp (S.I.); andokei@med.nagoya-u.ac.jp (K.A.); masaaki_machino_5445_2@yahoo.co.jp (M.M.); naoki.s.n@gmail.com (N.S.); hiro_tomi_1031@yahoo.co.jp (H.T.); love_derika@yahoo.co.jp (H.K.); imagama@med.nagoya-u.ac.jp (S.I.)
2. Department of Orthopedic Surgery, Okazaki City Hospital, Okazaki 444-8553, Japan; amlastregret@gmail.com
* Correspondence: hirospine@med.nagoya-u.ac.jp; Tel.: +81-52-741-2111

Abstract: Introduction: The T1 slope is important for cervical surgical planning, and it may be invisible on radiographic images. The prevalence of T1 invisible cases and the differences in demographic and radiographic characteristics between patients whose T1 slopes are visible or invisible remains unexplored. Methods: This pilot study aimed to evaluate the differences in these characteristics between outpatients whose T1 slopes were visible or invisible on radiographic images. Patients ($n = 60$) who underwent cervical radiography, whose T1 slope was confirmed clearly, were divided into the visible (V) group and invisible (I) group. The following radiographic parameters were measured: (1) C2-7 sagittal vertical axis (SVA), (2) C2-7 angle in neutral, flexion, and extension positions. Results: Based on the T1 slope visibility, 46.7% of patients were included in group I. The I group had significantly larger C2-7 SVA than the V group for males ($p < 0.05$). The C2-7 SVA tended to be larger in the I group, without significant difference for females ($p = 0.362$). Discussion: The mean C2-7 angle in neutral and flexion positions was not significantly different between the V and I groups for either sex. The mean C2-7 angle in the extension position was greater in the V group. The T1 slope was invisible in males with high C2-7 SVA.

Keywords: T1 slope; C2-7 SVA; C2-7 angle

1. Introduction

The T1 slope is defined as the angle between the horizontal line and superior endplate of the T1 vertebra [1]. It has been used to evaluate the sagittal balance of the cervical spine and has been reported to have a strong correlation with greater sagittal malalignment of the dens [1]. T1 slope angle, neck tilt, and thoracic inlet angle have been reported as significant cervical sagittal parameters, similar to the concept that pelvic incidence, pelvic tilt, and lumbar lordosis are important lumbosacral parameters in patients with adult spinal deformity [2–6]. The relationship between health-related quality of life and surgical outcomes and T1 slope has been examined in several studies [7,8].

T1 slope minus cervical lordosis can predict ideal cervical lordosis, and T1 slope plays an important role in planning cervical surgery: predicting the progression of kyphosis after cervical laminoplasty and the ideal correction angle in posterior cervical instrumentation [2,3,9]. However, the T1 vertical body is not always clearly visible on lateral cervical radiographic images because of interference by the shoulder and thoracic trunk in obese and short-necked patients [10,11]. Qiao et al. reported that the T1 upper endplate had poor visibility in 34% of cases with plain X-ray radiographs [12]. In such cases, appropriate surgical planning and clinical studies excluding cases with invisible T1 slopes have a selection bias and can be challenging.

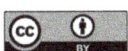

However, to the best of our knowledge, the percentage of patients with invisible T1 slopes and the difference in radiological characteristics between patients with visible or invisible T1 slopes remain unknown [13]. Therefore, this pilot study aimed to investigate the differences between these characteristics in outpatients with visible or invisible T1 slopes.

2. Materials and Methods

2.1. Study Design and Ethics Approval

Our study retrospectively included adult patients with neck pain who underwent lateral radiography with their necks in neutral, flexion, and extension positions from 2015 to 2016. The reason for radiography included spinal degenerative diseases, spinal tumors, and ossification of the posterior longitudinal ligament. Patients with a history of cervical infection, fractures, or surgery were excluded. This study was approved by the Research Ethics and Conflicts Committee of our University and was performed in accordance with the Declaration of Helsinki.

2.2. Radiological Assessment

Cervical lateral radiographs were obtained using standard radiographic techniques, in which the tube was centered on the level of the center of the xiphoid process. Lateral radiographic images were obtained with each participant standing and looking straight ahead. Flexion and extension radiographs were obtained with the neck in maximum flexion and extension. T1 slope angles were measured using these images, with the T1 slope defined as the superior endplate of the T1 vertebrae [12]. Three spine surgeons evaluated the visibility of the T1 slope. In cases where the surgeons disagreed regarding the visibility of the T1 slope, a discussion was held to reach a conclusion. Patients were divided into two groups based on whether the T1 slope was visible (V) or invisible (I), as decided by the three surgeons.

In this study, we used dynamic range control processing methods to improve the clarity of the radiographs. Dynamic range control processing can change the density and contrast of only low- and high-density areas [14].

The measured parameters in the radiographs were as follows: the Cobb angle from C2 to C7 (C2-7 angle) was defined as the angle between the inferior endplates of C2 and C7 on standing lateral radiographs. The C2-7 angle was measured in neutral, flexion, and extension positions. The C2-7 sagittal vertical axis (SVA) was defined as the deviation of the C2 plumb line (extending from the centroid of the C2 vertebra) from the superior posterior endplate of C7, with positive sagittal alignment defined as an anterior deviation. All parameters were measured twice by the same researcher independently using the same method.

2.3. Statistical Analyses

Sex was compared between the V and I groups using the Chi-square test. Patient age, body mass index (BMI), C2-7 SVA, and C2-7 angle measurements on radiographs were compared between the V and I groups using the Student's t-test. Each analysis was performed separately for men and women. For data aggregation and analyses, we used the IBM SPSS Statistics version 24.0 software (IBM Corp., Armonk, NY, USA), and $p < 0.05$ was considered statistically significant.

3. Results

The study population consisted of 60 consecutive patients with cervical spine disorders other than cervical spine trauma who visited our hospital between 2015 and 2016; of these, 30 (50.0%) were female, and the average age was 44.5 years (range: 34–81 years).

Among the 60 patients, 53.3% (32 patients; 10 men and 22 women) were included in the V group, and 46.7% (28 patients; 20 men and eight women) were included in the I group (Table 1, Figure 1).

Table 1. T1 slope visibility.

	Total (*n* = 60)	Male (*n* = 30)	Female (*n* = 30)	*p*-Value
T1 slope visibility (V group/I group)	53.3% (32/28)	33.3% (10/20)	73.3% (22/8)	<0.05

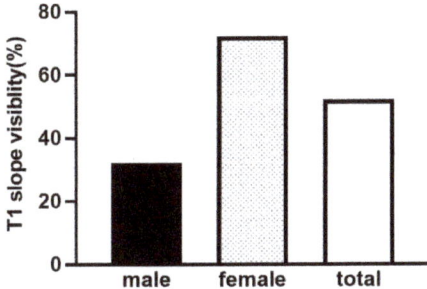

Figure 1. T1 slope visibility.

Among the 60 patients, there were spinal degenerative diseases (*n* = 28), spinal tumors (*n* = 9), ossification of the posterior longitudinal ligament (*n* = 14), and other conditions (*n* = 9). The V group included 16 patients with spinal degenerative diseases, 6 with spinal tumors, 10 with ossification of the posterior longitudinal ligament, and 5 with other conditions. The I group included 10 patients with spinal degenerative diseases, 4 with spinal tumors, 6 with ossification of the posterior longitudinal ligament, and 5 with other conditions. There was no significant difference between the V and I groups ($p = 0.943$) (Table 2).

Table 2. Cervical disorders in patients (*n* = 60).

Disorder	Total	No. of Patients V Group	I Group
Degenerative disorders	28	15	13
Spinal cord tumors	9	5	4
OPLL	14	8	6
Others	9	4	5

OPLL = ossification of the posterior longitudinal ligament. There was no significant difference between the V and I groups ($p = 0.943$).

Of the 60 patients, 23 and 37 received surgical and conservative treatment, respectively. In the V group, 12 patients received surgical treatment while 20 received conservative treatment. The I group included 11 patients who received surgical treatment and 17 who received conservative treatment. There was no significant difference between the V and I groups ($p = 0.887$) (Table 3).

Table 3. Treatment for patients (*n* = 60).

Treatment	Total	No. of Patients V Group	I Group
Surgical treatment	23	12	11
Conservative treatment	37	20	17

Surgical treatment: decompression, posterior fusion, anterior fusion, resection of tumors. Conservative treatment: medication, rehabilitation, observation. There was no significant difference between the V and I groups ($p = 0.887$).

There were significantly more males in the I group ($p < 0.05$) (Table 3). No significant differences were observed between the groups regarding age or BMI (Table 4). The mean age was 44.4 years (range: 35–78 years) in the V group, and 44.6 years (range: 34–81) in the I group. The mean BMI was 21.2 (range: 19.6–24.3) and 22.1 (range: 19.9–26.1) in the V and I groups, respectively.

Table 4. Baseline demographic characteristics of patients.

	Total	Visible (V group)	Invisible (I Group)	p-Value
Age (years)	44.5 ± 11.1	44.4 ± 12.5	44.6 ± 8.3	n.s.
BMI	21.6 ± 2.4	21.2 ± 2.3	22.1 ± 2.5	n.s.
Male:Female	30:30	10:22	20:8	<0.05

Values presented as mean ± SD; n.s., not significant; BMI, body mass index.

We compared the C2-7 SVA and C2-7 angles between the V and I groups for each sex. The mean C2-7 SVA was 16.0 mm in the V group and 28.9 mm in the I group for males. The I group had significantly greater C2-7 SVA than the V group ($p < 0.05$) (Figure 2). For females, the mean C2-7 SVA in the V group was 19.9 mm and 24.4 mm in the I group. Similar to males, there was a higher C2-7 SVA in the I group, but there was no significant difference ($p = 0.362$) (Figure 2).

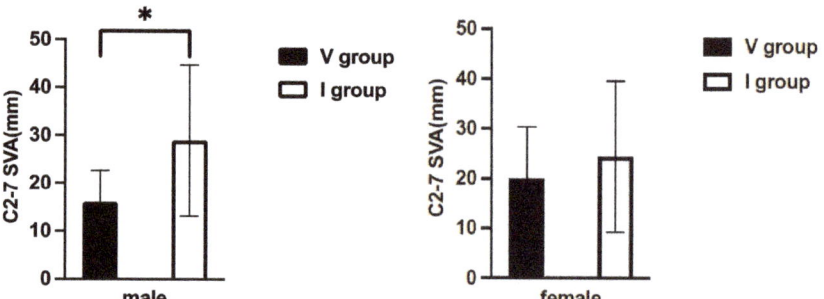

Figure 2. Comparison of the C2-7 SVA between the I and V groups in males and females. *: $p < 0.05$; V group: T1 slope visible; I group: T1 slope invisible; C2-7 SVA, C2-7 sagittal vertical axis.

In the neutral position, the mean C2-7 angle in males was 11.8° in the V group, and 12.1° in the I group, and the mean C2-7 angle in females was 11.0° and 10.4° in the V and I groups, respectively. There was no difference in the C2-7 angle in the neutral position for both males and females between the V and I groups (Figure 3).

Similar to the neutral position, there was no significant difference in the flexion position. In the flexion position, the mean C2-7 angle in males was −14.8° in the V group, and −14.0° in the I group, and the mean C2-7 angle in females was −9.4° in the V group and −8.7° in the I group. There was no significant difference in the flexion position in females: 39.2° in the V group and 30.7° in the I group ($p = 0.147$) (Figure 3). In contrast, in the extension position, the mean C2-7 angle in males was greater in the V group: 37.6° and 24.4° in the V and I groups, respectively ($p < 0.05$) (Figure 3).

Thus, male patients with greater C2-7 SVA had an invisible T1 slope, as shown in the representative cases in Figure 4A,B.

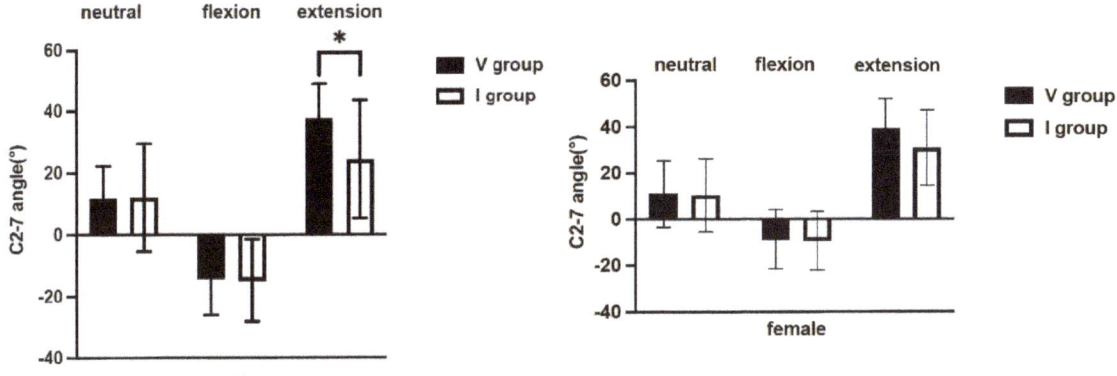

Figure 3. Comparison of the C2-7 angles between the I and V groups in neutral, flexion, and extension in males and females. *: $p < 0.05$; V group, T1 slope visible; I group, T1 slope invisible.

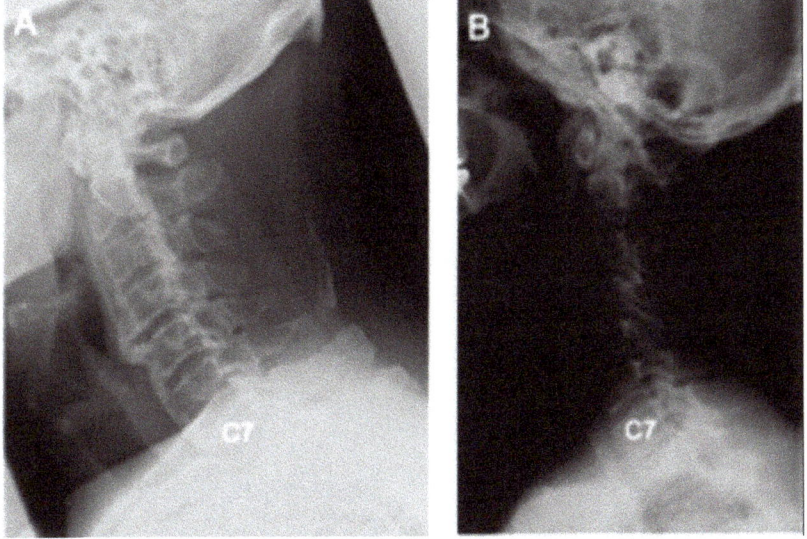

Figure 4. Comparison between invisible and visible T1 slopes of patients. (**A**) Patient with invisible T1 slope: 62 years old, male, ossification of the posterior longitudinal ligament, C2-7 SVA 58 mm, C2-7 angle 4°. (**B**) Patient with visible T1 slope: 63 years old, female, ossification of the posterior longitudinal ligament, C2-7 SVA 19 mm, C2-7 angle 22°.

In this study, some surgical cases were included. There was no clear difference in the imaging changes in surgical cases between both groups before and one year after surgery (Figure 5).

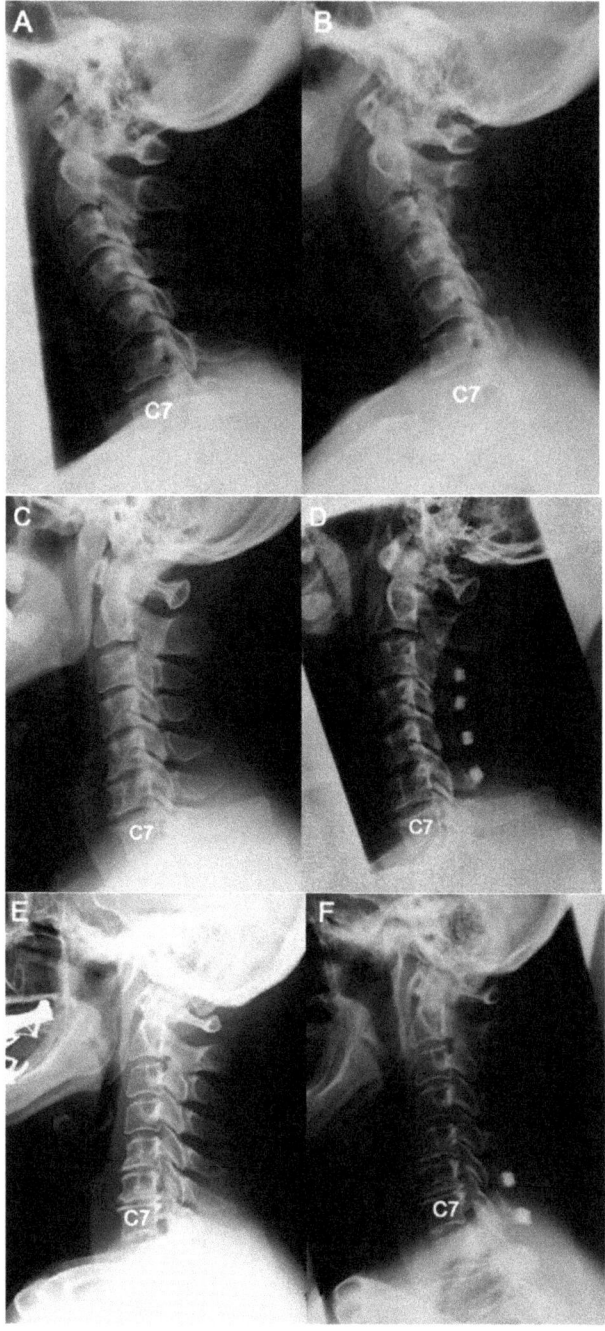

Figure 5. *Cont.*

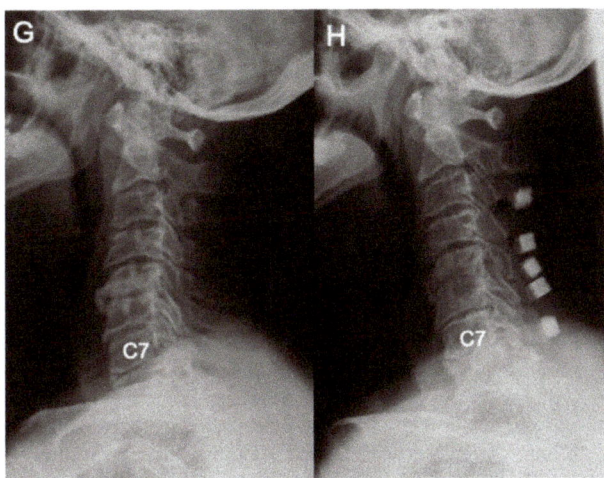

Figure 5. Pre and postoperative radiographs of patients with visible and invisible T1 slope. (**A,B**) Patient with invisible T1 slope: 50 years old, female, ossification of the posterior longitudinal ligament, C2-7 laminoplasty A; the preoperative radiograph, C2-7 SVA 39 mm, C2-7 angle 1°, C2 slope 27°, C7 slope 22°, B; the radiograph 1 year after surgery, C2-7 SVA 37 mm, C2-7 angle 11°, C2 slope 27°, C7 slope 17°. (**C,D**) Patient with invisible T1 slope: 51 years old, male, cervical spondylotic myelopathy, C3-7 laminoplasty A; the preoperative radiograph, C2-7 SVA 21 mm, C2-7 angle 15°, C2 slope 11°, C7 slope 22°, B; the radiograph 1 year after surgery, C2-7 SVA 18 mm, C2-7 angle 25°, C2 slope 5°, C7 slope 24. (**E,F**) Patient with visible T1 slope: 62 years old, female, ossification of the posterior longitudinal ligament, C5-7 laminoplasty A; the preoperative radiograph, C2-7 SVA 4 mm, C2-7 angle 7°, C2 slope 6°, C7 slope 7°, T1 slope 6°, B; the radiograph 1 year after surgery, C2-7 SVA 14 mm, C2-7 angle 2°, C2 slope 14°, C7 slope 16°, T1 slope 14°. (**G,H**) Patient with visible T1 slope: 44 years old, male, cervical spondylotic myelopathy, C3-7 laminoplasty A; the preoperative radiograph, C2-7 SVA 8 mm, C2-7 angle 12°, C2 slope 11°, C7 slope 17°, T1 slope 24°, B; the radiograph 1 year after surgery, C2-7 SVA 21 mm, C2-7 angle 1°, C2 slope 23°, C7 slope 18°, T1 slope 20°.

4. Discussion

To the best of our knowledge, this is the first study comparing the characteristics of patients with and without an identifiable T1 slope. This was a pilot study in outpatients as a preliminary step to determine the clinical significance of T1 slope visibility on surgery. In this study, the T1 slope could not be identified in 46.7% of the cases. T1 slope was invisible predominantly in males. In males, the C2-7 SVA was significantly larger, and the C2-7 angle in extension was significantly smaller in cases with an invisible T1 slope. The same trend was observed in females, but the difference was insignificant. Thus, the T1 slope was invisible in the male physique, and cases with anterior cervical shift characterized by larger C2-7 SVA.

The T1 slope was first reported by Knott et al. [1] in 2010 as the T1 sagittal angle. They noted that the T1 slope was positively correlated with the C2 SVA, influencing the global sagittal balance. Additionally, several other recent studies have addressed the relationship between the T1 slope and other parameters of the global sagittal balance of the spine. Patients with a large T1 slope require large cervical lordosis to preserve the sagittal balance of the cervical spine, suggesting that the T1 slope affects cervical sagittal alignment [14]. Furthermore, Lee et al. [3,15] reported a significant relationship between the T1 slope and thoracic kyphosis. A significant weak correlation between the T1 slope and lumbar lordosis was also reported [15]. These findings suggest that the T1 slope is associated with cervical sagittal alignment and thoracic and lumbar sagittal alignment, in addition to the fact that the T1 slope is an important factor for global sagittal alignment. However, it has been reported that upright cervical radiographs are more accurate than whole spine radiographs for evaluating cervical spine alignment, including T1 slope. This study used upright cervical spine radiographs instead of whole spine radiographs [16].

Despite the importance of the T1 slope, the T1 vertebral body is often unclear on cervical radiographic images due to interference of the shoulder contour, especially in obese or muscular individuals [11,17], resulting in difficulty in identifying the T1 slope. In previous reports, the T1 slope was difficult to identify in approximately one-third of the cases [12,17]. In this study, the T1 slope could not be identified in 46.7% of the cases, almost consistent with the previous observation.

Several alternative methods have been investigated in cases with an invisible T1 slope, including magnetic resonance imaging (MRI) or computed tomography (CT). T1s-CL is important for cervical spine postoperative alignment assessment. In a study examining alternative parameters to T1s-CL, the C2 slope was the parameter that correlated best with pre- and postoperative changes [18]. Supine MRI and CT images cannot be considered an alternative to the T1 slope on lateral radiographs as these images are not captured in the upright position [19]. Jun et al. reported that the T1 slope angle on radiographs was larger than on CT images. However, a significant correlation was noted between the T1 slope angles on radiographs and CT images [10]. Park et al. correlated C7 slope with T1 slope by measuring T1 slope on CT based on C7 slope on X-ray. However, they excluded cases where the T1 slope was not visible on the X-ray [13]. A strong correlation between C7 slope and T1 slope has been found in MRI studies with the patient seated in upright weight-bearing neutral positions. However, no comparison with x-rays has been made [20]. Ideally, the imaging modality enabling clear visualization of the T1 upper endplate in an upright position, such as EOS® (EOS® imaging, Paris, France), is generally desired [21]. EOS® is the EOS imaging system, a novel technique that allows for acquiring images of the body or of body sections in standing position and under normal weight-bearing conditions [22]. However, many facilities do not have access to EOS, and researchers have to exclude cases in which the T1 upper endplate is invisible. As an alternative to the T1 slope on lateral radiographs, the C7 slope reportedly correlated significantly with the T1 slope [12,17].

We showed that cases with invisible T1 slopes had some notable characteristics. First, the T1 slope was invisible in males. This may be affected by differences in body thickness and shoulder position between men and women: the T1 upper endplate could be affected by the shoulder and thoracic trunk, especially in obese and short-necked patients [10]. Furthermore, Reynolds et al. demonstrated that neck circumference influences cervical sagittal alignment [23]. Neck circumference is influenced by muscle or obesity [24]; thus, it can influence T1 slope visibility. Further, we found significant differences in extension (C2-7) angle and C2-7 SVA between patients in the I and V groups. In cases where the cervical vertebrae shift forward and the cervical backward bending angle is small, T1 is hidden under the soft tissue and appears invisible, as shown in Figure 4. The risk of kyphotic deformity after cervical decompression is high in cases with a large C2-7 SVA shift [25]. Many cases require deformity correction, and the T1 slope must be considered to achieve an ideal cervical lordosis. The classification of cervical spine deformity is based on the T1 slope [26]. However, it might be necessary to consider a new classification based on a reliably measurable index such as the C7 slope [12].

There are some limitations to this study. First, the number of patients included in this study was small. Further, this study was conducted on symptomatic patients, which may have affected the global alignments. To overcome this problem, clinicians should consider investigating the radiography of healthy individuals. However, these patients may be evaluated in clinical studies for surgical results. Furthermore, the condition of radiographic imaging was not completely unified; thus, it could affect T1 visibility. It would also have been desirable for the three surgeons to blindly classify the patients into the V and I groups before starting the study. However, since there were no numerical data, the three surgeons discussed the decision from the beginning. As a result, it was necessary to discuss and decide one way or the other, and the result would not have been different even if we had done it blindly at the beginning. In addition, C2-7 SVA and C2-7 angles were measured by a single person, and the validation is insufficient.

5. Conclusions

In summary, our study analyzed the differences in demographic and radiological characteristics between patients with visible or invisible T1 slopes. Our findings suggest that the T1 slope tends to be invisible in males with greater C2-7 SVA. This was a pilot study. Therefore, based on the results of this study, we would like to accumulate surgical cases in the future and further investigate the clinical significance of this study.

Author Contributions: Conceptualization, A.M.; methodology, S.I. (Sadayuki Ito); software, A.M.; validation, A.M.; formal analysis, S.I. (Sadayuki Ito); investigation, S.I. (Sadayuki Ito), H.N., A.M., K.A., M.M., N.S., H.T., H.K. and S.I. (Shiro Imagama); resources, S.I. (Sadayuki Ito), H.N., A.M., K.A., M.M., N.S., H.T., H.K. and S.I. (Shiro Imagama); data curation, A.M.; writing—original draft preparation, S.I. (Sadayuki Ito); writing—review and editing, S.I. (Sadayuki Ito) and H.N.; supervision, S.I. (Shiro Imagama); project administration, H.N. All authors have read and agreed to the published version of the manuscript.

Funding: This research did not receive any specific grant from funding agencies in the public, commercial, or not-for-profit sectors.

Institutional Review Board Statement: The research protocol was approved by the Human Research Ethics Committee and the University's Institutional Review Board (approval number: 2005-0354-3). All participants gave written informed consent prior to participation. The research procedure was carried out in accordance with the principles of the Declaration of Helsinki.

Informed Consent Statement: Informed consent was obtained from all subjects involved in the study.

Data Availability Statement: The data of this study are available from the corresponding author upon request.

Acknowledgments: We are grateful to the staff of the department of radiology at Nagoya University Hospital.

Conflicts of Interest: The authors declare that there is no conflict of interest regarding the publication of this paper.

References

1. Knott, P.T.; Mardjetko, S.M.; Techy, F. The use of the T1 sagittal angle in predicting overall sagittal balance of the spine. *Spine J.* **2010**, *10*, 994–998. [CrossRef] [PubMed]
2. Jun, H.S.; Kim, J.H.; Ahn, J.H.; Chang, I.B.; Song, J.H.; Kim, T.H.; Park, M.S.; Kim, Y.C.; Kim, S.W.; Oh, J.K. T1 slope and degenerative cervical spondylolisthesis. *Spine* **2015**, *40*, E220–E226. [CrossRef]
3. Lee, S.H.; Son, E.S.; Seo, E.M.; Suk, K.S.; Kim, K.T. Factors determining cervical spine sagittal balance in asymptomatic adults: Correlation with spinopelvic balance and thoracic inlet alignment. *Spine J.* **2015**, *15*, 705–712. [CrossRef]
4. Protopsaltis, T.S.; Soroceanu, A.; Tishelman, J.C.; Buckland, A.J.; Mundis, G.M., Jr.; Smith, J.S.; Daniels, A.; Lenke, L.G.; Kim, H.J.; Klineberg, E.O.; et al. Should Sagittal Spinal Alignment Targets for Adult Spinal Deformity Correction Depend on Pelvic Incidence and Age? *Spine* **2020**, *45*, 250–257. [CrossRef] [PubMed]
5. Terran, J.; Schwab, F.; Shaffrey, C.I.; Smith, J.S.; Devos, P.; Ames, C.P.; Fu, K.M.; Burton, D.; Hostin, R.; Klineberg, E.; et al. The SRS-Schwab adult spinal deformity classification: Assessment and clinical correlations based on a prospective operative and nonoperative cohort. *Neurosurgery* **2013**, *73*, 559–568. [CrossRef]
6. Protopsaltis, T.; Schwab, F.; Bronsard, N.; Smith, J.S.; Klineberg, E.; Mundis, G.; Ryan, D.J.; Hostin, R.; Hart, R.; Burton, D.; et al. TheT1 pelvic angle, a novel radiographic measure of global sagittal deformity, accounts for both spinal inclination and pelvic tilt and correlates with health-related quality of life. *J. Bone Jt. Surg. Am.* **2014**, *96*, 1631–1640. [CrossRef] [PubMed]
7. Kim, T.H.; Lee, S.Y.; Kim, Y.C.; Park, M.S.; Kim, S.W. T1 slope as a predictor of kyphotic alignment change after laminoplasty in patients with cervical myelopathy. *Spine* **2013**, *38*, E992–E997. [CrossRef] [PubMed]
8. Oe, S.; Yamato, Y.; Togawa, D.; Kurosu, K.; Mihara, Y.; Banno, T.; Yasuda, T.; Kobayashi, S.; Hasegawa, T.; Matsuyama, Y. Preoperative T1 Slope More Than 40° as a Risk Factor of Correction Loss in Patients with Adult Spinal Deformity. *Spine* **2016**, *41*, E1168–E1176. [CrossRef]
9. Cho, J.H.; Ha, J.K.; Kim, D.G.; Song, K.Y.; Kim, Y.T.; Hwang, C.J.; Lee, C.S.; Lee, D.H. Does preoperative T1 slope affect radiological and functional outcomes after cervical laminoplasty? *Spine* **2014**, *39*, E1575–E1581. [CrossRef]

10. Jun, H.S.; Chang, I.B.; Song, J.H.; Kim, T.H.; Park, M.S.; Kim, S.W.; Oh, J.K. Is it possible to evaluate the parameters of cervical sagittal alignment on cervical computed tomographic scans? *Spine* **2014**, *39*, E630–E636. [CrossRef]
11. Park, J.H.; Cho, C.B.; Song, J.H.; Kim, S.W.; Ha, Y.; Oh, J.K. T1 Slope and Cervical Sagittal Alignment on Cervical CT Radiographs of Asymptomatic Persons. *J. Korean Neurosurg. Soc.* **2013**, *53*, 356–359. [CrossRef] [PubMed]
12. Inoue, T.; Ando, K.; Kobayashi, K.; Nakashima, H.; Ito, K.; Katayama, Y.; Machino, M.; Kanbara, S.; Ito, S.; Yamaguchi, H.; et al. Age-related Changes in T1 and C7 Slope and the Correlation Between Them in More Than 300 Asymptomatic Subjects. *Spine* **2021**, *46*, E474–E481. [CrossRef] [PubMed]
13. Park, B.J.; Gold, C.J.; Woodroffe, R.W.; Yamaguchi, S. What is the most accurate substitute for an invisible T1 slope in cervical radiographs? A comparative study of a novel method with previously reported substitutes. *J. Neurosurg. Spine* **2021**, *1*, 1–7. [CrossRef] [PubMed]
14. Weng, C.; Wang, J.; Tuchman, A.; Wang, J.; Fu, C.; Hsieh, P.C.; Buser, Z.; Wang, J.C. Influence of T1 Slope on the Cervical Sagittal Balance in Degenerative Cervical Spine: An Analysis Using Kinematic MRI. *Spine* **2016**, *41*, 185–190. [CrossRef] [PubMed]
15. Yang, M.; Yang, C.; Zhai, X.; Zhao, J.; Zhu, X.; Li, M. Analysis of Factors Associated With Sagittal Balance in Normal Asymptomatic Individuals: A Retrospective Study in a Population of East China. *Spine* **2017**, *42*, E219–E225. [CrossRef]
16. Lee, D.H.; Park, S.; Kim, D.G.; Hwang, C.J.; Lee, C.S.; Hwang, E.S.; Cho, J.H. Cervical spine lateral radiograph versus whole spine lateral radiograph: A retrospective comparative study to identify a better modality to assess cervical sagittal alignment. *Medicine* **2021**, *100*, e25987. [CrossRef]
17. Gelb, D.E.; Lenke, L.G.; Bridwell, K.H.; Blanke, K.; McEnery, K.W. An analysis of sagittal spinal alignment in 100 asymptomatic middle and older aged volunteers. *Spine* **1995**, *20*, 1351–1358. [CrossRef]
18. Lee, H.J.; You, S.T.; Sung, J.H.; Kim, I.S.; Hong, J.T. Analyzing the Significance of T1 Slope minus Cervical Lordosis in Patients with Anterior Cervical Discectomy and Fusion Surgery. *J. Korean Neurosurg. Soc.* **2021**, *64*, 913–921. [CrossRef]
19. Xing, R.; Zhou, G.; Chen, Q.; Liang, Y.; Dong, J. MRI to measure cervical sagittal parameters: A comparison with plain radiographs. *Arch. Orthop. Trauma Surg.* **2017**, *137*, 451–455. [CrossRef]
20. Tamai, K.; Buser, Z.; Paholpak, P.; Sessumpun, K.; Nakamura, H.; Wang, J.C. Can C7 Slope Substitute the T1 slope?: An Analysis Using Cervical Radiographs and Kinematic MRIs. *Spine* **2018**, *43*, 520–525. [CrossRef]
21. Le Huec, J.C.; Demezon, H.; Aunoble, S. Sagittal parameters of global cervical balance using EOS imaging: Normative values from a prospective cohort of asymptomatic volunteers. *Eur. Spine J.* **2015**, *24*, 63–71. [CrossRef] [PubMed]
22. Garg, B.; Mehta, N.; Bansal, T.; Malhotra, R. EOS®imaging: Concept and current applications in spinal disorders. *J. Clin. Orthop. Trauma* **2020**, *11*, 786–793. [CrossRef] [PubMed]
23. Reynolds, J.; Marsh, D.; Koller, H.; Zenenr, J.; Bannister, G. Cervical range of movement in relation to neck dimension. *Eur. Spine J.* **2009**, *18*, 863–868. [CrossRef] [PubMed]
24. Ben-Noun, L.; Sohar, E.; Laor, A. Neck circumference as a simple screening measure for identifying overweight and obese patients. *Obes Res.* **2001**, *9*, 470–477. [CrossRef]
25. Kato, M.; Namikawa, T.; Matsumura, A.; Konishi, S.; Nakamura, H. Effect of Cervical Sagittal Balance on Laminoplasty in Patients With Cervical Myelopathy. *Glob. Spine J.* **2017**, *7*, 154–161. [CrossRef]
26. Ames, C.P.; Smith, J.S.; Eastlack, R.; Blaskiewicz, D.J.; Shaffrey, C.I.; Schwab, F.; Bess, S.; Kim, H.J.; Mundis, G.M., Jr.; Klineberg, E.; et al. Reliability assessment of a novel cervical spine deformity classification system. *J. Neurosurg. Spine* **2015**, *23*, 673–683. [CrossRef]

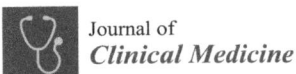

Article

An Indication-Based Concept for Stepwise Spinal Orthosis in Low Back Pain According to the Current Literature

Franz Landauer [1,*] and Klemens Trieb [1,2]

1. Department of Orthopaedic and Trauma Surgery, Paracelsus Medical University Salzburg, 5020 Salzburg, Austria; k.trieb@salk.at
2. Computed Tomography Research Group, University of Applied Sciences Upper Austria, 4600 Wels, Austria
* Correspondence: f.landauer@salk.at

Citation: Landauer, F.; Trieb, K. An Indication-Based Concept for Stepwise Spinal Orthosis in Low Back Pain According to the Current Literature. *J. Clin. Med.* **2022**, *13*, 510. https://doi.org/10.3390/jcm11030510

Academic Editors: Takashi Hirai, Hiroaki Nakashima, Masayuki Miyagi, Shinji Takahashi, Masashi Uehara and Panagiotis Korovessis

Received: 9 December 2021
Accepted: 17 January 2022
Published: 20 January 2022

Publisher's Note: MDPI stays neutral with regard to jurisdictional claims in published maps and institutional affiliations.

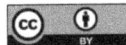

Copyright: © 2022 by the authors. Licensee MDPI, Basel, Switzerland. This article is an open access article distributed under the terms and conditions of the Creative Commons Attribution (CC BY) license (https://creativecommons.org/licenses/by/4.0/).

Abstract: Background: The current literature is not conclusive for spinal orthosis treatment in low back pain. Therefore, two questions have to be answered: Does the current literature support the indication of spinal orthosis treatment in low back pain? Which treatment concept can be derived from the result? Method: The 30 highest-rated literature citations (PubMed: best match, 30 December 2021) dealing with low back pain and spine orthosis were included in the study. Excluded were all articles related to Kinesio Taping, scoliosis, physical exercise, or dealing with side effects and unrelated to treatment effect. Thus, the literature list refers only to "low back pain and spine orthoses". These articles were analyzed according to the PRISMA criteria and divided according to "specific diagnosis", when the cause of pain was explained (group A), or when "specific diagnosis is not given" (group B). The articles were also distinguished by the information about the orthosis. Articles with biomechanical information about the function of the orthoses were called "diagnosis-based orthosis" (group C). All other articles were part of the group "unspecific orthotic treatment" (group D). The results were compared to each other in terms of effectiveness. According to anatomical causes, a concept of orthosis selection depending on diagnosis of low back pain for clinical practice was developed. The risk of bias lies in the choice of the MESH terms. The synthesis of the results was a clinical treatment concept based on findings from the current literature. Results: The literature citations with 1749 patients and 2160 citations of literature were processed; 21 prospective clinical or biomechanical studies and 9 review articles were included. The combination of literature citations according to "specific diagnosis" (group A) and "diagnosis based orthosis" (group C) was very likely to lead to a therapeutic effect (seven articles). No positive effect could be found in four articles, all dealing with postoperative treatment. When "specific diagnosis is not given" (group B) and combined with "unspecific orthotic treatment" (group D), therapy remained without measurable effect (15 articles). An effect was described in four articles (three biomechanical studies and one postoperative study). In review articles, according to specific diagnosis, only one article dealt with fractures and another with stenosis. In all review articles where specific diagnosis was not given, no effect with spine orthoses could be found. Using this knowledge, we created a clinical treatment concept. The structure was based on diagnosis and standardized orthoses. According to pain location and pathology (muscle, intervertebral disc, bone, statics, postoperative) the orthoses were classified to anatomical extent and the mechanical limitation (bandage, bodice, corset, orthosis with shoulder straps and erecting orthosis). Conclusion: The effectiveness of spinal orthoses could not be deduced from the current literature. The most serious limitation was the inconsistency of the complaint and the imprecise designation of the orthoses. Interpretation: Articles with a precise allocation of the complaint and a description of the orthosis showed a positive effect. The treatment concept presented here is intended to provide a basis for answering the question concerning the effectiveness of spinal orthoses as an accompanying treatment option in low back pain.

Keywords: back pain; low back pain; brace; spine orthoses; lumbar support; spine support

1. Introduction

Spinal orthoses are used for spinal complaints in a very undifferentiated manner. This concerns the medical clarification as well as the selection of the aids. The international literature has referred to the clarification of a treatment algorithm.

The goal of orthotic care for spinal disorders is to reduce discomfort while activating the patient. This is achieved by segmental spinal stabilization and/or position correction. However, a targeted reduction of discomfort is only possible if the cause of the discomfort is known. This results in the requirement for a structured clinical examination, followed by imaging procedures.

A structured treatment concept is required for orthotic care, comparable to surgical planning. Undifferentiated indications bring orthotic treatment into disrepute, and the opinion of physicians regarding this form of treatment may be classified as negative. Nevertheless, the prescribing behavior is surprisingly generous in, for example, Austria. It is not the intention of this article to present this discrepancy. Rather, it aims to provide a guideline for structured care. The structure of this article is based on orthotics of the thoraco-lumbo-sacral spine.

The current literature is focused on lumbar complaints and thus on quickly available adaptable orthoses (adaptable device = industrial products).

This article attempts to reconcile the medical indications with the biomechanical criteria for orthotic fitting, and to address the following questions: does the current literature support the indication of spinal orthosis treatment in low back pain, and what treatment concept can be derived from the result? We hypothesized that if the cause of low back pain is not clarified and differentiated, no targeted effect may be expected from orthotic fitting.

2. Methods

The present article follows the current PRISMA criteria from 2020. This report comprises a literature review for which the current literature was first searched in PubMed on 30 October 2021 for the MESH terms "low back pain and spine orthoses", then updated on 30 December 2021. Excluded were all articles related to Kinesio Taping, scoliosis, physical exercise programs and articles unrelated to treatment effect. Papers related only to a side effect were not included in the literature list. A general definition of low back pain and spine orthoses is given. Thus, the literature list refers only to "low back pain and spine orthoses" and resulted in 30 matches [1–30]. If the cause of the complaints was mentioned in an article, said article was assigned to group (A) with specific diagnosis.

Papers that did not provide a definite indication of the cause of pain were assigned to group (B), "specific diagnosis is not given". Orthoses were differentiated in the same way. Articles with clear biomechanical information about the orthosis were called "diagnosis based orthosis" (group C). All other articles with only general biomechanical information were assigned to the group "unspecific orthotic treatment" (group D).

For the treatment concept, the next step was to create a structured differentiation of the orthoses. The differentiation was made in accordance with colloquial terms because a generally accepted definition or classification does not exist. In a further step, a standardization of the orthotic indication was created in accordance with the different causes of pain. This resulted in a clarification concept for the cause of pain and subsequently a functional, biomechanical treatment goal for the orthosis selection. This concept was summarized in tabular form.

The risk of bias lies in the choice of the MESH terms. The synthesis of the results yielded a clinical treatment concept based on findings from the current literature.

3. Results

In the first search, 43,153 papers ("low back pain") were found; when adding "brace", 318 remained, 4949 for "spine support" and 3623 for "lumbar support". For "orthoses", 391 papers remained. The abstracts were searched for the exclusion criteria as described above. Thereafter, 54 papers remained for full-text screening, which resulted in full-text analysis of the 30 papers presented here with clinical relevance ([1–30], Figure 1).

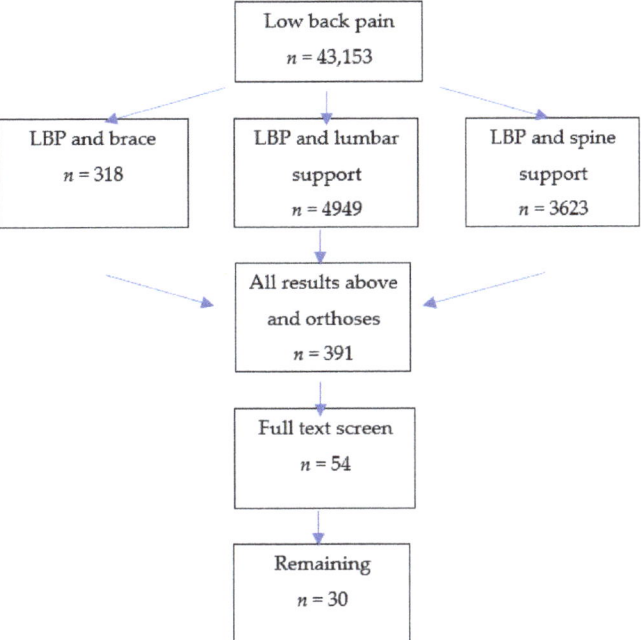

Figure 1. Flow diagram.

Literature citations with 1749 patients and 2160 citations were processed. Ultimately, 21 prospective clinical or biomechanical studies and 9 review articles were included.

The following definitions of low back pain and spine orthoses were used:

Low back pain was defined as pain of musculoskeletal origin extending from the lowest rib to the gluteal fold that may at times extend as somatic referred pain into the thigh (above the knee). The definition of the North American Spine Society (978-1-929988-65-5) of an orthosis is as follows: A brace, splint, or other artificial external device serving to support the limbs or spine or to prevent or assist relative movement [13].

Many different terms are used for back orthoses (spinal orthoses, spine support, back supports, braces, bandage, girdle spine support, bodice, corsage, corset etc.).

This concerns the choice of words used, the indication for the orthotic fitting as well as its mode of action and design. A generally valid definition is lacking. There is only a general classification in ISO 8549-3:2020(en) (see Tables 1–3).

3.1. Overview of the Current Literature

The cause of the complaint must be diagnostically narrowed down.

The orthosis must be clearly defined in terms and function (Table 1).

Only when a differentiated cause of the complaint according to "specific diagnosis" was determined (group A) and the appropriately adapted "diagnosis based orthosis" was used (group C), were positive effects found in prospective studies ([2,5,9,22,28,30], Table 1), one retrospective study ([28], Table 1) and one review article ([10], Table 2).

No positive effect was prescribed in postoperative prospective studies ([20,23,25], Table 1) and one review article ([29], Table 2).

When no specific diagnosis is given (group B) and nonspecific orthotic treatment is administered (group D), no consistent result can be expected. The listed prospective studies ([1,6,8,11,14,17–19], Table 1) and review articles ([12,13,15,16,24,26,27], Table 2) demonstrated no positive effect. An effect was described in three biomechanical studies ([3,4,7], Table 1) and one postoperative study [21].

All meta-analyses and literature research reviewed did not provide medical or technical differentiation [1,6,8,11–19,24,26,27]. Thus, general orthotic designations such as "lumbar support" are used in the following. A general conclusion could not be found.

No review articles were identified where specific diagnosis was not given and orthosis with unspecific treatment was combined.

Table 1. Therapy effect in the literature for prospective studies and one retrospective study, depending on cause of complaint and orthosis.

Diagnosis		Orthosis
Group A According to specific diagnosis	With effect [2,5,9,22,30] (retrospective study 28)	Group C Diagnosis based Orthosis
	Without effect [20,23,25]	
Group B Specific diagnosis is not given	With effect [3,4,7,21]	Group D Orthosis as unspecific treatment
	Without effect [1,6,8,11,14,17–19]	

Table 2. Therapy effect in the literature for review articles depending on cause of complaint and orthosis.

Diagnosis		Orthosis
Group A According to specific diagnosis	With effect [10]	Group C Diagnosis based Orthosis
	Without effect [29]	
Group B Specific diagnosis is not given	With effect -	Group D Orthosis as unspecific treatment
	Without effect [12,13,15,16,24,26,27]	

3.2. Summary of the Literature and Whether It Supports the Indication of Spinal Orthosis Treatment in Low Back Pain

In the examined scientific literature we found a wide range of terms for orthoses. The terms did not give a clear indication of the orthosis used (orthosis, lumbar support, lumbar belt, brace, bandage, bodice, corset, pelvic orthosis, LSO (lumbosacral orthosis), low-profile exosuit, TLSO (thoraco-lumbar orthosis), hip orthosis, lumbar corset, bracing, back belt, rigid brace). Conversely, in biomechanical studies, clear descriptions could be found ([1–5,7,11], Table 1).

The medical descriptions of the complaint did not always indicate the cause of pain. Wordings were non-specific with regard to low back pain, back pain, etc. [6,8,14,17–19,22,27,28]. Within meta-analyses, review articles and an online survey, the causes of the pain were not differentiated [10,12,15,16,24,26,29]. In all cases of postoperative treatment, clear information about the clinical situation was given [20,21,23,25,29]. Only in one clinical study was clear information (MRI-Modic 1) given [28].

3.3. Differentiation of Spine Orthoses

In the following we make an effort to systematize the different terms used to describe orthoses and to link them to complaints and diagnostics.

Bandage (Soft orthosis with or without pads):
Protective, supporting bandage, soft/elastic (i.e., encompassing body parts with/without pads).

The indications for fitting are acute or chronic complaints diagnosed by clinical examination.

The mode of action is through a circular socket and force application via a pad.

The diagnosis is considered to be mild, chronic or recurrent pain in the lumbar region (back support brace with dynamic pad, Figure 2).

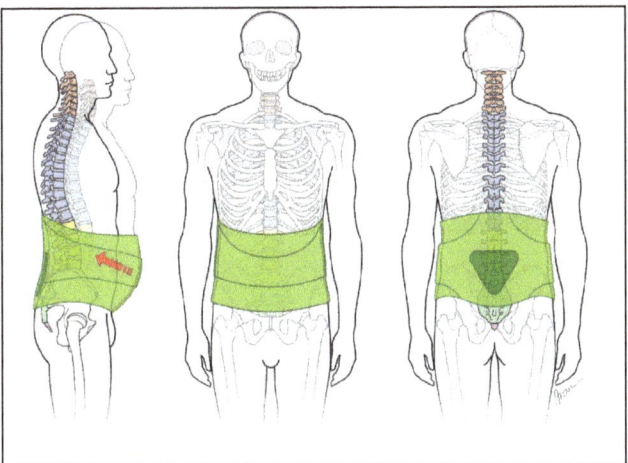

Figure 2. Bandage "Soft orthosis with or without pads".

Furthermore, spinal pain with moderate instability and lumbalgia are specified (lordosis/correction/bandage).

Bodice (girdle spine support, soft orthoses with struts, spine support, corsage):
Locally differentiated diagnoses are defined as indications for bodices. X-ray imaging is recommended for indication.

The mode of action is via stiffening elements that overlap and stabilize body regions. Delordosing of the lumbar spine is the major goal.

The diagnosis of recurrent pain in the lumbar spine or at the thoraco-lumbar transition is the primary focus (e.g., lumbalgia, dorsalgia), postnucleotomy syndrome and for postoperative immobilization, but also instability, etc. (spine support with struts, Figure 3).

A distinction must be made between height differentiations with anatomical assignment as stretching only the lumbar spine (LSO) or including the thoracic spine (TLSO), etc.

Spine support with abdominal sling for delordosis and relief of the segments of the lumbar spine (in case of highly protruding abdomen, pregnancy, etc.).

Corset (soft orthoses with a rigid part to encompass the pelvis or a rigid orthoses):
Diagnosis of ailments that can be treated by correction and/or stabilization over the pelvic area form the indication for corsets.

Their mode of action is the correction in the sagittal and frontal planes and the limitation of rotation. This results in a degree of limitation that recommends slice imaging (CT or MRI) in most cases.

Segmental instabilities, spondylitis or spondylodiscitis, tumors and metastases, fractures without significant change in shape etc. are the most common indications.

A special form of indication is a bridging corset with the possibility of gradual release of movement (e.g., as postoperative care; Figure 4). The corset becomes a bodice by removing the pelvic frame and a bandage by removing the stiffening elements. This gradually increases mobility.

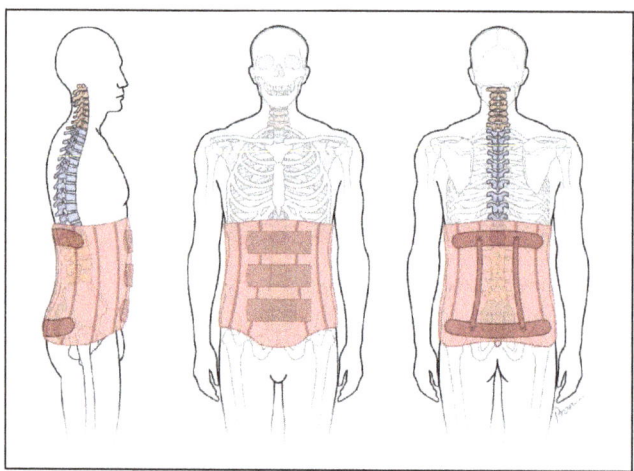

Figure 3. Bodice "soft orthosis with struts".

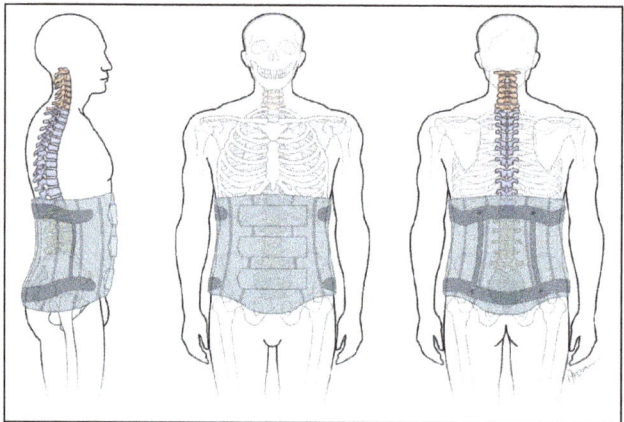

Figure 4. Corset "Soft orthoses with a rigid part encompass the pelvis".

Back brace with shoulder straps to erect the spine: dorsal struts with shoulder straps to erect the thoracic spine.

Symptomatic osteoporosis and hyperkyphosis in seniors are the most common indication for this treatment (Figure 5) [30].

Spinal orthosis which does not encompass the body to relieve spine: orthoses that do not encircle the trunk in a circular manner. Their aim is correction, especially in the sagittal plane. Thus, the indication for straightening the spine is in the primary focus. Vertebral fracture treatment without significant bony deformity forms the main indication (Figure 6).

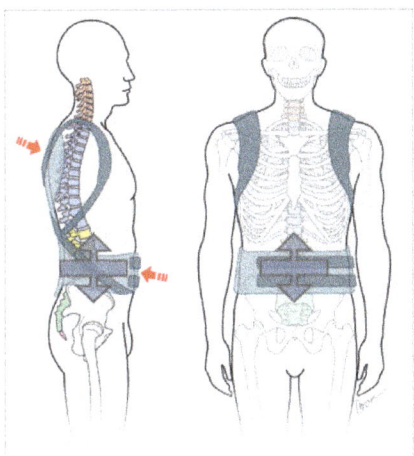

Figure 5. Back brace with shoulder straps to erect spine.

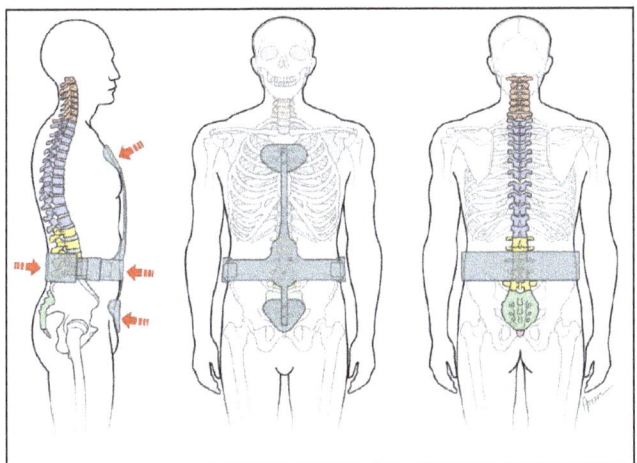

Figure 6. Spinal orthosis to relieve the spine.

Our goal was to derive a treatment concept on the basis of a delineation of the indications for different orthoses.

According to the results of the literature review and classification of spinal orthosis, we made a standardization of indication. A clarification concept of the complaints followed by the orthosis selection depending on anatomical cause of the complaint was an element of the treatment concept.

In Table 3, pain localization is linked to pathology and orthosis selection is based on the anatomical localization and cause of the complaint. Table 3 gives an overview for a basic concept.

The result of a clinical examination is sufficient for the prescription of a bandage. Bandages can relieve pressure through the circular socket and, through the use of pads, provide targeted force application and thus pain relief (Figure 2).

Diagnoses derived from X-ray findings allow segmental assignment. Thus, a segmental force application or change in position of the spine is required to alleviate the symptoms. This correction can be achieved by a bodice (girdle spine support) (Figure 3).

A differentiated diagnosis by means of CT or MRI provides information that can be assigned to segmental anatomical structures. Only wearing a corset can provide the resulting stabilization or change of spine positioning (Figure 4).

In everyday use, there are overlaps between bodices and corsets.

A back brace with shoulder straps is indicated to erect the spine without affecting breathing. A fragile kyphotic spine, especially in elderly people, is the main indication (osteoporosis, metastasis, etc.) (Figure 5).

Spine supports which do not encompass the body are a possible treatment of vertebral body fractures without loss of stability, and support the healing conservatively (according to AO classifications A0 and A1) (Figure 6).

For prevention, wearables have become increasingly available as a training device for postoperative treatment and to avoid discomfort. The line between medical treatment and sports equipment is becoming increasingly blurred.

Table 3. Standardization of indication and therapy goals.

	Diagnosis		Orthosis		
Summary	Back pain		Spinal orthosis		
Local distribution	Cervical syndrome Dorsalgia Lumbalgia Sacralgia Combination		Cervical orthosis (CO) Thoracic orthosis (TO) Lumbo-sacral orthosis (LSO) Sacro-iliac orthosis (SIO) Thoraco-lumbar-sacral orthosis (TLSO) Cervico-thoraco-lumbo-sacral orthosis (CTLSO)		
Pathology	Diagnosis	Therapy	Mode of action	Product	
Muscle	Lumbalgia	Relief	Targeted force application via pads	Bandage	
Disc	Lumbalgia Lumboischialgia Instability	Stabilization Positioning	Delordosization through dorsal bridging		
Bone	Spondylarthrosis Baastrup Osteochondrosis Osteoporosis Fracture Metastases	Position change Stabilization Stabilization Prevention	Delordosis	Bodice Corset Back brace Spinal orthosis	Depending on the necessary stability
Static	Hyperkyphosis Hyperlordosis Scoliosis	Position correction			
Postoperative	Post segmental fusion	Stabilization Protect the adjacent segment Rapid mobilization	Local relief	Soft orthosis with struts	
Training device	Long-term treatment or prevention	Activation	Stimulators Assistive products	Wearables	

4. Discussion

This manuscript demonstrates missing links between low back pain and orthotic fitting. As a result of these findings, we developed a concept for orthotic selection depending on the pathological source. This could be considered a step towards improving the accompanying treatment options and therapeutic accuracy.

Spinal orthoses can limit range of motion, and can stabilize or reposition spinal segments. In the case of obesity or during pregnancy, the circular design can relieve the spine through targeted application of ventral forces. Other local effects are described, but not well studied. For temporary orthotic treatment, the effects must be consistent with the cause of the complaint.

One prospective study did not show any effectiveness of lumbar supports in 28 assembly-line workers, with respect to low back functionality and disability [1]. In contrast, another reported positive effects of wearing a lumbar belt in workers [4]. An in vitro biomechanical study investigating the effects on posterior pelvis kinematics reported an altered lumbosacral transition and increased movement in the sacroiliac joint by pelvic orthosis [5].

Two prospective reports dealt with postoperative bracing including 119 patients. No indication for postoperative bracing regarding pain relief or quality of life was observed [22,23]. The same was true for 96 patients with conservatively treated thoracolumbar burst fractures [9] or following single-level lumbar discectomy in 54 patients [20].

Regarding low back pain, different study protocols reported a positive effect of lumbar orthosis in 115 patients [2,6,18,21]. In contrast, four different randomized studies did not provide any pain relief after six months observation of 266 patients [8,14,17,30]. No positive effect of wearing a lumbar orthosis on muscle thickness measured by ultrasound was reported in 44 patients [19]. Reduced back muscle fatigue was reported in six healthy participants after wearing a low-profile elastic exosuit [7].

Here we only individually discuss those contributions that describe no effect despite differentiated cause of pain and differentiated orthotic fitting. In total, 30 studies were identified, of which 20 were prospective studies (Table 1) and nine were reviews or meta-analyses (Table 2). The remaining paper was a retrospective analysis of treating chronic lumbar back pain with a rigid lumbar brace [28]. The literature selection process is presented in the flow diagram in Figure 6.

Zoia et al. investigated postoperative orthotic fitting after monosegmental disc surgery. Their highly structured study concluded that after monosegmental disc surgery, the short-term and mid-term outcomes displayed no difference to orthosis-free care [20].

It should be noted that all patients displayed monoradicular lumboischialgia and were surgically treated by only two surgeons using microscopes. The corresponding pain reduction did not suggest an effect of additional orthoses, since a sufficient postoperative pain treatment would be expected. The question about a possible reduction of pain medication, recurrence frequency or longer-term instability has not been answered.

Fujiwara et al. reported that orthotic fitting after PLIF (posterior lumbar interbody fusion) resulted in no benefit compared to orthotic-free fitting. Severe osteoporosis was mentioned as an exception [23].

Neither a benefit nor a disadvantage in terms of complaints was recorded in the control period of 3 months. In this case, it was also true that drug therapy was not answered. A long-term effect on follow-up degeneration was not discussed.

Orthotic fitting after posterior instrumented fusion did not improve quality of life or complaints, as reported by Soliman. The number of complications and reoperations in the brace group (7 out of 25) and in the control group (5 out of 18) must be seen as a limitation on the outcome [25].

Disc surgery, or segmental fusion, should not require additional external stabilization. However, this only applies to the surgically treated segment. The protection of the adjacent segment and thus the reduction of connecting degenerations cannot be derived from this.

It must also be considered that a sufficient postoperative medicinal pain treatment excludes the discomfort as a measure for an indication of the orthotic fitting.

From this perspective, local wound treatment, reduction of complications and, in the long term, prevention of follow-up degeneration should be cited as measures of treatment success with spine orthoses.

In a Cochrane Database of Systematic Reviews from 2016, the "Surgical versus non-surgical treatment for lumbar spinal stenosis" was treated. The authors concluded that they had very little confidence to confirm whether surgical treatment or a conservative approach is better for lumbar spinal stenosis, and they could not provide any new recommendations to guide clinical practice [29].

The results of the current literature are presented in a structured manner. Overall, there are no general statements for or against treatment with orthoses in low back pain.

The simple systematic structuring of orthoses forms the basis for finding promising treatments, but also forms a basis for contraindications.

Strict scientific statements cannot be provided. The structure of the orthoses is influenced by clinical application, since neither the nomenclature for orthoses nor a recommendation for indications is currently available.

This manuscript highlights the weakness of the current indications for orthotic provision in low back pain.

Accordingly, we can conclude that the current literature gives no recommendations to guide clinical practice.

The effectiveness of spine orthoses cannot be deduced from the current literature. The most serious limitation is the inconsistency of the complaints and orthoses. Furthermore, the imprecise designation of the orthoses is an additional limitation.

5. Conclusions

The effectiveness of spinal orthoses cannot be determined on the basis of the current literature. A major limitation is the lack of standardized nomenclature.

The lack of differentiation of the causes of pain is another weakness in many scientific papers. This limitation cannot be overcome by statistical methods or meta-analyses.

Additionally, in the case of postoperative treatments, pain reduction cannot be applied as a measure of therapeutic success in the presence of sufficient medicinal pain management.

The categorization of spinal orthoses demonstrated in this manuscript should be an impetus for further efforts to standardize products. These suggestions can provide the basis for answering the question of the effectiveness of spinal orthoses in conjunction with a differentiated cause of complaints. Spinal orthoses are an additional treatment option in limited indication of medication or surgery.

We found that articles with a precise allocation of the complaint and a description of the orthosis showed a positive effect. The treatment concept presented here is intended to provide a basis for answering the question concerning the effectiveness of spinal orthoses as an accompanying treatment option.

Author Contributions: Conceptualization, F.L. and K.T.; methodology, F.L. and K.T.; validation, F.L. and K.T.; formal analysis, F.L. and K.T.; writing—original draft preparation, F.L. and K.T.; writing—review and editing, F.L. and K.T. All authors have read and agreed to the published version of the manuscript.

Funding: This research received no external funding.

Institutional Review Board Statement: Not applicable for studies not involving humans or animals.

Informed Consent Statement: Not applicable.

Data Availability Statement: The study did not report any data.

Conflicts of Interest: The authors declare no conflict of interest.

References

1. Bataller-Cervero, A.V.; Rabal-Pelay, J.; Roche-Seruendo, L.E.; Lacárcel-Tejero, B.; Alcázar-Crevillén, A.; Villalba-Ruete, J.A.; Cimarras-Otal, C. Effectiveness of lumbar supports in low back functionality and disability in assembly-line workers. *Ind. Health* **2019**, *57*, 588–595. [CrossRef]
2. Junji, K.; Ko, M.; Tadashi, Y.; Shinno, I.; Akihiro, I. Efficacy of a trunk orthosis with joints providing resistive force on low-back load in elderly persons during static standing. *Clin. Interv. Aging.* **2015**, *10*, 1413–1420.
3. Pape, J.L.; Brism, J.M.; Sizer, P.S.; Matthijs, O.C.; Browne, K.L.; Dewan, B.M.; Sobczak, S. Increased spinal height using propped slouched sitting postures: Innovative ways to rehydrate intervertebral discs. *Appl. Ergon.* **2018**, *66*, 9–17. [CrossRef] [PubMed]

4. Shahvarpoura, A.; Preuss, R.; Sullivanc, M.J.; Negrinia, A.; Larivièrea, C. The effect of wearing a lumbar belt on biomechanical and psychological outcomes related to maximal flexion-extension motion and manual material handling. *Appl. Ergon.* **2018**, *69*, 17–24. [CrossRef] [PubMed]
5. Klima, S.; Grunert, R.; Ondruschka, B.; Scholze, M.; Seidel, T.; Werner, M.; Hammer, N. Pelvic orthosis effects on posterior pelvis kinematics: An in-vitro biomechanical study. *Sci. Rep.* **2018**, *8*, 15980. [CrossRef] [PubMed]
6. Mi, J.; Ye, J.; Zhao, X.; Zhao, J. Effects of lumbosacral orthoses on postural control in individuals with or without non-specific low back pain. *Eur. Spine J.* **2018**, *27*, 180–186. [CrossRef] [PubMed]
7. Lamers, E.P.; Soltys, J.C.; Keaton, L.; Scherpereel, K.L.; Yang, A.J.; Zelik, K.E. Low-profile elastic exosuit reduces back muscle fatigue. *Sci. Rep.* **2020**, *10*, 15958. [CrossRef]
8. Annaswamy, T.; Cunniff, K.; Kroll, M.; Yap, L.; Hasley, M.; Lin, C.; Petrasic, J. Lumbar Bracing for Chronic Low Back Pain. *Am. J. Phys. Med. Rehabil.* **2021**, *100*, 742–749. [CrossRef]
9. Urquhart, J.C.; Alrehaili, O.A.; Fisher, C.G.; Fleming, A.; Rasoulinejad, P.; Gurr, K.; Bailey, S.I.; Siddiqi, F.; Bailey, C.S. Treatment of thoracolumbar burst fractures: Extended follow-up of a randomized clinical trial comparing orthosis versus no orthosis. *J. Neurosurg. Spine* **2017**, *27*, 42–47. [CrossRef] [PubMed]
10. Mulcahy, M.J.; Dower, A.; Tait, M. Orthosis versus no orthosis for the treatment of thoracolumbar burst fractures: A systematic review. *J. Clin. Neurosci.* **2021**, *85*, 49–56. [CrossRef]
11. Ballard, M.T.; Drury, C.; Bazrgari, B. Changes in Lumbo-Pelvic Coordination of Individuals with and without Low Back Pain When Wearing a Hip Orthosis Frontiers in Sports and Active Living. Available online: www.frontiersin.org (accessed on 1 July 2020).
12. Krismer, M.; van Tulder, M. Low back pain (non-specific). *Best Pract. Res. Clin. Rheumatol.* **2007**, *21*, 77–91. [CrossRef]
13. Kreiner, D.S.; Matz, P.; Bono, C.M.; Cho, C.H.; Easa, J.E.; Ghiselli, G.; Ghogawala, Z.; Reitman, C.A.; Resnick, D.K.; Watters, W.C., III; et al. Guideline summary review: An evidence-based clinical guideline for the diagnosis and treatment of low back pain. *Spine J.* **2020**, *20*, 998–1024. [CrossRef]
14. Azadinia, F.; Ebrahimi-Takamjani, I.; Kamyab, M.; Asgari, M.; Parnianpour, M. Effects of lumbosacral orthosis on dynamical structure of center of pressure fluctuations in patients with non-specific chronic low back pain: A randomized controlled trial. *J. Bodyw. Mov. Ther.* **2019**, *23*, 930–936. [CrossRef] [PubMed]
15. Van Duijvenbode, I.; Jellema, P.; van Poppel, M.; van Tulder, M.W. Lumbar supports for prevention and treatment of low back pain. *Cochrane Database Syst. Rev.* **2008**, *2*, CD001823. [CrossRef] [PubMed]
16. Takasaki, H.; Miki, T. The impact of continuous use of lumbosacral orthoses on trunk motor performance: A systematic review with meta-analysis. *Spine J.* **2017**, *17*, 889–900. [CrossRef] [PubMed]
17. Samania, M.; Shirazib, Z.R.; Hadadic, M.; Sobhanib, S. A randomized controlled trial comparing the long-term use of soft lumbosacral orthoses at two different pressures in patients with chronic nonspecific low back pain. *Clin. Biomech.* **2019**, *69*, 87–95. [CrossRef] [PubMed]
18. Anders, C.; Agnes Hübner, A. Influence of elastic lumbar support belts on trunk muscle function in patients with nonspecific acute lumbar back pain. *PLoS ONE* **2019**, *14*, e0211042. [CrossRef]
19. Azadinia, F.; Takamjani, I.E.; Kamyab, M.; Kalbassi, G.; Sarrafzadeh, J.; Parnianpour, M. The Effect of Lumbosacral Orthosis on the Thickness of Deep Trunk Muscles Using Ultrasound Imaging. *Am. J. Phys. Med. Rehabil.* **2019**, *98*, 536–544. [CrossRef]
20. Zoia, C.; Bongetta, D.; Alicino, C.; Chimenti, M.; Pugliese, R.; Gaetani, P. Usefulness of corset adoption after single-level lumbar discectomy: A randomized controlled trial. *J. Neurosurg. Spine* **2018**, *28*, 481–485. [CrossRef]
21. Goto, T.; Sakai, T.; Sugiura, K.; Manabe, H.; Tezuka, F.; Yamashita, K.; Takata, Y.; Katoh, S.; Sairyo, K. A semi-rigid thoracolumbar orthosis fitted immediately after spinal surgery: Stabilizing effects and patient satisfaction. *J. Med. Investig.* **2019**, *66*, 275–279. [CrossRef]
22. Smits, A.J.; Deunk, J.; Stadhouder, A.; Altena, M.C.; Hendrik, D.; Kempen, R.; Willem Bloemers, F.W. Is postoperative bracing after pedicle screw fixation of spine fractures necessary? Study protocol of the ORNOT study: A randomised controlled multicentre trial. *BMJ Open* **2018**, *8*, 1–8. [CrossRef]
23. Fujiwara, H.; Makino, T.; Yonenobu, K.; Moriguchi, Y.; Oda, T.; Kaito, T. Efficacy of lumbar orthoses after posterior lumbar interbody fusion—a prospective randomized study. *Medicine* **2019**, *98*, 1–7. [CrossRef]
24. Bogaert, L.; Van Wambeke, P.; Thys, T.; Swinnen, T.W.; Dankaerts, W.; Brumagne, S.; Moke, L.; Peers, K.; Depreitere, B.; Janssens, L. Postoperative bracing after lumbar surgery: A survey amongst spinal surgeons in Belgium. *Eur. Spine J.* **2019**, *28*, 442–449. [CrossRef] [PubMed]
25. Soliman, H.A.; Barchi, S.; Parent, S.; Maurais, G.; Jodoin, A.; Mac-Thiong, J.M. Early Impact of Postoperative Bracing on Pain and Quality of Life After Posterior Instrumented Fusion for Lumbar Degenerative Conditions. *Spine J.* **2018**, *43*, 155–160. [CrossRef]
26. Myung, E.; Neto, J.D.; Murta, G.A.; Vieira, A.; de Lima, P.R.G.; Lessa, L.; Bernardo, W.M. ANAMT Technical Guideline (DT 05): Prevention of occupational low back pain through back belts, lumbar support or braces. *Rev. Bras. Med. Trab.* **2018**, *16*, 524–531. [CrossRef] [PubMed]
27. Schott, C.; Zirke, S.; Schmelzle, J.M.; Kaiser, C.; Fernández, L.A. Effectiveness of lumbar orthoses in low back pain: Review of the literature and our results. *Orthop. Rev.* **2018**, *10*, 7791. [CrossRef]

28. Boutevillain, L.; Bonnin, A.; Chabaud, A.; Morel, C.; Giustiniani, M.; Pereira, B.; Soubrier, M.; Coudeyre, E. Short-term pain evolution in chronic low back pain with Modic type 1 changes treated by a lumbar rigid brace: A retrospective study. *Ann. Phys. Rehabil. Med.* **2019**, *62*, 3–7. [CrossRef]
29. Zaina, F.; Tomkins-Lane, C.; Carragee, E.; Negrini, S. Surgical versus non-surgical treatment for lumbar spinal stenosis. *Cochrane Database Syst. Rev.* **2016**, *1*, 1–49. [CrossRef]
30. Alin, C.K.; Uzunel, E.; Kronhed, A.-C.G.; Alinaghizadeh, H.; Salminen, H. Effect of treatment on back pain and back extensor strength with a spinal orthosis in older women with osteoporosis: A randomized controlled trial. *Arch. Osteoporos.* **2019**, *14*, 5. [CrossRef] [PubMed]

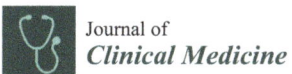 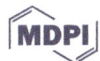

Article

Impact of the COVID-19 Pandemic on Elderly Patients with Spinal Disorders

Hidetomi Terai [1], Shinji Takahashi [1,*], Koji Tamai [1], Yusuke Hori [1], Masayoshi Iwamae [2], Masatoshi Hoshino [3], Shoichiro Ohyama [4], Akito Yabu [1] and Hiroaki Nakamura [1]

1. Department of Orthopaedic Surgery, Osaka City University Graduate School of Medicine, Osaka 545-8585, Japan; hterai@med.osaka-cu.ac.jp (H.T.); koji.tamai.707@gmail.com (K.T.); yusukehori0702@gmail.com (Y.H.); yabuakito@gmail.com (A.Y.); hnakamura@med.osaka-cu.ac.jp (H.N.)
2. Department of Orthopaedic Surgery, Shimada Hospital, Osaka 583-0875, Japan; iwamae0519@gmail.com
3. Department of Orthopaedic Surgery, Osaka City General Hospital, Osaka 534-0021, Japan; hoshino717@gmail.com
4. Department of Orthopaedic Surgery, Nishinomiya Watanabe Hospital, Nishinomiya 662-0863, Japan; a03ma012@yahoo.co.jp
* Correspondence: shinji@med.osaka-cu.ac.jp; Tel.: +81-06-6645-3851

Citation: Terai, H.; Takahashi, S.; Tamai, K.; Hori, Y.; Iwamae, M.; Hoshino, M.; Ohyama, S.; Yabu, A.; Nakamura, H. Impact of the COVID-19 Pandemic on Elderly Patients with Spinal Disorders. *J. Clin. Med.* **2022**, *11*, 602. https://doi.org/10.3390/jcm11030602

Academic Editor: Panagiotis Korovessis

Received: 3 December 2021
Accepted: 25 January 2022
Published: 25 January 2022

Publisher's Note: MDPI stays neutral with regard to jurisdictional claims in published maps and institutional affiliations.

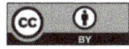

Copyright: © 2022 by the authors. Licensee MDPI, Basel, Switzerland. This article is an open access article distributed under the terms and conditions of the Creative Commons Attribution (CC BY) license (https://creativecommons.org/licenses/by/4.0/).

Abstract: During the ongoing coronavirus disease 2019 (COVID-19) pandemic, home-quarantine has been necessary, resulting in lifestyle changes that might negatively affect patients with spinal disorders, including a reduction in their quality of life (QoL) and activities of daily living (ADLs). However, studies on this impact are lacking. This study aimed to investigate the age-related changes in QoL and ADLs in patients with spinal disorders, and also identify factors associated with decline in ADLs. This multicenter cross-sectional study included patients who visited four private spine clinics for any symptoms. The study participants either had a clinic reservation, were first-time clinic visitors, or had a return visit to the clinic. The participants completed several questionnaires at two points: pre-pandemic and post-second wave. Changes in patient symptoms, exercise habits, ADLs, and health-related QoL were assessed. A logistic regression model was used to calculate the odds ratio (OR) of each variable for decline in ADLs. We included 606 patients; among them, 281 and 325 patients were aged <65 and ≥65 years, respectively. Regarding exercise habits, 46% and 48% of the patients in the <65 and ≥65-year age groups, respectively, did not change their exercise habits. In contrast, 40% and 32% of the patients in the <65 and ≥65-year age groups, respectively, decreased their exercise habits. In the multivariate analysis, the adjusted ORs for sex (female), decreased exercise habit, and age >65 years were 1.7 (1.1–2.9), 2.4 (1.4–3.9), and 2.7 (1.6–4.4), respectively. In conclusion, there was a decline in the ADLs and QoL after the COVID-19 outbreak in patients with spinal disorders. Aging, reduction of exercise habits, and female sex were independent factors related to decline in ADLs.

Keywords: COVID-19; pandemic; spinal disorder; elderly; exercise habit; female; quality of life; activities of daily living

1. Introduction

The coronavirus disease 2019 (COVID-19) pandemic has continued worldwide since early 2020 [1]. The pandemic was declared by the World Health Organization on 11 March 2020, with alarming levels of spread and severity [2]. In Japan, a state of emergency in response to the COVID-19 pandemic was declared between 7 April and 25 May 2020. People were required to stay at home during this period, with their lifestyles changing even after the end of the declaration. During this period, most gyms for elderly people were closed because the novel severe acute respiratory syndrome coronavirus 2 (SARS-CoV-2) is primarily transmitted through direct routes, including respiratory droplets and direct person-to-person contact [3,4]. Specifically, age ≥ 65 years is a known risk factor for severe acute respiratory infection by COVID-19 [5]. Consequently, people within that age category have more compromised activity compared with younger adults. Additionally, disuse in the elderly population increases their vulnerability to rapid skeletal muscle atrophy, functional strength loss, and multiple related negative health consequences [6].

The Japanese Orthopedic Association recommends the guidelines of the Centers for Medicare and Medicaid Services and American College of Surgeons [7,8], that is, that low acuity and intermediate acuity practice should be postponed or rescheduled. The North American Spine Society has provided guidelines for applying injections, interventional procedures, and surgeries, with the understanding that decision-making is strongly influenced by multiple factors, as follows [9]. The current pandemic might negatively affect patients with spinal disorders, including by reducing quality of life (QoL) and activities of daily living (ADLs), especially in the elderly population. However, there has been no study of this impact. Therefore, the present study aimed to reveal the changes in the QoL and ADLs of patients with spinal disorders after the first and second waves of the pandemic according to age, and to investigate the factors related to deterioration in ADLs.

2. Materials and Methods

2.1. Study Design

This was a multicenter cross-sectional study in four spine clinics. All patients who visited the spine clinics for any symptoms were asked to participate in a survey. Patients who provided informed consent were enrolled and were allowed to withdraw at any point if they wished (i.e., during or after completing the questionnaire). The participants were asked to answer questions from several questionnaires at two points: pre-pandemic and post-second wave. This survey was conducted between 1 November 2020 and 31 December 2020 in Osaka, Japan. In Japan, the first and second waves of the COVID-19 pandemic occurred in April and August, respectively, and the third wave occurred during the study period.

All study participants provided written informed consent. The study protocol was approved by the Institutional Review Board of the representative institution (approval No: 2020-242).

2.2. Patients

Patients who had a reservation in the clinic, were visiting our spine clinic for the first time, or had a return visit to the clinic were enrolled in this study after providing written informed consent. Patients who could not understand the questionnaires were excluded from the analysis in order to ensure that the data obtained was accurate. Patients with new symptoms after the outbreak were excluded from the analysis investigating outcome changes.

Among 1103 patients who visited our spine clinics, 747 patients were enrolled in this study. Among those 747 patients with spinal disorders, 141 patients were excluded since their symptoms had developed after the COVID-19 outbreak. Therefore, we included 606 patients in the analysis. There were 281 and 325 patients in the <65- and ≥65-year groups, respectively (Table 1); the respective average ages were 49.0 (standard deviation, SD: 10.7) and 75.9 (6.3) years. The proportion of females was higher in the <65-year group (45%) than in the ≥65-year group (53%) (p = 0.039). There was no between-group difference in the ratio of patients who refrained from visiting clinics (37% and 32%, p-value = 0.228). Regarding exercise habits, 46% and 48% of patients in the <65- and ≥65-year groups, respectively, did not change their exercise habits. In contrast, 40% and 32% of patients in the <65- and ≥65-year groups, respectively, decreased their exercise habits. Compared with pre-pandemic symptoms, the current symptoms were worse in 8% and 7% of patients in the <65- and ≥65-year groups, respectively, with no significant between-group difference (p-value = 0.988).

Table 1. Comparison of the patient characteristics between individuals aged <65 and ≥65 years.

	Age < 65 Years n = 281 n (%) or Mean (SD)	Age ≥ 65 Years n = 325 n (%) or Mean (SD)	p-Value
Age	49.0 (10.7)	75.9 (6.3)	<0.001
Sex (female)	126 (45)	173 (53)	0.039
Patients who refrained from visiting clinics due to the pandemic			
	103 (37)	104 (32)	0.228
Frequency of change of exercise habits before and after the outbreak			
No change	129 (46)	157 (48)	<0.001
More	17 (6)	3 (0.9)	
Less	89 (32)	130 (40)	
No exercise before or after the pandemic	46 (16)	35 (11)	
Comparison of the current and pre-outbreak symptoms			
Worse	19 (8)	20 (7)	0.988
Little worse	26 (11)	31 (11)	
No change	162 (71)	194 (71)	
Little better	11 (5)	15 (6)	
Better	9 (4)	12 (4)	

2.3. Procedures for Data Collection

The study coordinator gave short instructions and the patients filled out the paper questionnaire forms with pencils. The paper questionnaires were returned on the day of the clinic visit. To deal with the risk of social-desirability bias, the questionnaires guaranteed anonymity and responses were compiled [10].

2.4. Instruments

The authors worked independently and then agreed on the final questionnaire design by proving feedback on content accuracy, wording, question order, and survey structure. Adjustments were progressively included by considering the feedback that emerged [11]. When full agreement among experts was achieved, the survey was started.

2.4.1. General Information

The questions requested participants' date of birth, sex, and whether they were reluctant (whether they had hesitated or not hesitated) to visit the hospital (Questionnaire items in Supplementary Materials).

2.4.2. Changes after the COVID-19 Pandemic

Changes after the COVID-19 pandemic were assessed with respect to changes in patient symptoms (improved, deteriorated, stable, or newly occurred after the pandemic), exercise habits (increased, decreased, stable, or no exercise habit), ADLs, and health-related QoL (HRQoL).

ADLs were evaluated using the criteria proposed by the long-term care insurance system of the Japanese Health and Welfare Ministry for evaluation of the degree of independence of disabled elderly individuals [12]. In rank J, despite the presence of disability, daily life is almost independent, and patients can leave the home without assistance from other individuals. In rank A, patients live independently indoors but require assistance to leave the home. In rank B, patients require some assistance living indoors and spend most of the day in bed, though they can sit up. Finally, in rank C, the patients spend all day in bed and require assistance with urination/defecation, dressing, and eating. We divided the ranks into two groups, that is, J, A (dependent or requires assistance to leave home) and B, C (bedridden or nearly bedridden).

HRQoL at both time points (pre-pandemic and post-second wave) was cross-sectionally assessed using the EuroQoL 5-dimension 5-level (EQ-5D) descriptive system in one survey. The EQ-5D measures HRQoL on a 1—5 scale of five severity levels in five dimensions, including Mobility, Self-Care, Usual Activities, Pain/Discomfort, and Anxiety/Depression. The Japanese version of the EQ-5D-5L was used in this survey. Subsequently, the domain scores were converted into a summarized index based on previously published values [13].

2.5. Statistical Analysis

A restricted maximum-likelihood mixed-model regression was used to establish whether there was a significant difference in HRQoL between pre-pandemic and post-second wave. The model was used to assess the difference in HRQoL post-second wave between the <65- and ≥65-year groups. Additionally, we compared the number of patients who reached the minimum clinically important difference (MCID) between the <65- and ≥65-year groups. The index score required a change of at least 0.08 decline to reach the MCID [14] using a chi-square test. Each ADL at pre-pandemic and post-second wave was compared using Fisher's exact test. Change in ADLs between pre-pandemic and post-second wave was compared using a chi-square test. Next, a binomial logistic regression model was used to calculate the odds ratio (OR) of each variable for ADLs decline (ADLs decline/no ADLs decline). The model was adjusted for potential confounding factors with a p-value < 0.05 in the univariate analysis, including age (<65/≥65 years), sex, regular exercise (decrease/no change after the outbreak), and ADLs status pre-pandemic. In the sensitivity analysis, the Mobility and Self-Care dimensions of the EQ-5D-5L were used to evaluate decline in ADLs. We defined decline in ADLs as one rank reduction of Mobility or Self-Care in EQ-5D-5L. Statistical significance was set at p < 0.05. Between-group comparisons of continuous and categorical variables were performed using t-tests and chi-square/Fisher's exact tests, respectively. All p-values were two-sided. All statistical analyses were performed using SAS version 9.4 (SAS Institute Inc., Cary, NC, USA).

3. Results

3.1. Change in QoL and ADLs after the First and Second Waves of the Pandemic between the <65- and ≥65-Year Groups

Figure 1 shows the between-group comparison of the pre- and post-outbreak HRQoL measured using EQ-5D. The pre-outbreak EQ-5D scores in the <65- and ≥65-year groups were 0.89 (0.14) and 0.85 (0.17), respectively. The post-outbreak EQ-5D scores in the <65- and ≥65-year groups were 0.85 (0.15) and 0.79 (0.19), respectively. The mixed-effect model revealed a significant between-group difference, as well as between before and after the pandemic (both p-values < 0.001). There was no interaction between age (<65/≥65 years) and time (before and after the pandemic) (p-value = 0.139). The number of patients who reached the MCID were 47 (17%) vs. 51 (16%), respectively (p-value = 0.734).

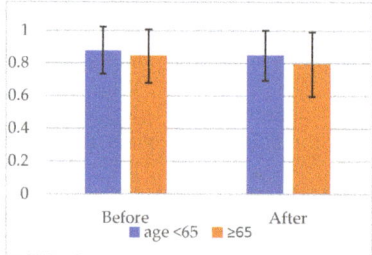

Figure 1. Comparison of pre- and post-pandemic health-related quality of life measured using the EQ-5D between patients aged <65 and ≥65 years. A mixed-effect model showed a significant difference between patients aged <65 and ≥65 years (p-value < 0.001), as well as before and after the pandemic (p-value < 0.001). There was no interaction between age (<65/≥65 years) and time (pre- and post-pandemic) (p-value = 0.139).

Table 2 shows the between-group comparison of ADLs. Compared with the ≥65-year group, the <65-year group showed better pre-outbreak ADLs ($p < 0.001$). The pre-outbreak proportion of rank J1 was 77% and 58% in the <65- and ≥65-year groups, respectively. Moreover, the post-outbreak ADLs in the <65-year group was better than the pre-outbreak ADLs in the ≥65-year group ($p < 0.001$). However, the post-outbreak proportion of rank J1 decreased to 68% and 46% in the <65- and ≥65-year groups, respectively. Contrastingly, after the outbreak, the proportion of rank J2 increased from 21% to 29% and from 30% to 38% in the <65- and ≥65-year groups, respectively. There was greater deterioration in ADLs in the ≥65-year group than in the <65-year group (10% vs. 18%, p-value < 0.001).

Table 2. Comparison of activities of daily living before and after the pandemic between patients aged <65 and ≥65 years.

	Pre-Pandemic			Post-Pandemic		
	Age < 65 Years	Age ≥ 65 Years	p-Value	Age < 65 Years	Age ≥ 65 Years	p-Value
	n (%)	n (%)		n (%)	n (%)	
ADLs rank						
Rank J1	215 (77)	189 (58)	<0.001	192 (68)	149 (46)	<0.001
Rank J2	60 (21)	96 (30)		81 (29)	124 (38)	
Rank A1	0	26 (8)		1 (0.4)	30 (9)	
Rank A2	5 (2)	13 (4)		7 (2)	22 (7)	
Rank B	1 (0.4)	1 (0.3)		0	0	
ADLs change	<65	≥65				
	n (%)	n (%)				
Improved	5 (2)	9 (3)	<0.001			
No change	249 (89)	258 (79)				
Deteriorated	27 (10)	58 (18)				

Rank J1: Daily life is almost independent, and patients can go outside using different means of transportation without assistance from other individuals. Rank J2: Patients can go outside in the home vicinity without assistance from other individuals. Rank A1: Patients live independently indoors but require assistance to go out, and they stay out of bed for most of the day. Rank A2: Patients live independently indoors but require assistance to go out; however, they seldom go out and take several bed rests during the day. Rank B: Patients require some assistance living indoors and spend most of the day in bed; however, they can sit up.

3.2. Factors Related to Decline in ADLs

Table 3 shows the univariate and multivariate ORs for reduction in ADLs. The univariate analysis showed that for female patients, the OR of a reduction in ADLs was significantly increased in comparison to the male patients. The OR of a reduction in ADLs was also significantly increased in patients whose exercise habit had declined after the COVID-19 pandemic in comparison to the patients whose exercise habit had not changed or had improved. Additionally, the OR of a reduction in ADLs was significantly increased for the patients aged ≥65 years in comparison to the patients aged <65 years. There was no association between hesitation of visiting clinics and reduction in ADLs (p-value = 0.221). The pre-outbreak ADLs rank (per 1 rank increase) decreased the risk of reduction in ADLs. In the multivariate analysis, the adjusted ORs for sex (female), decrease of exercise habit, and age ≥ 65 years were 1.7 (1.1–2.9), 2.4 (1.4–3.9), and 2.7 (1.6–4.4), respectively. The adjusted OR for pre-outbreak ADLs rank (per 1 rank increase) was 0.3 (0.2–0.5).

Table 4 shows the univariate and multivariate ORs for reduction in ADLs using the Mobility or Self-care dimensions of EQ-5D-5L. There were 234 patients (39%) with reductions in ADLs. In the multivariate analysis, the adjusted ORs for decrease of exercise habit and age ≥65 years were 2.5 (1.5–4.1) and 1.9 (1.1–3.1), respectively.

Table 3. Factors associated with reduction in ADLs using the long-term care insurance system of the Japanese Health and Welfare Ministry.

	Univariate ORs (95% CI)	p-Value	Adjusted ORs (95% CI)	p-Value
Sex (female)	1.7 (1.1–2.8)	0.020	1.7 (1.1–2.9)	0.025
Hesitated to visit the clinic (yes)	1.3 (0.8–2.1)	0.221		
Decrease in exercise habits	2.2 (1.4–3.5)	0.001	2.4 (1.4–3.9)	<0.001
Age >65 years	2.0 (1.3–3.3)	0.004	2.7 (1.6–4.4)	<0.001
ADLs pre-pandemic (per 1 rank increase)	0.4 (0.2–0.6)	<0.001	0.3 (0.2–0.5)	<0.001

OR, odds ratio; CI, confidence interval; ADLs, activities of daily living.

Table 4. Factors associated with reduction in ADLs using the Mobility or Self-Care dimensions of EQ-5D-5L.

	Univariate ORs (95% CI)	p-Value	Adjusted ORs (95% CI)	p-Value
Sex (female)	1.3 (0.97–1.9)	0.079	1.5 (0.90–2.4)	0.124
Hesitated to visit the clinic (yes)	1.0 (0.7–1.5)	0.851		
Decrease in exercise habits	1.4 (0.98–1.9)	0.063	2.5 (1.5–4.1)	<0.001
Age > 65 years	1.5 (1.1–2.1)	0.015	1.9 (1.1–3.1)	0.016
Mobility dimension before pandemic (per 1 rank increase)	0.7 (0.5–0.92)	0.011	0.5 (0.3–0.7)	<0.001
Self-Care dimension before pandemic (per 1 rank increase)	0.7 (0.4–1.3)	0.315	1.4 (0.7–3.0)	0.294

OR, odds ratio; CI, confidence interval; ADLs, activities of daily living.

4. Discussion

This is the first report to reveal the impact of the COVID-19 outbreak on status changes in patients with spinal disorders. This study sought to elucidate patients' behavioral changes and the impact on their functional status during this pandemic. The patients' HRQoL and ADLs were worse after the outbreak. There were physical and mental factors related to the decline in the HRQoL. Staying at home led to loss of opportunity to exercise and loneliness among individuals. This study reported a significant decrease in the EQ-5D by 0.04–0.06. Additionally, 16–17% of patients reached the MCID of EQ-5D. Upon the announcement of the first pandemic wave, leisure activities were closed for >1 month from March to May. Moreover, even after the end of the emergency declaration, lifestyles dramatically changed. Public health restrictions affect the physical activity of the elderly, especially those with pre-pandemic higher exercise/sports activity levels and lower HRQoL [15]. In the Chinese population, there were significant correlations among physical activity levels, HRQoL, and perceived stress levels [15]. Additionally, prolonged sitting time was found to negatively affect the HRQoL [15].

There was an obvious pandemic effect on ADLs, especially in elderly patients. This is consistent with a previous report detailing that muscle atrophy by disuse was more rapid and greater in elderly individuals than in young individuals [6]. This negative impact caused by the outbreak was more apparent in the elderly population. Additionally, they displayed a more significant decrease in exercise habits. During this pandemic period, there was a greater need for enforcing exercise programs for elderly people. Moreover, pandemic-related anxiety was found to be highest among citizens aged ≥65 years [16].

In our study, female sex was an independent risk factor for reduction in ADLs. Kim et al. [17] reported that disability in ADLs was more common in females (20.8% of the patients aged >65 years) than in males (13.3%). Moreover, compared with males, females showed a higher prevalence of chronic diseases, including arthritis, osteoporosis, and disc degeneration, which were risk factors for disability in ADLs. Furthermore, low back pain is more common in women [18]. Low physical activity might enforce back pain, which worsens chronic pain and results in low activity. In addition, the differences that exist between males and females in perception, expression, and pain tolerance are influenced by a wide variety of social and psychological factors [19]. Further, the incidence of knee osteoarthritis was much higher in females (71.9% of the patients aged 70–79 years) than in males (48.2%) [20]. Muscle weakness is a primary risk factor for pain, disability, and joint damage progression [21]. There might be sex differences in disuse muscle atrophy.

This study reported a positive relationship between exercise habits and decline in ADLs. Therefore, maintaining exercise habits is crucial for risk reduction. A recent systematic review highlighted that running may be a protective factor against the onset of low back pain based on studies investigating the incidence of low back pain in runners [22]. In this study, effective and safe remote rehabilitation was performed in 41.9% of patients with COVID-19, which facilitated rehabilitation in COVID-19-specialized general wards [23]. Additionally, telemedicine can provide very effective and satisfactory care in physical medicine and rehabilitative spine practice [24]. During the COVID-19 pandemic, there is a need for health services involving an integrated rehabilitation pathway to not only manage the numerous survivors, but also patients with spinal disease.

There was no association between hesitation in visiting clinics and decline in ADLs. Telemedicine might help to minimize risk of exposure for providers, in addition to allowing patients to stay at home and comply with public health recommendations during the pandemic, yet might have limited capability for thorough physical examination. However, Iyer et al. [25] proposed a simple remote examination method for use by spinal healthcare providers during telemedicine appointments to facilitate their ability to diagnose and treat patients. In Japan, spine surgeons performed interventions based on the prescription given at the last visit. Additionally, most patients who refrained from visiting might have had lower disease severity. Even during the emergency declaration, surgery was performed for emergent or urgent cases, including severe neurologic deficits, intractable pain, spinal trauma, and spinal infection.

This study has several limitations. First, recall bias should be considered since the questionnaire was completed after the outbreak [26]. Therefore, a simple question commonly used to determine ADLs in Japanese elderly individuals was used in order to prevent ambiguous answers. In addition, we confirmed the results of the sensitivity analysis using EQ-5D-5L Mobility and Self-Care dimensions. Second, in order to ensure that the questionnaire was easy for elderly participants to complete, it was designed such that it did not comprise detailed information. Therefore, we could not collect details regarding comorbidities and spine diseases, and did not collect information on treatment including medication, physical therapy, and surgery. This could be crucial for assessing patient status. Third, the sample size might be too small to analyze the association of 'Hesitated to visit the clinic' with reduction in ADLs. Fourth, this study involved only Japanese participants. Therefore, the results may not be generalizable to other populations. Finally, this study design could have led to a selection bias since the patients whose symptoms improved did not revisit the hospitals. This might have resulted in overestimates of reduction in ADLs and QoL. However, we believe that this did not affect the relationship between the factors and decline in ADLs.

5. Conclusions

This study revealed the decline in ADLs and QoL after the COVID-19 outbreak in patients with spinal disorders. Moreover, aging, reduction of exercise habits, and female sex were independent related factors for decline in ADLs. Therefore, there is an increased need for encouraging exercise for elderly people when the number of COVID-19 infections is remittent. In addition, we need safe and sustainable exercise programs for elderly people, even during the pandemic.

Supplementary Materials: The following supporting information can be downloaded at: https://www.mdpi.com/article/10.3390/jcm11030602/s1, Questionnaire items.

Author Contributions: Conceptualization, K.T. and H.N.; methodology, M.H.; formal analysis, S.T.; investigation, Y.H. and M.I.; data curation, S.O. and A.Y.; writing—original draft preparation, H.T.; writing—review and editing, S.T.; supervision, H.N. All authors have read and agreed to the published version of the manuscript.

Funding: This research received no external funding.

Institutional Review Board Statement: The study protocol was approved by the Institutional Review Board of the representative institution (Osaka City University: No. R02996). All information was handled in accordance with the standards for privacy of individually identifiable health information of the Health Insurance Portability and Accountability Act in Japan.

Informed Consent Statement: Informed consent was obtained from all subjects involved in the study.

Conflicts of Interest: The authors declare no conflict of interest.

References

1. Chandrasekaran, B.; Fernandes, S. Since January 2020 Elsevier Has Created a COVID-19 Resource Centre with Free Information in English and Mandarin on the Novel Coronavirus. The COVID-19 Resource Centre Is Hosted on Elsevier Connect, the Company's Public News and Information Website. *Diabetes Metab. Syndr.* **2020**, *14*, 337–339.
2. World Health Organization. WHO Director-General's Opening Remarks at the Media Briefing on COVID-19—11 March 2020. Available online: https://www.who.int/director-general/speeches/detail/who-director-general-s-opening-remarks-at-the-media-briefing-on-covid-19---11-march-2020 (accessed on 27 February 2021).
3. Jain, N.S.; Alluri, R.K.; Schopler, S.S.; Hah, R.; Wang, J.C. COVID-19 and Spine Surgery: A Review and Evolving Recommendations. *Glob. Spine J.* **2020**, *10*, 528–533. [CrossRef] [PubMed]
4. Jayaweera, M.; Perera, H.; Gunawardana, B.; Manatunge, J. Transmission of COVID-19 Virus by Droplets and Aerosols: A Critical Review on the Unresolved Dichotomy. *Environ. Res.* **2020**, *188*, 109819. [CrossRef] [PubMed]
5. Du, R.-H.; Liang, L.-R.; Yang, C.-Q.; Wang, W.; Cao, T.-Z.; Li, M.; Guo, G.-Y.; Du, J.; Zheng, C.-L.; Zhu, Q.; et al. Predictors of Mortality for Patients with COVID-19 Pneumonia Caused by SARS-CoV-2: A Prospective Cohort Study. *Eur. Respir. J.* **2020**, *55*, 2000524. [CrossRef] [PubMed]
6. Wall, B.T.; Dirks, M.L.; Van Loon, L.J.C. Skeletal Muscle Atrophy during Short-Term Disuse: Implications for Age-Related Sarcopenia. *Ageing Res. Rev.* **2013**, *12*, 898–906. [CrossRef] [PubMed]
7. Centers for Medicare & Medicaid Services Non-Emergent, Elective Medical Services, and Treatment Recommendations. Available online: https://www.cms.gov/files/document/cms-non-emergent-elective-medical-recommendations.pdf (accessed on 27 February 2021).
8. College of Surgeons, A. COVID-19: Elective Case Triage Guidelines for Surgical Care Orthopaedics. Available online: https://www.facs.org/-/media/files/covid19/guidance_for_triage_of_nonemergent_surgical_procedures_orthopaedics.ashx (accessed on 27 February 2021).
9. North American Spine Society. NASS Guidance Document on Elective, Emergent and Urgent Procedures. Available online: https://www.spine.org/Portals/0/assets/downloads/Publications/NASSInsider/NASSGuidanceDocument040320.pdf (accessed on 28 February 2021).
10. Maselli, F.; Esculier, J.F.; Storari, L.; Mourad, F.; Rossettini, G.; Barbari, V.; Pennella, D.; Cataldi, F.; Viceconti, A.; Geri, T.; et al. Low back pain among Italian runners: A cross-sectional survey. *Phys. Ther. Sport* **2021**, *48*, 136–145. [CrossRef]
11. Rossettini, G.; Palese, A.; Geri, T.; Fiorio, M.; Colloca, L.; Testa, M. Physical therapists' perspectives on using contextual factors in clinical practice: Findings from an Italian national survey. *PLoS ONE* **2018**, *30*, e0208159. [CrossRef]
12. Takahashi, S.; Hoshino, M.; Takayama, K.; Iseki, K.; Sasaoka, R.; Tsujio, T.; Yasuda, H.; Sasaki, T.; Kanematsu, F.; Kono, H.; et al. Predicting Delayed Union in Osteoporotic Vertebral Fractures with Consecutive Magnetic Resonance Imaging in the Acute Phase: A Multicenter Cohort Study. *Osteoporos. Int.* **2016**, *27*, 3567–3575. [CrossRef]
13. EuroQol. Crosswalk Index Value Calculator. 2018. Available online: https://euroqol.org/eq-5d-instruments/eq-5d-5l-about/valuation-standard-value-sets/crosswalk-index-value-calculator/ (accessed on 28 February 2021).
14. Pickard, A.S.; Neary, M.P.; Cella, D. Estimation of Minimally Important Differences in EQ-5D Utility and VAS Scores in Cancer. *Health Qual. Life Outcomes* **2007**, *5*, 70. [CrossRef]
15. Suzuki, Y.; Maeda, N.; Hirado, D.; Shirakawa, T.; Urabe, Y. Physical Activity Changes and Its Risk Factors among Community-Dwelling Japanese Older Adults during the COVID-19 Epidemic: Associations with Subjective Well-Being and Health-Related Quality of Life. *Int. J. Environ. Res. Public Health* **2020**, *17*, 6591. [CrossRef]
16. Hyland, P.; Shevlin, M.; McBride, O.; Murphy, J.; Karatzias, T.; Bentall, R.P.; Martinez, A.; Vallières, F. Anxiety and Depression in the Republic of Ireland during the COVID-19 Pandemic. *Acta Psychiatr. Scand.* **2020**, *142*, 249–256. [CrossRef] [PubMed]
17. Kim, I.H. Age and Gender Differences in the Relation of Chronic Diseases to Activity of Daily Living (ADL) Disability for Elderly South Koreans: Based on Representative Data. *J. Prev. Med. Public Health* **2011**, *44*, 32–40. [CrossRef] [PubMed]
18. De Schepper, E.I.T.; Damen, J.; Van Meurs, J.B.J.; Ginai, A.Z.; Popham, M.; Hofman, A.; Koes, B.W.; Bierma-Zeinstra, S.M. The Association between Lumbar Disc Degeneration and Low Back Pain: The Influence of Age, Gender, and Individual Radiographic Features. *Spine* **2010**, *35*, 531–536. [CrossRef] [PubMed]
19. Bisconti, M.; Brindisino, F.; Maselli, F. Gender Medicine and Physiotherapy: A Need for Education. Findings from an Italian National Survey. *Healthcare* **2020**, *8*, 516. [CrossRef] [PubMed]

20. Yoshimura, N.; Muraki, S.; Oka, H.; Mabuchi, A.; En-Yo, Y.; Yoshida, M.; Saika, A.; Yoshida, H.; Suzuki, T.; Yamamoto, S.; et al. Prevalence of Knee Osteoarthritis, Lumbar Spondylosis, and Osteoporosis in Japanese Men and Women: The Research on Osteoarthritis/Osteoporosis against Disability Study. *J. Bone Miner. Metab.* **2009**, *27*, 620–628. [CrossRef] [PubMed]
21. Slemenda, C.; Brandt, K.D.; Heilman, D.K.; Mazzuca, S.; Braunstein, E.M.; Katz, B.P.; Wolinsky, F.D. Quadriceps Weakness and Osteoarthritis of the Knee. *Ann. Intern. Med.* **1997**, *127*, 97–104. [CrossRef] [PubMed]
22. Maselli, F.; Storari, L.; Barbari, V.; Colombi, A.; Turolla, A.; Gianola, S.; Rossettini, G.; Testa, M. Prevalence and incidence of low back pain among runners: A systematic review. *BMC Musculoskelet. Disord.* **2020**, *21*, 343. [CrossRef]
23. Sakai, T.; Hoshino, C.; Yamaguchi, R.; Hirao, M.; Nakahara, R.; Okawa, A. Remote Rehabilitation for Patients with COVID-19. *J. Rehabil. Med.* **2020**, *52*, jrm00095. [CrossRef]
24. Bhuva, S.; Lankford, C.; Patel, N.; Haddas, R. Implementation and Patient Satisfaction of Telemedicine in Spine Physical Medicine and Rehabilitation Patients during the COVID-19 Shutdown. *Am. J. Phys. Med. Rehabil.* **2020**, *99*, 1079–1085. [CrossRef]
25. Iyer, S.; Shafi, K.; Lovecchio, F.; Turner, R.; Albert, T.J.; Kim, H.J.; Press, J.; Katsuura, Y.; Sandhu, H.; Schwab, F.; et al. The Spine Physical Examination Using Telemedicine: Strategies and Best Practices. *Glob. Spine J.* **2020**, *12*, 8–14. [CrossRef]
26. Howick, J.; Bishopm, F.L.; Heneghan, C.; Wolstenholme, J.; Stevens, S.; Hobbs, F.D.; Lewith, G. Placebo use in the United Kingdom: Results from a national survey of primary care practitioners. *PLoS ONE* **2013**, *8*, e58247. [CrossRef] [PubMed]

Article

Nutritional Influences on Locomotive Syndrome

Sadayuki Ito [1], Hiroaki Nakashima [1,*], Kei Ando [1], Masaaki Machino [1], Taisuke Seki [1], Shinya Ishizuka [1], Yasuhiko Takegami [1], Kenji Wakai [2], Yukiharu Hasegawa [3] and Shiro Imagama [1]

[1] Department of Orthopedic Surgery, Nagoya University Graduate School of Medicine, Nagoya 466-8560, Japan; sadaito@med.nagoya-u.ac.jp (S.I.); andokei@med.nagoya-u.ac.jp (K.A.); masaaki_machino_5445_2@yahoo.co.jp (M.M.); taiseki@med.nagoya-u.ac.jp (T.S.); shinyai@med.nagoya-u.ac.jp (S.I.); takegami@med.nagoya-u.ac.jp (Y.T.); imagama@med.nagoya-u.ac.jp (S.I.)

[2] Department of Preventive Medicine, Nagoya University Graduate School of Medicine, Nagoya 466-8550, Japan; wakai@med.nagoya-u.ac.jp

[3] Department of Rehabilitation, Kansai University of Welfare Science, Osaka 582-0026, Japan; hasegawa@tamateyama.ac.jp

* Correspondence: hirospine@med.nagoya-u.ac.jp; Tel.: +81-52-741-2111

Abstract: Healthy dietary habits are important to prevent locomotive syndrome (LS). We investigated the relationship between LS and nutritional intake using community health checkup data. We included 368 participants who underwent LS staging, blood sampling, and nutritional intake assessments. Participants (163 adults < 65; 205 older adults ≥ 65) were divided into normal (N; LS stage 0) and LS (L; LS stage 1–2) groups, and blood sample data and nutritional intake were compared between groups. Among adults (N group, 71; L group, 92), low-density lipoprotein cholesterol (LDL-C) was significantly lower, and Vitamin B_1 intake was significantly higher in the L than in the N group; LDL-C, $p = 0.033$; Vitamin B1, 0.029. Among older adults (N group, 85; L group, 120), hemoglobin (Hb), albumin, and calcium levels were significantly lower, and sodium, monounsaturated fatty acids (MUFA), and n-6 polyunsaturated fatty acids (n-6 PUFA) were significantly higher in the L than the N group; Hb, $p = 0.036$; albumin, 0.030; calcium, 0.025; sodium, 0.029; MUFA, 0.047; n-6 PUFA, 0.0233). Logistic regression analysis indicated that sodium was the risk factor for the L group (exp (B) 1.001, 95% CI: 1–1.001, $p = 0.032$). In conclusion, salt intake was associated with LS.

Keywords: locomotive syndrome; nutrition; health checkup data

1. Introduction

Most developed countries are facing an aging society [1], and the number of people who need support and care in daily life due to musculoskeletal disorders is increasing [2]. Locomotive syndrome (LS) has been proposed by the Japanese Orthopaedic Association (JOA) as an umbrella term to refer to the condition of reduced mobility due to musculoskeletal disorders [2]. Details of the LS can be viewed at the following website; https://locomo-joa.jp/assets/pdf/index_english.pdf (accessed on 23 January 2022). Locomotive syndrome is defined as a condition of reduced mobility due to the impairment of locomotive organs. LS is assessed by evaluating the degree of motor function via the two-step test, stand-up test, and 25-question Geriatric Locomotive Function Scale (GLFS-25). LS has received worldwide attention for assessing motor function in musculoskeletal diseases [3]. LS is associated with a significantly lower quality of life (QOL) [4] and shorter life expectancy. Prevention of LS has long been advocated for maintaining and improving physical function in middle-aged and older adults [5]. In recent years, there have been reports using LS as an index of postoperative outcome. [6,7].

Visceral diseases and genetic factors can also contribute to LS. Variable factors, such as habitual inactivity, sedentary lifestyle, and inadequate nutrition contribute to the progression of LS [8]. Therefore, the JOA proposed an exercise for LS called locomotion training

(LT), which consists of standing on one leg with the eyes open and performing squats, heel raises, and front lunges [9].

In addition to reduced mobility, malnutrition is a common condition in older adults and is associated with morbidity, mortality, and reduced quality of life [10,11]. Malnutrition also affects musculoskeletal health and has been associated with chronic musculoskeletal pain in older adults [12]. Malnutrition in older adults can progress through a variety of mechanisms. Immobility due to musculoskeletal conditions has been associated with sarcopenia and decreased oral intake [13]. Impaired mobility and malnutrition, two conditions prevalent among older individuals, may be correlated and may potentiate each other, resulting in poor health-related outcomes [10]. Muscle strength is the direct key that links impaired mobility to malnutrition. Decreased muscle strength has been reported to be an indicator of impaired mobility [14], and decreased muscle mass has been reported to be a consequence of malnutrition [15].

There are no reports directly examining the relationship between LS and dietary habits. This study aimed to examine the relationship between LS and nutritional intake and identify the nutrients and dietary habits that influence LS.

2. Materials and Methods

2.1. Study Participants

The individuals surveyed were volunteers who underwent a municipal-supported health checkup in Yakumo in 2016 and 2017. Data from 2016 were used for those who participated in two consecutive years (2016 and 2017). Yakumo has a population of approximately 17,000, of whom 28% are >65 years old. More people in this town engage in agriculture and fishing than those in urban areas. Yakumo has conducted annual health checkups since 1982. Physical examinations included voluntary orthopedic and physical function tests and internal examinations. Psychological examinations and a health-related QOL survey (SF-36) were also conducted [16]. This study included all participants who completed an assessment of the LS risk stage, bioelectrical impedance analysis (BIA), fasting blood samples, and nutritional intake status. The exclusion criteria were as follows: history of spine or joint surgery, severe knee injury, severe hip osteoarthritis, history of hip or spine fractures, neuropathy, severe mental illness, diabetes that was diagnosed and treated by a physician, kidney or heart disease, nonfasting, severe impairment of walking or standing, and impairment of the central or peripheral nervous system.

Of the 758 participants who underwent health checks, 368 (154 men; 214 women) met the inclusion criteria. The research protocol was approved by the Human Research Ethics Committee and the university's institutional review board (No. 2014-0207). All participants provided written informed consent before participation. The research procedure was conducted in accordance with the principles of the Declaration of Helsinki.

2.2. Examination of Motor Function

Grip strength in the standing position was measured once in each hand using a handgrip dynamometer (Toei Light Co., Ltd., Saitama, Japan). The mean value was used for analysis [17]. Participants walked a 10 m straight course once at their fastest pace, and the time taken to complete the course was recorded as the 10 m walking time [18].

2.3. LS Stage Tests

The JOA proposes three tests to assess the risk of LS by evaluating the degree of motor function: the two-step test, stand-up test, and 25-question Geriatric Locomotive Function Scale (GLFS-25) [2]. LS is classified into stages 1 and 2. These stages are defined as follows: stage 1 indicates that motor function is beginning to decline and stage 2 indicates that motor function is progressing toward decline. Three tests were conducted according to the JOA guidelines [2].

The standing test assessed the ability to stand on one or both feet from stools of 40, 30, 20, and 10 cm height. The difficulty rating from easy to difficult was based on standing on both legs from stools of 40, 30, 20, and 10 cm, followed by standing on one leg from stools of 40, 30, 20, and 10 cm. The test results were expressed as the minimum height of the stool that the participant could stand on.

In the two-step test, the physical therapist measured the length of two steps from the starting line to the tip of the toes. The score was calculated by normalizing the maximum length of the two steps by the height.

The GLFS-25 is a comprehensive self-report survey that refers to the previous month [19]. The method consists of four questions on pain, 16 questions on activities of daily living (ADL), three questions on social functioning, and two questions on mental status. Each item was rated from no disability (0 points) to severe disability (4 points).

LS 0, 1, and 2 were defined as follows:

LS 0

The participant was categorized as Stage 0 if all of the three following conditions were met:

1. Stand-up test, ability in one-leg standing from a 40 cm-high seat (both legs).
2. Two-step test, >1.3.
3. 25-question GLFS score, <7.

LS1

The participant was categorized as Stage 1 if any of the three following conditions were met:

1. Stand-up test, difficulty in one-leg standing from a 40 cm-high seat (either leg).
2. Two-step test, <1.3.
3. 25-question GLFS score, ≥7.

LS2

The participant was categorized as Stage 2 if any of the three following conditions were met:

1. Stand-up test, difficulty in standing from a 20 cm-high seat using both legs.
2. Two-step test, <1.1.
3. 25-question GLFS score, ≥16 [20].

We divided the participants into two groups: the normal (N) group (LS 0) and the locomotive syndrome (L) group (LS1,2).

2.4. Bioelectrical Impedance Analysis (BIA)

BIA was used to analyze the participants' body composition. The participants underwent the BIA on an empty stomach. The conditions of BIA measurement, such as consumption of food and beverages, were similar to those reported earlier [21]. Anthropometric data, including height, weight, body mass index (BMI), body fat percentage (BFP), and appendicular skeletal muscle mass index (SMI), were measured using the BIA. The Inbody 770 BIA device (Inbody Co., Ltd., Seoul, Korea), which can differentiate between tissues (such as fat, muscle, and bone) based on their electrical impedance, was used for the participants' body composition [16]. The accuracy of this device has been reported previously [22]. Participants grasped the handles of the analyzer, which have embedded electrodes, and stood on the platform with the soles of their feet in contact with the electrodes. There were two electrodes for each foot and hand. The BMI was calculated using the following formula: weight (kg)/height^2 (m^2). The muscle mass of each limb was automatically calculated by BIA using the Inbody 770 BIA device. The SMI was calculated using the following formula: SMI = appendicular skeletal muscle mass (kg)/height^2 (m^2) [23].

2.5. Blood Sample Assessment

At the checkup, fasting blood samples were collected by venipuncture and centrifuged within 1 h of collection. Serum samples were stored at −80 °C until measurements were taken. Routine biochemical analysis was performed in the laboratory of Yakumo Town Hospital [24]. The following items were investigated; white blood cell, hemoglobin, platelet,

HbA1c, total protein, serum albumin, alkaline phosphatase (ALP), aspartate transaminase (AST), alanine aminotransferase (ALT), γ-glutamyltranspeptidase, total cholesterol, triglyceride, high-density lipoprotein cholesterol (HDL-C), low-density lipoprotein cholesterol (LDL-C), blood urea nitrogen, creatinine, uric acid, calcium, C-reactive protein.

2.6. Lifestyle Habits

Trained nurses administered a questionnaire on health and daily lifestyle habits, including smoking (current smoker, ex-smoker, or nonsmoker), alcohol consumption (regular drinkers, ex-drinkers, or nondrinkers), nutritional intake status, menopausal status (yes or no), and history of major illness. Anthropometric indices (height and weight) and blood pressure were measured during the health examination. Body mass index (BMI) was calculated as body weight (kg) divided by height (m) squared.

Hypertension was defined as systolic blood pressure of 140 mmHg or higher or diastolic blood pressure of 90 mmHg or higher (based on the Japanese Society of Hypertension guidelines) [25] or the use of antihypertensive medications. Diabetes mellitus was defined as a fasting blood glucose level of 126 mg/dL or higher or a glycated hemoglobin (HbA1c) level of 6.5% or higher or use of antidiabetic drugs. The Japanese Diabetes Society (JDS) HbA1c value (%) was converted to the equivalent National Glycohemoglobin Standardization Program (NGSP) value (%) using the formula HbA1c (NGSP) = HbA1c (JDS) + 0.4% [26]. Dyslipidemia was defined as a triglyceride level of $\geq$150 mg/dL, high-density lipoprotein cholesterol (HDL-C) level of < 40 mg/dL, or a low-density lipoprotein cholesterol (LDL-C) level of $\geq$140 mg/dL (based on the Japan Atherosclerosis Society guidelines) [27], or use of antidyslipidemic drugs.

2.7. Nutritional Intake Status

Dietary information was obtained using a validated food frequency questionnaire (FFQ), which asked about the intake of 188 food and beverage items, excluding supplements. Food and beverage items were grouped into nine categories ranging in frequency from "rarely" to "7 or more times a day" (or "10 or more drinks a day" for beverages). The question asked about usual consumption of the listed foods over the past year. The food list was initially developed from the 1989–1991 weighed food record according to contribution rates based on absolute values of energy and intake of 14 target nutrients, and was used in a prospective Japan Health Center-based study 8–12 [28] modified for middle-aged and older residents in a wide range of regions in Japan. In doing so, we took into account 17 additional nutrients, such as dietary fiber and folate, changes in foods contributing to the absolute nutrient intake due to updates to the Standard Tables of Food Composition in Japan [29], and regional and generational changes in diet in the current cohort. Energy and nutrient intakes were calculated by summing the product of the frequency of eating, portion size, energy, and nutrient content of each food item, referring to the Fifth Revised and Expanded Standard Tables of Food Composition in Japan [30]. Nutrients included protein, fat, carbohydrate, minerals (sodium, potassium, calcium, and iron), vitamins (carotene, Vitamins A, D, E, B_1, B_2, folate, and C), and total dietary fiber (TDF) (soluble DF and insoluble DF). Fat was divided into saturated fatty acids, monounsaturated fatty acids (MUFA), n-6 and n-3 polyunsaturated fatty acids (PUFAs), and n-3 highly unsaturated fatty acids (n-3 HUFAs, including eicosapentaenoic acid (20:5), docosapentaenoic acid (22:5), docosahexaenoic acid (22:6)), and cholesterol [31].

2.8. Statistical Analyses

We divided all participants into adults (< 65 years old) and older adults ($\geq$ 65 years old). Continuous variables were expressed as mean $\pm$ standard deviation (SD). We compared continuous variables of the L group to those of the N group using the Student's *t*-test and categorical variables using the chi-square test. These analyses were conducted for total adult and older adult, respectively. Statistical significance was set at $p < 0.05$. All the parameters listed in the supplement tables were examined. In addition, the table shows the parameters that showed significant differences and their related parameters.

Logistic regression analysis was performed on each adult and older adult to evaluate the important risk factors in the L group. In the logistic regression analyses, we defined that the dependent variable was the group and that the covariables were the parameters that showed significant differences in the Student t-test and the chi-square test comparing the L Group and N Group. All statistical analyses were performed using SPSS Statistics v.28.0 software for Mac (IBM Corp., Armonk, NY, USA). Statistical significance was set at $p < 0.05$.

3. Results

Participant characteristics are shown in Table 1 and Supplemental Table S1. There were 154 men and 214 women, with an average age of 63.8 ± 10.5 years. There were 156 (76 male; 80 female) and 212 (78 male; 134 female) participants in the N and L groups, respectively.

3.1. Adult Participants

The average age of the adult group was 54.3 ± 7.3 years. In total, 71 (28 male; 43 female) and 92 (24 male; 68 female) participants were included in the N and L groups, respectively (Table 2, Supplemental Table S2). The body fat percentage (BFP) was significantly higher and the grip strength and gait speed were significantly lower in the L than in the N group (BFP; N: 28.2 ± 5.1, L: 31.0 ± 6.8, $p = 0.005$, grip strength; N: 29.6 ± 9.8, L: 25.1 ± 8.7, $p = 0.002$, gait speed; N: 2.4 ± 0.3, L: 2.3 ± 0.5, $p = 0.04$).

Analyses of the laboratory data and nutrient intakes indicated that LDL-C was significantly lower and Vitamin B_1 was significantly higher in the L than in the N group (LDL-C; N: 132.1 ± 32.4, L: 121.8 ± 28.5, $p = 0.033$, Vitamin B_1; N: 0.66 ± 0.07, L: 0.69 ± 0.09, $p = 0.029$). There were no significant between-group differences in the other laboratory data, nutrient intake, SMI, or history of metabolic diseases (Table 2, Supplemental Table S2).

As significant differences were observed among several factors, they were examined as covariates for risk factors of the L group in the logistic regression analysis. BFP and LDL-C were risk factors (BFP; exp (B) 1.068, 95% CI: 1.003–1.127, $p = 0.038$, LDL-C; exp (B) 0.988, 95% CI: 0.977–1, $p = 0.042$) (Table 3).

3.2. Older Adult Participants

The average age of older adult participants was 71.3 ± 5.3 years. The N and L groups contained 85 (48 male: 37 female) and 120 (54 male: 66 female) participants, respectively (Table 4, Supplemental Table S3). The average age of participants was significantly higher in the L than in the N group (N: 70.2 ± 4.7; L: 72.2 ± 5.6, $p = 0.008$). The BFP was significantly higher and the grip strength was significantly lower in the L than in the N group (BFP; N: 26.7 ± 6.3, L: 29.7 ± 6.9, $p = 0.002$, grip strength; N: 29.0 ± 8.0, L: 25.1 ± 8.0, $p = 0.001$).

Analyses of laboratory data indicated that Hb, albumin, and calcium levels were significantly lower in the L than in the N group (Hb: 13.8 ± 1.0, L: 13.4 ± 1.1, $p = 0.036$, albumin; N: 4.4 ± 0.2, L: 4.3 ± 0.2, $p = 0.030$, calcium; N: 9.2 ± 0.3, L: 9.1 ± 0.3, $p = 0.025$). Regarding nutrient intake, sodium, MUFA, and n-6 PUFA were significantly higher in the L than in the N group (sodium: N: 1961.1 ± 586.7, L: 2183.1 ± 789.0, $p = 0.029$; MUFA: N: 15.8 ± 3.8, L: 17.2 ± 5.4, $p = 0.047$, n-6 PUFA; N: 10,898.3 ± 2808.4, L: 12,149.4 ± 4807.4, $p = 0.0233$). The prevalence of hypertension was higher in the L group than in the N group (N: 42.3%, L: 60.8%, $p = 0.007$). There were no significant between-group differences in gait speed, SMI, other laboratory data, nutrient intake, or history of metabolic diseases between the N and L groups (Table 4).

Factors for which significant between-group differences were observed were examined as covariates for the risk factors of the L group in the logistic regression analysis. BFP, sodium, and hypertension were risk factors (exp (B) 1.073, 95% CI: 1.017–1.132, $p = 0.011$, sodium; exp (B) 1.001, 95% CI: 1–1.001, $p = 0.032$, hypertension; exp (B) 2.288, 95% CI: 1.186–4.412, $p = 0.014$) (Table 5).

Table 1. The comparison of each parameter between nonolder adult and older adult participants.

	All (n = 368)	Adult (n = 163)	Older Adult (n = 205)	p
Male/Female	154/214	52/111	102/103	0.001 *
Age (yrs)	63.8 ± 10.5	54.3 ± 7.3	71.3 ± 5.3	<0.001 *
Height (cm)	158.1 ± 8.1	159.4 ± 7.8	157 ± 8.2	0.006 *
Weight (kg)	59.2 ± 11.5	59.6 ± 12.3	58.9 ± 10.8	0.553
BMI (kg/m^2)	23.5 ± 3.5	23.3 ± 3.6	23.7 ± 3.4	0.231
BFP (%)	29.1 ± 6.6	29.8 ± 6.3	28.5 ± 6.8	0.057
SMI (kg/m^2)	6.70 ± 1.03	6.65 ± 1.07	6.73 ± 1.00	0.477
Grip strength (kg)	26.9 ± 8.8	27.1 ± 9.4	26.7 ± 8.2	0.730
N/L	156/212	71/92	85/120	0.383
Hypertension (y/n)	140/228	31/132	109/96	<0.001 *
Diabetes (y/n)	24/344	3/160	21/184	0.001 *
Hypertension (y/n)	140/228	31/132	109/96	<0.001 *
Laboratory data				
Hemoglobin (g/dL)	13.5 ± 1.2	13.4 ± 1.3	13.6 ± 1.1	0.175
Serum Albumin (g/dL)	4.4 ± 0.2	4.4 ± 0.2	4.3 ± 0.2	0.183
Total-cholesterol (mg/dL)	207.2 ± 33.2	212.6 ± 31.8	202.9 ± 33.7	0.005 *
Triglyceride (mg/dL)	111.2 ± 69.5	103.7 ± 59.9	117.1 ± 75.8	0.067
HDL-C (mg/dL)	61.5 ± 14.9	62.9 ± 14.5	60.4 ± 15.1	0.103
LDL-C (mg/dL)	120.5 ± 30.7	126.3 ± 30.6	115.8 ± 30	0.001 *
Calcium (mg/dL)	9.2 ± 0.3	9.2 ± 0.3	9.2 ± 0.3	0.726
Nutritional intake				
Energy (kcal/day)	1644.1 ± 389.5	1591.1 ± 351.2	1686.3 ± 413.4	0.020 *
Protein (g/day)	53.3 ± 13.7	51.5 ± 10.8	54.8 ± 15.6	0.022 *
Fat (g/day)	44.6 ± 13.5	42.9 ± 12.2	46 ± 14.3	0.031 *
Carbohydrate (g/day)	229.1 ± 69.5	221.1 ± 67.6	235.4 ± 70.6	0.050
Sodium (mg/day)	1972.3 ± 689.4	1822.9 ± 620.8	2091.1 ± 719	<0.001 *
Calcium (mg/day)	543.9 ± 191.6	502.7 ± 150.7	576.7 ± 213.5	<0.001 *
SFA (g/day)	11.6 ± 2.9	11.1 ± 2.4	11.9 ± 3.2	0.011 *
MUFAd (g/day)	16.4 ± 4.8	16.1 ± 4.8	16.6 ± 4.8	0.293
PUFA (g/day)	13.2 ± 4.5	12.5 ± 4.0	13.8 ± 4.9	0.009 *
Cholesterol (mg/day)	241.6 ± 79.1	238.9 ± 78.4	243.7 ± 79.8	0.560
n-3 PUFA (g/day)	2299.2 ± 750.9	2195 ± 764.7	2382 ± 731	0.017 *
n-6 PUFA (g/day)	11,206.8 ± 3901.2	10,673.7 ± 3523.9	11,630.7 ± 4136.5	0.019 *
Energy from alcohol (kcal/day)	47.2 ± 96.7	49 ± 101.5	45.7 ± 92.9	0.742
n-3 HUFA (g/day)	754.6 ± 403.1	682.2 ± 344.5	812.1 ± 436.5	0.002 *

Values are expressed as means ± standard deviations; BMI: body mass index, BFP: body fat percentage, SMI: skeletal muscle mass index, y/n: yes/no; SMI: skeletal muscle mass index, N/L: normal group/locomotive syndrome group, y/n: yes/no; HDL-C: high-density lipoprotein cholesterol, LDL-C: low-density lipoprotein cholesterol; SFA: saturated fatty acid, MUFA: monounsaturated fatty acid, PUFA: polyunsaturated fatty acid, HUFA: highly unsaturated fatty acid. All analyses are comparisons between adults and older adults. The comparison of male/female was conducted by a chi-square test, and the comparisons of the others were conducted by a Student t-test. *: $p < 0.05$.

Table 2. The comparison of each parameter between the N and L groups in adult participants.

	Adult (n = 163)	N (n = 71)	L (n = 92)	p
Male/Female	52/111	28/43	24/68	0.090
Age (yrs)	54.3 ± 7.3	53.2 ± 8	55.1 ± 6.7	0.094
BMI (kg/m^2)	23.3 ± 3.6	22.8 ± 3.3	23.7 ± 3.8	0.164
BFP (%)	29.8 ± 6.3	28.2 ± 5.1	31.0 ± 6.8	0.005 *
SMI (kg/m^2)	6.65 ± 1.07	6.72 ± 1.04	6.60 ± 1.09	0.489
Grip strength (kg)	27.1 ± 9.4	29.6 ± 9.8	25.1 ± 8.7	0.002 *

Table 2. Cont.

	Adult (n = 163)	N (n = 71)	L (n = 92)	p
Hypertension (y/n)	31/132	9/62	22/70	0.075
Diabetes (y/n)	3/160	3/68	0/92	0.081
Hyperlipidemia (y/n)	27/136	11/60	16/76	0.833
Laboratory data				
Hemoglobin (g/dL)	13.4 ± 1.3	13.5 ± 1.5	13.3 ± 1.1	0.268
Serum Albumin (g/dL)	4.4 ± 0.2	4.4 ± 0.2	4.4 ± 0.2	0.139
Total-cholesterol (mg/dL)	212.6 ± 31.8	216.2 ± 36.9	209.8 ± 27.2	0.205
Triglyceride (mg/dL)	103.7 ± 59.9	104.6 ± 69.8	103.1 ± 51.5	0.879
HDL-C (mg/dL)	62.9 ± 14.5	61.8 ± 14.7	63.8 ± 14.4	0.397
LDL-C (mg/dL)	126.3 ± 30.6	132.1 ± 32.4	121.8 ± 28.5	0.033
Calcium (mg/dL)	9.2 ± 0.3	9.2 ± 0.3	9.2 ± 0.3	0.962
Nutritional intake				
energy (kcal/day)	1591.1 ± 351.2	1617.7 ± 360.7	1570.6 ± 344.4	0.397
protein (g/day)	51.5 ± 10.8	51.3 ± 9	51.7 ± 12	0.808
fat (g/day)	42.9 ± 12.2	42.0 ± 9.2	43.6 ± 14.1	0.408
carbohydrate (g/day)	221.1 ± 67.6	228 ± 71.9	215.7 ± 63.9	0.251
Sodium (mg/day)	1822.9 ± 620.8	1879.4 ± 612.3	1779.3 ± 627.2	0.309
Calcium (mg/day)	502.7 ± 150.7	507.8 ± 152.7	498.8 ± 149.8	0.708
SFA (g/day)	11.1 ± 2.4	11.2 ± 2.6	11.1 ± 2.2	0.903
MUFAd (g/day)	16.1 ± 4.8	15.5 ± 3.3	16.5 ± 5.7	0.170
PUFA (g/day)	12.5 ± 4	12.3 ± 2.9	12.7 ± 4.6	0.571
Cholesterol (mg/day)	238.9 ± 78.4	222.6 ± 50.9	251.4 ± 92.7	0.020 *
n-3 PUFA (g/day)	2195 ± 764.7	2100.3 ± 481.5	2268 ± 922.2	0.166
n-6 PUFA (g/day)	10,673.7 ± 3523.9	10,579.5 ± 2506.8	10,746.4 ± 4154.5	0.765
Energy from alcohol (kcal/day)	49.0 ± 101.5	39.2 ± 67.3	56.6 ± 121.4	0.280
n-3 HUFA (g/day)	682.2 ± 344.5	640 ± 274.9	714.8 ± 388.1	0.170

Values are expressed as means ± standard deviations. BMI: body mass index, BFP: body fat percentage, SMI: skeletal muscle mass index, y/n: yes/no, HDL-C: high-density lipoprotein cholesterol, LDL-C: low-density lipoprotein cholesterol, SFA: saturated fatty acid, MUFA: monounsaturated fatty acid, PUFA: polyunsaturated fatty acid, HUFA: highly unsaturated fatty acid. All analyses are comparisons between the N and L group. The comparisons of male/female, hypertension, diabetes, and hyperlipidemia were conducted by a chi-square test, and the comparison of the others were conducted by a Student t-test. *: $p < 0.05$. There were significant differences in BFP, grip strength, gait speed, LDL-C, and Vitamin B_1 between the N and L groups.

Table 3. Logistic regression analysis for risk factors of the locomotive syndrome (L group) in adult participants.

	B	SE	Wald	df	p	Exp(B)	95% CI
BFP	0.061	0.030	4.287	1	0.038 *	1.063	1.003–1.127
Grip strength	−0.036	0.019	3.624	1	0.057	0.964	0.929–1.001
Gait speed	−0.686	0.377	3.308	1	0.069	0.504	0.240–1.055
LDL-C	−0.012	0.006	4.128	1	0.042 *	0.988	0.977–1.000
Vitamin B1	3.799	2.140	3.150	1	0.076	44.639	0.673–2961.192

BFP: body fat percentage, LDL-C: low-density lipoprotein cholesterol. *: $p < 0.05$. Covariates: BFP, grip strength, gait speed, LDL-C, Vitamin B_1. There were significant differences in BFP and LDL-C.

Table 4. The comparison of each parameter between the N and L groups in older adult participants.

	Older Adult (n = 205)	N (n = 85)	L (n = 120)	p
male/female	102/103	48/37	54/66	0.120
Age (yrs)	71.3 ± 5.3	70.2 ± 4.7	72.2 ± 5.6	0.008 *
BMI (kg/m^2)	23.7 ± 3.4	23.2 ± 3.4	24.1 ± 3.3	0.061
BFP (%)	28.5 ± 6.8	26.7 ± 6.3	29.7 ± 6.9	0.002 *
SMI (kg/m^2)	6.73 ± 1.00	6.86 ± 1.06	6.64 ± 0.95	0.140
grip strength (kg)	26.7 ± 8.2	29.0 ± 8.0	25.1 ± 8.0	0.001 *

Table 4. Cont.

	Older Adult (n = 205)	N (n = 85)	L (n = 120)	p
Hypertension (y/n)	109/96	36/49	73/47	0.007 *
Diabetes (y/n)	21/184	6/79	15/105	0.157
Hyperlipidemia (y/n)	81/124	36/49	45/75	0.305
Laboratory data				
Hemoglobin (g/dL)	13.6 ± 1.1	13.8 ± 1.0	13.4 ± 1.1	0.036 *
Serum Albumin (g/dL)	4.3 ± 0.2	4.4 ± 0.2	4.3 ± 0.2	0.030 *
Total-cholesterol (mg/dL)	202.9 ± 33.7	205.3 ± 35	201.2 ± 32.8	0.399
Triglyceride (mg/dL)	117.1 ± 75.8	112.6 ± 59.9	120.3 ± 85.4	0.479
HDL-C (mg/dL)	60.4 ± 15.1	61.1 ± 15.3	59.8 ± 15.0	0.55
LDL-C (mg/dL)	115.8 ± 30	118.4 ± 28.2	114 ± 31.3	0.305
Calcium (mg/dL)	9.2 ± 0.3	9.2 ± 0.3	9.1 ± 0.3	0.025 *
Nutritional intake				
energy (kcal/day)	1686.3 ± 413.4	1638.8 ± 348.7	1719.9 ± 452	0.167
protein (g/day)	54.8 ± 15.6	52.9 ± 11.6	56.2 ± 17.8	0.132
fat (g/day)	46 ± 14.3	44 ± 12.1	47.4 ± 15.6	0.090
carbohydrate (g/day)	235.4 ± 70.6	227.2 ± 62	241.2 ± 75.8	0.162
Sodium (mg/day)	2091.1 ± 719	1961.1 ± 586.7	2183.1 ± 789	0.029 *
Calcium (mg/day)	576.7 ± 213.5	565.9 ± 182.2	584.4 ± 233.7	0.543
SFA (g/day)	11.9 ± 3.2	11.8 ± 3.1	12.0 ± 3.3	0.720
MUFAd (g/day)	16.6 ± 4.8	15.8 ± 3.8	17.2 ± 5.4	0.047 *
PUFA (g/day)	13.8 ± 4.9	13.0 ± 3.3	14.3 ± 5.7	0.063
Cholesterol (mg/day)	243.7 ± 79.8	234.4 ± 64.3	250.3 ± 88.9	0.161
n-3 PUFA (g/day)	2382 ± 731	2271.3 ± 518.1	2460.4 ± 843.6	0.068
n-6 PUFA (g/day)	11,630.7 ± 4136.5	10,898.3 ± 2808.4	12,149.4 ± 4807.4	0.033 *
Energy from alcohol (kcal/day)	45.7 ± 92.9	51.9 ± 87.2	41.3 ± 96.9	0.426
n-3 HUFA (g/day)	812.1 ± 436.5	781 ± 274.1	834.1 ± 522	0.393

Values are expressed as means ± standard deviations. BMI: body mass index, BFP: body fat percentage, SMI: skeletal muscle mass index, y/n: yes/no, HDL-C: high-density lipoprotein cholesterol, LDL-C: low-density lipoprotein cholesterol, SFA: saturated fatty acid, MUFA: monounsaturated fatty acid, PUFA: polyunsaturated fatty acid, HUFA: highly unsaturated fatty acid. All analyses are comparisons between N and L group. The comparisons of male/female, hypertension, diabetes, and hyperlipidemia were conducted by a chi-square test, and the others were conducted by a Student t-test. *: $p < 0.05$. There were significant differences in age, BFP, grip strength, hemoglobin, albumin, calcium, sodium, MUFA, n-6 PUFA, and hypertension between the N and L groups.

Table 5. Logistic regression analysis for risk factors of the locomotive syndrome (L group) in older adult participants.

	B	SE	Wald	df	p	Exp(B)	95% CI
Age (yrs)	0.057	0.035	2.633	1	0.105	1.059	0.988–1.135
BFP (%)	0.070	0.027	6.534	1	0.011 *	1.073	1.017–1.132
Grip strength (kg)	−0.036	0.023	2.514	1	0.113	0.964	0.922–1.009
Hb (g/dL)	−0.008	0.161	0.003	1	0.959	0.992	0.724–1.359
Albumin (g/dL)	−0.622	0.807	0.594	1	0.441	0.537	0.111–2.610
Calcium (mg/dL)	−1.115	0.594	3.525	1	0.060	0.328	0.102–1.050
Sodium (mg/day)	0.001	0.000	4.625	1	0.032 *	1.001	1.000–1.001
MUFA (g/day)	0.050	0.075	0.445	1	0.505	1.051	0.908–1.218
n-6 PUFA (g/day)	0.000	0.000	0.277	1	0.598	1.000	1.000–1.000
Hypertension	0.828	0.335	6.100	1	0.014 *	2.288	1.186–4.412

BFP: body fat percentage, MUFA: monounsaturated fatty acid, PUFA: polyunsaturated fatty acid, *: $p < 0.05$. Covariates: age, BFP, grip strength, hemoglobin, albumin, calcium, sodium, MUFA, n-6 PUFA, and hypertension. There were significant differences in BFP, sodium, and hypertension.

4. Discussion

There have been several reports on the relationship between motor function and muscle and nutrition [10,11]. However, to our knowledge, no study has directly examined the relationship between nutritional intake status and LS. In this study, salt, MUFA, and n-6 PUFA intakes were significantly higher in group L among older adults. Multivariate analysis indicated that higher salt intake was particularly associated with LS.

In an aging society, the rate of LS is increasing, and the number of people who have difficulty leading independent daily lives is increasing [4]. Therefore, preventing LS plays a vital role in preventing the need for nursing care. In this study, a significant decrease in grip strength was observed in the L group in both adults and older adults. This suggests that a decline in muscle strength accompanies the functional decline in LS and that the influence of muscle strength on LS is significant and closely related to sarcopenia. Exercise and nutrition are important factors in preventing sarcopenia [32] and are thought to be equally important in influencing LS. Exercise therapy has been advocated for LS prevention [9]. However, there have been no detailed studies on the effects of nutrition on LS. Thus, there is no specific diet therapy for LS prevention.

BFP and LDL-C levels were lower in group L among adults, according to the multivariate analysis. Higher body fat may reflect lower physical activity, such as lack of exercise, in group L. High LDL cholesterol is associated with a higher percentage of fat than muscle [33]. However, in this study, LDL-C levels of both groups were within the normal range, so the difference was not clinically significant.

Vitamin B_1 intake was lower in group L among adults, according to the univariate analysis. Vitamin B_1 is active in glucose metabolism, and its deficiency can lead to poor conversion of sugar to energy and increased fatigue [34]. In this study, the intake of Vitamin B_1 was higher in group L, but both groups had deficient Vitamin B_1 intake compared to the daily recommended amount [35], and the difference in intake was small and not significant for LS.

Among older adults, group L had higher salt intake and hypertension, according to the multivariate analysis. Excessive salt intake is one of the causes of various diseases, such as hypertension [36,37], where sodium in the skeletal muscle accumulates more in older than in younger people, and patients with refractory hypertension have increased tissue sodium (Na^+) content compared to normotensive controls [38]. Moreover, the sodium-potassium-chloride symporter 1 (NKCC1) is highly expressed in mammalian skeletal muscles. The physiological function of NKCC1 in myogenesis remains unclear. However, NKCC1 protein levels increase skeletal myoblast differentiation, and NKCC1 inhibitors markedly suppress skeletal myoblast differentiation [39]. It has also been reported that excess sodium leads to downregulation of NKCC expression [40]. Further, the risk of sarcopenia, which is associated with decreased muscle mass and strength, is related to the amount of salt intake because Na^+ is stored in tissues, and NKCC1 is involved in muscle hypertrophy and suppression [41]. Here, salt intake was higher in the L group.

Regarding hypertension and muscle, hypertension reduces muscle blood flow [42] and correlates with low muscle mass [43]. Arterial stiffness and age-related hormonal decline are risk factors for hypertension and muscle loss [44]. Similar to these observations, this study also detected an association between hypertension and LS. Thus, higher salt intake and hypertension were associated with muscle metabolism and sarcopenia, which may be associated with the locomotive syndrome. In this study, we found that the locomotive syndrome group had weaker grip strength, which may be due to muscle weakness and sarcopenia. Therefore, it can be said that factors related to muscle mass loss are closely related to the locomotive syndrome.

In contrast, even after multivariate analysis of confounding factors involved in locomotive syndrome, including grip strength, higher salt intake was significantly associated with locomotive syndrome. Higher salt intake may also be related to motor nerves, sensory nerves that control balance, and other factors, in addition to its effect on muscle mass. There are many unclear points regarding the relationship between higher salt intake and nonmuscle factors; thus, further basic research is needed in the future.

Among older adults, there were no significant differences except for salt intake and hypertension in multivariate analysis. However, there were significant differences in MUFA and PUFA intake, hemoglobin, serum albumin, and calcium in the univariate analysis.

Although there was no significant multivariate difference between n-6 and n-3 PUFA levels and locomotive syndrome, there may be a small relationship with locomotive function. In recent years, several studies have reported that n-6 and n-3 PUFAs have opposite effects on insulin resistance (IR) and body homeostasis [45]. It is postulated that n-3 PUFAs attenuate the development of IR by reducing inflammation, whereas n-6 PUFAs promote IR [46]. More recent evidence indicates that n-6 PUFAs play a key role in the inflammatory process and are associated with various metabolic diseases [47]. Therefore, it seems reasonable to control the dietary ratios of n-6/n-3 PUFAs to ameliorate obesity-related IR, which is beneficial for protection against chronic and metabolic diseases. A study of rats fed a high-fat diet demonstrated that the accumulation of fatty acids in various lipid fractions increased in the gastrocnemius red muscle when there was a shift in the n-6/n-3 PUFA balance in favor of n-6 PUFAs. The increases in n-6 PUFAs are associated with fat accumulation in muscle [48]. A high percentage of n-6 PUFAs was also associated with LS in this study.

This study had several limitations. First, the participants were middle-aged and older adults who lived in a relatively rural area and were employed in agriculture or fishing. Thus, the differences in lifestyles between these participants and people in an urban environment may limit the generalizability of our results. Second, the participants attended annual health examinations, suggesting that they may be more health-conscious than other people. Third, this was a cross-sectional, single-center study. In the future, longitudinal and multicenter collaborative research is needed to verify our findings. Fourth, BIA is not the gold standard assessment for body composition (the 4-compartment model or DXA are better).

5. Conclusions

In conclusion, this study examined the relationship between LS and nutrition. Salt intake and hypertension were associated with locomotive syndrome. Thus, we suggest that limiting salt intake may effectively prevent LS.

Supplementary Materials: The following supporting information can be downloaded at: https://www.mdpi.com/article/10.3390/jcm11030610/s1, Table S1: The comparison of all parameters between non-elderly and elderly participants; Table S2: The comparison of all parameters between the N group and L group in adult participants; Table S3: The comparison of all parameters between the N group and L group in older adult participants.

Author Contributions: Conceptualization, S.I. (Sadayuki Ito); methodology, S.I. (Sadayuki Ito); software, K.W.; validation, K.W.; formal analysis, S.I. (Sadayuki Ito); investigation, S.I. (Sadayuki Ito), H.N., K.A., M.M., T.S., S.I. (Shinya Ishizuka), Y.T., Y.H., and S.I. (Shiro Imagama); resources, S.I. (Sadayuki Ito); investigation, S.I. (Sadayuki Ito); H.N., K.A., M.M., T.S., S.I. (Shinya Ishizuka), Y.T., Y.H., and S.I. (Shiro Imagama); data curation, S.I. (Sadayuki Ito); writing—original draft preparation, S.I. (Sadayuki Ito); writing—review and editing, S.I. (Sadayuki Ito) and H.N.; supervision, S.I. (Shiro Imagama); project administration, H.N. All authors have read and agreed to the published version of the manuscript.

Funding: This research did not receive any specific grant from funding agencies in the public, commercial, or not-for-profit sectors.

Institutional Review Board Statement: The research protocol was approved by the Human Research Ethics Committee and the university's Institutional Review Board (No. 2014-0207). All participants gave written informed consent prior to participation. The research procedure was carried out in accordance with the principles of the Declaration of Helsinki.

Informed Consent Statement: All participants gave written informed consent prior to participation.

Data Availability Statement: The data of health check-ups used to support the findings of this study are available from the corresponding author upon request.

Acknowledgments: We are grateful to the staff of the Comprehensive Health Care Program held in Yakumo, Hokkaido, and Aya Henmi and Hiroko Ino of Nagoya University for their assistance throughout this study.

Conflicts of Interest: The authors declare no conflict of interest.

References

1. Preston, S.H.; Stokes, A. Sources of Population Aging in More and Less Developed Countries. *Popul. Dev. Rev.* **2012**, *38*, 221–236. [CrossRef]
2. Nakamura, K.; Ogata, T. Locomotive Syndrome: Definition and Management. *Clin. Rev. Bone Miner. Metab.* **2016**, *14*, 56–67. [CrossRef]
3. Yi, H.-S.; Lee, S. Overcoming osteoporosis and beyond: Locomotive syndrome or dysmobility syndrome. *Osteoporos. Sarcopenia* **2018**, *4*, 77–78. [CrossRef]
4. Hirano, K.; Imagama, S.; Hasegawa, Y.; Ito, Z.; Muramoto, A.; Ishiguro, N. The influence of locomotive syndrome on health-related quality of life in a community-living population. *Mod. Rheumatol.* **2013**, *23*, 939–944. [CrossRef]
5. Muramoto, A.; Imagama, S.; Ito, Z.; Hirano, K.; Ishiguro, N.; Hasegawa, Y. Spinal sagittal balance substantially influences locomotive syndrome and physical performance in community-living middle-aged and elderly women. *J. Orthop. Sci.* **2016**, *21*, 216–221. [CrossRef]
6. Ohba, T.; Oba, H.; Koyama, K.; Oda, K.; Tanaka, N.; Fujita, K.; Haro, H. Locomotive syndrome: Prevalence, surgical outcomes, and physical performance of patients treated to correct adult spinal deformity. *J. Orthop. Sci.* **2021**, *26*, 678–683. [CrossRef]
7. Kato, S.; Kurokawa, Y.; Kabata, T.; Demura, S.; Matsubara, H.; Kajino, Y.; Okamoto, Y.; Kimura, H.; Shinmura, K.; Igarashi, K.; et al. Improvement of locomotive syndrome with surgical treatment in patients with degenerative diseases in the lumbar spine and lower extremities: A prospective cohort study. *BMC Musculoskelet. Disord.* **2020**, *21*, 515. [CrossRef]
8. Ishibashi, H. Locomotive syndrome in Japan. *Osteoporos. Sarcopenia* **2018**, *4*, 86–94. [CrossRef]
9. Aoki, K.; Sakuma, M.; Ogisho, N.; Nakamura, K.; Chosa, E.; Endo, N. The effects of self-directed home exercise with serial telephone contacts on physical functions and quality of life in elderly people at high risk of locomotor dysfunction. *Acta Med. Okayama* **2015**, *69*, 245–253. [CrossRef]
10. Saka, B.; Kaya, O.; Ozturk, G.B.; Erten, N.; Karan, M.A. Malnutrition in the elderly and its relationship with other geriatric syndromes. *Clin. Nutr.* **2010**, *29*, 745–748. [CrossRef]
11. Jiménez-Redondo, S.; Beltrán de Miguel, B.; Gavidia Banegas, J.; Guzmán Mercedes, L.; Gómez-Pavón, J.; Cuadrado Vives, C. Influence of nutritional status on health-related quality of life of non-institutionalized older people. *J. Nutr. Health Aging* **2014**, *18*, 359–364. [CrossRef]
12. Ramsey, K.A.; Meskers, C.G.M.; Trappenburg, M.C.; Verlaan, S.; Reijnierse, E.M.; Whittaker, A.C.; Maier, A.B. Malnutrition is associated with dynamic physical performance. *Aging Clin. Exp. Res.* **2020**, *32*, 1085–1092. [CrossRef]
13. Visvanathan, R. Under-nutrition in older people: A serious and growing global problem! *J. Postgrad. Med.* **2003**, *49*, 352–360.
14. Reid, K.F.; Fielding, R.A. Skeletal muscle power: A critical determinant of physical functioning in older adults. *Exerc. Sport Sci. Rev.* **2012**, *40*, 4–12. [CrossRef]
15. Jensen, G.L.; Cederholm, T.; Correia, M.; Gonzalez, M.C.; Fukushima, R.; Higashiguchi, T.; de Baptista, G.A.; Barazzoni, R.; Blaauw, R.; Coats, A.J.S.; et al. GLIM Criteria for the Diagnosis of Malnutrition: A Consensus Report From the Global Clinical Nutrition Community. *JPEN J. Parenter. Enteral Nutr.* **2019**, *43*, 32–40. [CrossRef]
16. Tanaka, S.; Ando, K.; Kobayashi, K.; Hida, T.; Ito, K.; Tsushima, M.; Morozumi, M.; Machino, M.; Ota, K.; Suzuki, K.; et al. Utility of the Serum Cystatin C Level for Diagnosis of Osteoporosis among Middle-Aged and Elderly People. *Biomed. Res. Int.* **2019**, *2019*, 5046852. [CrossRef]
17. Muramoto, A.; Imagama, S.; Ito, Z.; Hirano, K.; Tauchi, R.; Ishiguro, N.; Hasegawa, Y. Threshold values of physical performance tests for locomotive syndrome. *J. Orthop. Sci.* **2013**, *18*, 618–626. [CrossRef]
18. Imagama, S.; Hasegawa, Y.; Ando, K.; Kobayashi, K.; Hida, T.; Ito, K.; Tsushima, M.; Nishida, Y.; Ishiguro, N. Staged decrease of physical ability on the locomotive syndrome risk test is related to neuropathic pain, nociceptive pain, shoulder complaints, and quality of life in middle-aged and elderly people—The utility of the locomotive syndrome risk test. *Mod. Rheumatol.* **2017**, *27*, 1051–1056. [CrossRef]
19. Seichi, A.; Hoshino, Y.; Doi, T.; Akai, M.; Tobimatsu, Y.; Iwaya, T. Development of a screening tool for risk of locomotive syndrome in the elderly: The 25-question Geriatric Locomotive Function Scale. *J. Orthop. Sci.* **2012**, *17*, 163–172. [CrossRef]
20. Suzuki, K.; Honjo, H.; Ichino, N.; Osakabe, K.; Sugimoto, K.; Yamada, H.; Kusuhara, Y.; Watarai, R.; Hamajima, T.; Hamajima, N.; et al. Association of serum carotenoid levels with urinary albumin excretion in a general Japanese population: The Yakumo study. *J. Epidemiol.* **2013**, *23*, 451–456. [CrossRef]
21. Kyle, U.G.; Bosaeus, I.; De Lorenzo, A.D.; Deurenberg, P.; Elia, M.; Manuel Gómez, J.; Lilienthal Heitmann, B.; Kent-Smith, L.; Melchior, J.-C.; Pirlich, M.; et al. Bioelectrical impedance analysis-part II: Utilization in clinical practice. *Clin. Nutr.* **2004**, *23*, 1430–1453. [CrossRef]
22. Park, K.S.; Lee, D.-H.; Lee, J.; Kim, Y.J.; Jung, K.Y.; Kim, K.M.; Kwak, S.H.; Choi, S.H.; Park, K.S.; Jang, H.C.; et al. Comparison between two methods of bioelectrical impedance analyses for accuracy in measuring abdominal visceral fat area. *J. Diabetes Complicat.* **2016**, *30*, 343–349. [CrossRef] [PubMed]
23. Hida, T.; Imagama, S.; Ando, K.; Kobayashi, K.; Muramoto, A.; Ito, K.; Ishikawa, Y.; Tsushima, M.; Nishida, Y.; Ishiguro, N.; et al. Sarcopenia and physical function are associated with inflammation and arteriosclerosis in community-dwelling people: The Yakumo study. *Mod. Rheumatol.* **2018**, *28*, 345–350. [CrossRef] [PubMed]

24. Ito, S.; Nakashima, H.; Ando, K.; Kobayashi, K.; Machino, M.; Seki, T.; Ishizuka, S.; Fujii, R.; Takegami, Y.; Yamada, H.; et al. Association between Low Muscle Mass and Inflammatory Cytokines. *Biomed. Res. Int.* **2021**, *2021*, 5572742. [CrossRef] [PubMed]
25. Ogihara, T.; Kikuchi, K.; Matsuoka, H.; Fujita, T.; Higaki, J.; Horiuchi, M.; Imai, Y.; Imaizumi, T.; Ito, S.; Iwao, H.; et al. The Japanese Society of Hypertension Guidelines for the Management of Hypertension (JSH 2009). *Hypertens. Res.* **2009**, *32*, 3–107. [CrossRef] [PubMed]
26. Seino, Y.; Nanjo, K.; Tajima, N.; Kadowaki, T.; Kashiwagi, A.; Araki, E.; Ito, C.; Inagaki, N.; Iwamoto, Y.; Kasuga, M.; et al. Report of the Committee on the classification and diagnostic criteria of diabetes mellitus. *Diabetol. Int.* **2010**, *1*, 2–20. [CrossRef]
27. Japan Atherosclerosis Society (JAS) guidelines for prevention of atherosclerotic cardiovascular diseases. *J Atheroscler. Thromb.* **2007**, *16*, 5–57.
28. Tsubono, Y.; Takamori, S.; Kobayashi, M.; Takahashi, T.; Iwase, Y.; Iitoi, Y.; Akabane, M.; Yamaguchi, M.; Tsugane, S. A data-based approach for designing a semiquantitative food frequency questionnaire for a population-based prospective study in Japan. *J. Epidemiol.* **1996**, *6*, 45–53. [CrossRef]
29. Science and Technology Agency. *Standard Tables of Food Composition in Japan*, 7th ed.; Printing Bureau, Ministry of Finance: Tokyo, Japan, 2015.
30. Watanabe, T. Food Composition Tables of Japan and the Nutrient Table/Database. *J. Nutr. Sci. Vitaminol.* **2015**, *61*, S25–S27. [CrossRef]
31. Yokoyama, Y.; Takachi, R.; Ishihara, J.; Ishii, Y.; Sasazuki, S.; Sawada, N.; Shinozawa, Y.; Tanaka, J.; Kato, E.; Kitamura, K.; et al. Validity of Short and Long Self-Administered Food Frequency Questionnaires in Ranking Dietary Intake in Middle-Aged and Elderly Japanese in the Japan Public Health Center-Based Prospective Study for the Next Generation (JPHC-NEXT) Protocol Area. *J. Epidemiol.* **2016**, *26*, 420–432. [CrossRef]
32. Anton, S.D.; Hida, A.; Mankowski, R.; Layne, A.; Solberg, L.M.; Mainous, A.G.; Buford, T. Nutrition and Exercise in Sarcopenia. *Curr. Protein Pept. Sci.* **2018**, *19*, 649–667. [CrossRef] [PubMed]
33. Cho, A.R.; Lee, J.H.; Kwon, Y.J. Fat-to-Muscle Ratios and the Non-Achievement of LDL Cholesterol Targets: Analysis of the Korean Genome and Epidemiology Study. *J. Cardiovasc. Dev. Dis.* **2021**, *8*, 96. [CrossRef] [PubMed]
34. Manzetti, S.; Zhang, J.; van der Spoel, D. Thiamin function, metabolism, uptake, and transport. *Biochemistry* **2014**, *53*, 821–835. [CrossRef]
35. Yates, A.A.; Schlicker, S.A.; Suitor, C.W. Dietary Reference Intakes: The new basis for recommendations for calcium and related nutrients, B vitamins, and choline. *J. Am. Diet Assoc.* **1998**, *98*, 699–706. [CrossRef]
36. Rust, P.; Ekmekcioglu, C. Impact of Salt Intake on the Pathogenesis and Treatment of Hypertension. *Adv. Exp. Med. Biol.* **2017**, *956*, 61–84. [CrossRef]
37. Aaron, K.J.; Sanders, P.W. Role of dietary salt and potassium intake in cardiovascular health and disease: A review of the evidence. *Mayo Clin. Proc.* **2013**, *88*, 987–995. [CrossRef] [PubMed]
38. Kopp, C.; Linz, P.; Dahlmann, A.; Hammon, M.; Jantsch, J.; Müller, D.N.; Schmieder, R.E.; Cavallaro, A.; Eckardt, K.U.; Uder, M.; et al. 23Na magnetic resonance imaging-determined tissue sodium in healthy subjects and hypertensive patients. *Hypertension* **2013**, *61*, 635–640. [CrossRef]
39. Mandai, S.; Furukawa, S.; Kodaka, M.; Hata, Y.; Mori, T.; Nomura, N.; Ando, F.; Mori, Y.; Takahashi, D.; Yoshizaki, Y.; et al. Loop diuretics affect skeletal myoblast differentiation and exercise-induced muscle hypertrophy. *Sci. Rep.* **2017**, *7*, 46369. [CrossRef]
40. Tsuchiya, Y.; Nakashima, S.; Banno, Y.; Suzuki, Y.; Morita, H. Effect of high-NaCl or high-KCl diet on hepatic Na^+- and K^+-receptor sensitivity and NKCC1 expression in rats. *Am. J. Physiol. Regul. Integr. Comp. Physiol.* **2004**, *286*, R591–R596. [CrossRef]
41. Yoshida, Y.; Kosaki, K.; Sugasawa, T.; Matsui, M.; Yoshioka, M.; Aoki, K.; Kuji, T.; Mizuno, R.; Kuro, O.M.; Yamagata, K.; et al. High Salt Diet Impacts the Risk of Sarcopenia Associated with Reduction of Skeletal Muscle Performance in the Japanese Population. *Nutrients* **2020**, *12*, 3474. [CrossRef]
42. Gueugneau, M.; Coudy-Gandilhon, C.; Meunier, B.; Combaret, L.; Taillandier, D.; Polge, C.; Attaix, D.; Roche, F.; Féasson, L.; Barthélémy, J.C.; et al. Lower skeletal muscle capillarization in hypertensive elderly men. *Exp. Gerontol.* **2016**, *76*, 80–88. [CrossRef] [PubMed]
43. Han, J.M.; Lee, M.-Y.; Lee, K.-B.; Kim, H.; Hyun, Y.Y. Low relative skeletal muscle mass predicts incident hypertension in Korean men: A prospective cohort study. *J. Hypertens.* **2020**, *38*, 2223–2229. [CrossRef] [PubMed]
44. Anderson, L.J.; Liu, H.; Garcia, J.M. Sex Differences in Muscle Wasting. *Adv. Exp. Med. Biol.* **2017**, *1043*, 153–197. [CrossRef] [PubMed]
45. Saini, R.K.; Keum, Y.S. Omega-3 and omega-6 polyunsaturated fatty acids: Dietary sources, metabolism, and significance—A review. *Life Sci.* **2018**, *203*, 255–267. [CrossRef] [PubMed]
46. Liu, H.Q.; Qiu, Y.; Mu, Y.; Zhang, X.J.; Liu, L.; Hou, X.H.; Zhang, L.; Xu, X.N.; Ji, A.L.; Cao, R.; et al. A high ratio of dietary n-3/n-6 polyunsaturated fatty acids improves obesity-linked inflammation and insulin resistance through suppressing activation of TLR4 in SD rats. *Nutr. Res.* **2013**, *33*, 849–858. [CrossRef]
47. Sonnweber, T.; Pizzini, A.; Nairz, M.; Weiss, G.; Tancevski, I. Arachidonic Acid Metabolites in Cardiovascular and Metabolic Diseases. *Int. J. Mol. Sci.* **2018**, *19*, 3285. [CrossRef]
48. Bielawiec, P.; Harasim-Symbor, E.; Sztolsztener, K.; Konstantynowicz-Nowicka, K.; Chabowski, A. Attenuation of Oxidative Stress and Inflammatory Response by Chronic Cannabidiol Administration Is Associated with Improved n-6/n-3 PUFA Ratio in the White and Red Skeletal Muscle in a Rat Model of High-Fat Diet-Induced Obesity. *Nutrients* **2021**, *13*, 1603. [CrossRef]

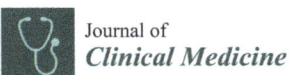

Article

Risk Factors and Surgical Management of Recurrent Herniation after Full-Endoscopic Lumbar Discectomy Using Interlaminar Approach

Koichiro Ono [1,2,*], Kazuo Ohmori [2], Reiko Yoneyama [2], Osamu Matsushige [2] and Tokifumi Majima [1]

1. Department of Orthopedic Surgery, Nippon Medical School, 1-1-5 Sendagi, Bunkyo-ku, Tokyo 113-8603, Japan; t-majima@nms.ac.jp
2. Center for Spinal Surgery, Nippon Koukan Hospital, 1-2-1 Koukandori, Kawasaki-ku, Kawasaki-shi 210-0852, Japan; kazuospine@gmail.com (K.O.); reikothjk@gmail.com (R.Y.); omatsushige@yahoo.co.jp (O.M.)
* Correspondence: koichiro-ono@nms.ac.jp

Citation: Ono, K.; Ohmori, K.; Yoneyama, R.; Matsushige, O.; Majima, T. Risk Factors and Surgical Management of Recurrent Herniation after Full-Endoscopic Lumbar Discectomy Using Interlaminar Approach. *J. Clin. Med.* **2022**, *11*, 748. https://doi.org/10.3390/jcm11030748

Academic Editors: Takashi Hirai, Hiroaki Nakashima, Masayuki Miyagi, Shinji Takahashi and Masashi Uehara

Received: 8 December 2021
Accepted: 25 January 2022
Published: 29 January 2022

Publisher's Note: MDPI stays neutral with regard to jurisdictional claims in published maps and institutional affiliations.

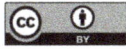

Copyright: © 2022 by the authors. Licensee MDPI, Basel, Switzerland. This article is an open access article distributed under the terms and conditions of the Creative Commons Attribution (CC BY) license (https://creativecommons.org/licenses/by/4.0/).

Abstract: Full-endoscopic lumbar discectomy (FED) is one of the least invasive procedures for lumbar disc herniation. Patients who receive FED for lumbar disc herniation may develop recurrent herniation at a frequency similar to conventional procedures. Reoperation and risk factors of recurrent lumbar disc herniation were investigated among 909 patients who received FED using an interlaminar approach (FED-IL). Sixty-five of the 909 patients received reoperation for recurrent herniation. Disc height, smoking, diabetes mellitus (DM), subligamentous extrusion (SE) type, and Modic change were identified as the risk factors for recurrence. Other indicators such as LL, Cobb angle, disc migration, age, sex, and body mass index (BMI) did not reach significance. Among 65 patients, reoperation was performed within 14 days following FED-IL (very early) in 7 patients, from 15 days to 3 months (early) in 14 patients, from 3 months to 1 year (midterm) in 17 patients, and after more than 1 year (late) in 27 patients. The very early group included a greater number of males, and the mean age was significantly lower in comparison to other groups. All patients in the very early group received FED-IL for reoperation. Reoperation within 2 weeks allows FED-IL to be performed without adhesion. Fusion surgery was performed on three cases in the early and midterm groups and on 10 cases in the late group, which increased over time as degenerative change and adhesion progressed. The procedure selected to treat recurrent herniation mostly depends on the surgeon's preference. Revision FED-IL is the first choice for recurrent herniation in terms of minimizing surgical burden, whereas fusion surgery offers the advantage that discectomy can be performed through unscarred tissues. FED-IL is recommended for recurrent herniation within 2 weeks before adhesion progresses.

Keywords: full-endoscopic lumbar discectomy; recurrent herniation; early recurrence

1. Introduction

Patients with lumbar disc herniation experience acute leg pain and disturbance in activities of daily living. Conservative management, in the form of medication and rest, is generally the first choice for this pathology. However, patients with intolerable pain for whom conservative treatment fails or who develop paralysis of limb muscles are considered for earlier surgical intervention. Patients who desire to return to work earlier are also candidates for discectomy. Moreover, patients who have received surgery for lumbar disc herniation show greater improvement in function and satisfaction regarding treatment than non-surgically managed patients [1], so discectomy can be recommended. Several surgical options are available for lumbar disc herniation, including open microdiscectomy [2], microendoscopic discectomy [3], and full-endoscopic lumbar discectomy (FED) [4–7]. Among these, FED is the most minimally invasive surgery as the cannula only has a diameter of 8 mm, and posterior structures are preserved [5]. The minimal trauma of

FED results in a shorter operation time and hospital stay [2,8]. FED is a new technique of which the frequency and risk factors of recurrent herniation following FED remain to be elucidated. With developments in instruments and techniques, patients who have undergone FED for lumbar disc herniation may still develop recurrent herniation at a frequency similar to conventional discectomy [8]. Here, we retrospectively investigated recurrent lumbar disc herniation after FED using an interlaminar approach (FED-IL). Risk factors and surgical procedures for recurrent lumbar disc herniation that are dependent on the postoperative period are also discussed.

2. Materials and Methods

2.1. Patient Population

A total of 909 patients (630 males, 279 females) who underwent FED for lumbar disc herniation at Nippon Koukan Hospital and were followed-up for at least 1 year after primary FED-IL were retrospectively reviewed. Mean age was 49.2 years (range, 12–90 years) and mean follow-up was 46.3 months (range, 12–90.1 months). Recurrence of lumbar disc herniation was defined as relapsed disc herniation at the same disc level and on the same side as the herniation treated by the initial FED, leading to reoperation. According to these criteria, 65 patients were diagnosed with recurrent herniation (recurrent group) and the other 844 patients were registered into the non-recurrent group (Table 1). Patients with recurrent disc herniation were allocated to groups according to the interval from primary FED to reoperation: very early (VE) group, up to 14 days post-FED; early (E) group, 15 days to 3 months post-FED; midterm (M) group, 3 months to 1-year post-FED; and long-term (L) group, more than 1-year post-FED (Table 2). The mean interval from primary FED-IL to reoperation for the VE, E, M and L groups was 0.3, 1.3, 6.9, and 27.7 months, respectively (Table 2).

Table 1. Comparison between the recurrent and non-recurrent groups. Case number, disc height, lumbar lordosis, PI-LL, Cobb angle, migration, type of herniation (SE: subligamentous extrusion, TE: transligamentous extrusion, SQ: sequestration), Modic change, mean age, sex, mean BMI, smoking, and diabetes mellitus (DM) are shown. The recurrent group had lower disc height, higher rate of Modic change, smoking, and DM compared to the non-recurrent group. Moreover, the recurrent group tended to have more SE-type herniation than the non-recurrent group ($p = 0.076$).

Groups		Recurrent	Non-Recurrent	p Value
Cases (total 909)		65	844	
Mean age (years)		50.3	48.4	0.42
Sex (Male:Female)		44:21	590:254	0.71
Mean BMI (kg/m^2)		24	26	0.36
Smoking	+	31	288	0.027
	−	34	556	
DM	+	13	84	0.011
	−	52	760	
Disc height		9.6	11.9	<0.01
Lumbar lordosis (LL)		32	34.5	0.16
Cobb angle		3.0	3.3	0.66
Migration	+	22	362	0.15
	−	43	482	
Type	SE	47	517	0.076
	non-SE (TE or SQ)	18	327	
Modic	+	31	112	<0.01
	−	34	732	

Table 2. Groups of recurrent lumbar disc herniation. Patients are sorted into 4 groups depending on the interval from primary FED-IL (1st OP) to reoperation (2nd OP). Mean age, sex, mean BMI, reoperation procedure, mean 1st OP time, mean post 1st OP hospitalization days, mean 2nd OP time, and mean post 2nd OP hospitalization days are shown. * Mean age differs significantly between L and VE groups ($p < 0.05$). ** Mean 2nd OP time was significantly shorter compared to the other groups ($p < 0.01$). *** Mean post 2nd OP hospitalization days was significantly shorter compared to the other groups ($p < 0.01$). OP = operation, FEDIL = full-endoscopic lumbar discectomy, interlaminar approach, TF = transforaminal approach, MEL = microendoscopic lumbar discectomy, BMI = body mass index.

Groups	Very Early (VE)	Early (E)	Midterm (M)	Long-Term (L)
Cases (total 65)	7	14	17	27
Period from 1st to 2nd OP	0–14 days	15 days–3 months	3 months–1 year	>1 year
Mean period from 1st to 2nd OP	0.3 months	1.3 months	6.9 months	27.7 months
Mean age (years)	42.9	49.6	47.8	54.1 *
Sex (Male:Female)	6:1	9:5	9:8	20:7
Mean BMI (kg/m^2)	23.9	22.9	24.1	24.6
Reoperation procedure (FEDIL/TF/MEL/Open/Fusion)	7/0/0/0/0	9/2/0/1/3	12/2/0/0/3	15/1/1/0/10
Mean 1st OP time (min)	59.1	61.7	71.3	72.4
Mean post-1st OP hospitalization days	7.4	3.3	3.1	4.3
Mean 2nd OP time	26.4 **	66.7	74.9	73.0
Mean post-2nd OP hospitalization days	4.0 ***	7.7	6.5	10.7

2.2. Surgical Procedures and Data Collection

2.2.1. Surgical Procedure for Primary FED-IL

In all cases, primary FED-IL was performed under general anesthesia with the patient in a prone position. The entry point was marked on the symptomatic side about 1 cm lateral from the midline and caudal to the affected disc level to best utilize the interlaminar window (Figure 1a–d). After draping, a spinal needle was introduced under fluoroscopic guidance from the marked point to the caudal part of the upper lamina (Figure 1e,f). A small skin incision was made on the marked point, and the fascia was cut simultaneously (Figure 1g). A pencil dilator was inserted into the caudal part of the upper lamina (Figure 1e), and this was followed by a cannula and rigid endoscope (RIWOspine GmbH, Knittlingen, Germany). Finally, the endoscope procedure was initiated.

Soft tissues were removed using a bipolar probe (Trigger-Flex Bipolar System; Elliquence, New York, NY, USA) and forceps (Figure 2a) to expose the ligamentum flavum of the interlaminar window (Figure 2b). Drilling of the inner edge of the lamina and facet joint was performed when the interlaminar window was too narrow for cannula insertion. The ligamentum flavum was cut with an angled cutter to reach the spinal canal (Figure 2b) with additional resection to detect the lateral edge of the nerve root. The perineural membrane was removed using micro-rongeurs to precisely identify the structures (Figure 2c,d). The annulus fibrosus was opened by the dissector or bipolar probe (Figure 2e), and herniated disc material was removed piece by piece (Figure 2f). Turning the cannula prevented neural structures from causing damage during resecting herniated material (Figure 2g). After the relaxation of the nerve structure was observed (Figure 2h), the endoscope was removed, and a drainage tube was inserted through the cannula under fluoroscopic guidance. Finally, the cannula was removed.

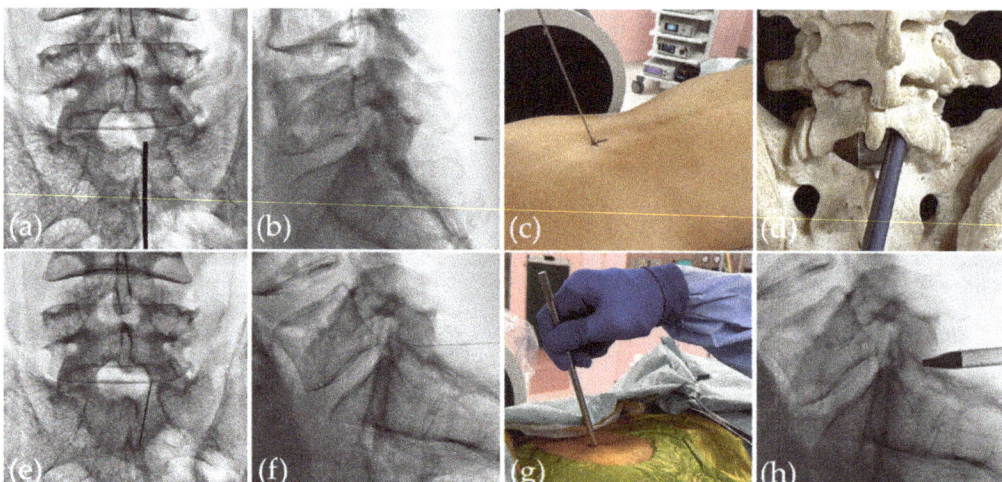

Figure 1. Entry point was indicated by the metal rod: (**a**) frontal view; (**b**) lateral view; (**c**) direction of endoscope on the skin; (**d**) through the interlaminar window. After draping, a spinal needle was introduced under fluoroscopic guidance from the marked point to the caudal part of the upper lamina: (**e**) anteroposterior view; (**f**) lateral view; (**g**) picture of the operative field. (**h**) Pencil dilator was inserted and placed into the interlaminar window.

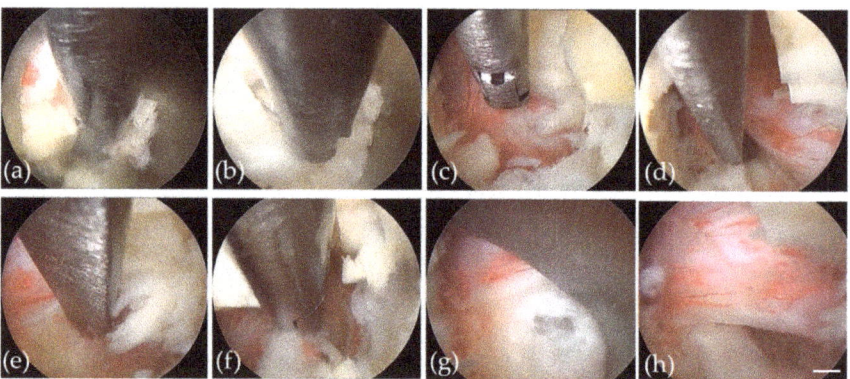

Figure 2. (**a**) Removal of soft tissues using Trigger-Flex Bipolar and forceps to expose the ligamentum flavum of the interlaminar window. (**b**) The ligamentum flavum was cut with an angled cutter to reach the spinal canal. (**c**) Perineural membrane was removed using micro-rongeurs. (**d**) Identification of the lateral edge of the nerve using a dissector. (**e**) The annulus was opened using a dissector or bipolar probe. (**f**) Resection of herniated disc material. (**g**) The cannula was turned to search for residual herniation. (**h**) Loosening of nerve structure was confirmed. Scale bar of 1 mm is shown as white bar.

2.2.2. Re-FED-IL for Very Early Recurrent Herniation

During re-FED-IL, the endoscope was inserted using the same skin incision made for primary FED-IL. The hematoma (Figure 3a*) was removed, and relapsed herniated disc material (Figure 3b**) was detected with no adhesions. Loosening of the nerve structure marked the end of the procedure (Figure 3c***).

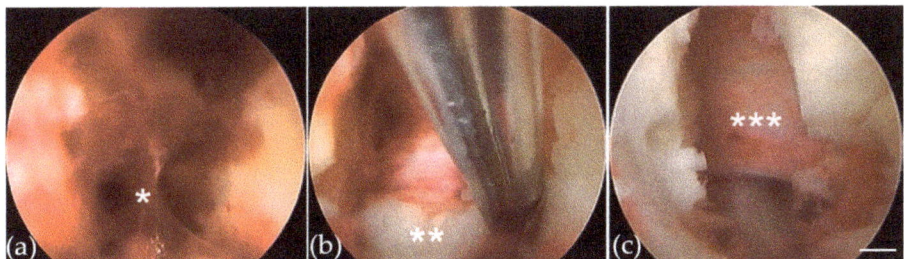

Figure 3. Endoscopic views of Re-FED-IL. (**a**) Hematoma (*) around the ligamentum flavum. (**b**) Relapsed herniated disc material (**) appeared from the lateral edge of the nerve root. There was no adhesion around herniation. (**c**) Loosening of nerve structure was confirmed. FED-IL = full-endoscopic discectomy, interlaminar approach. Scale bar of 1 mm is shown as white bar.

2.2.3. Re-FED-IL for Early-to-Late Recurrent Herniation

Re-FED-IL for early-to-late recurrent herniation needs to deal with adhesion. Under endoscopic and fluoroscopic guidance, drill descending facet or lamina to reach the bottom of the spinal canal from the fresh part to avoid adhesion. Careful exposure of disc herniation was indispensable, while the adhesive nerve root and dura matter remained untouched to avoid damaging neural structures. Loosening of the structures marked the end of the procedure.

2.2.4. Minimally Invasive Surgery (MIS) Posterior Lumbar Interbody Fusion (PLIF) for Recurrent Herniation

MIS-PLIF was performed as described elsewhere [9]. In brief, recurrent herniation removal and the insertion of interbody cages were performed 3–5 cm from the midline incision. Resecting the lamina or facet joint and approaching from the fresh part helped to avoid adhesion. After the midline incision closed, percutaneous pedicle screws (PPS)-rod fixation was performed.

2.3. Evaluated Data

Age, sex, body mass index (BMI), smoking, diabetes mellitus (DM), disc height, lumbar lordosis (LL), Cobb angle, migration, type of herniation (SE: subligamentous extrusion, TE: transligamentous extrusion, SQ: sequestration), and Modic change were compared between recurrent and non-recurrent groups. In addition, age, sex, BMI, reoperation procedure, 1st and 2nd operation time, and duration of postoperative hospitalization were compared among the four subgroups of recurrence. Disc height was obtained from the average of the anterior and posterior disc heights according to the Dabbs method [10]. Lumbar lordosis was measured as the angle between the superior of L1 and S1 [11].

2.4. Clinical Assessment

Clinical outcomes in the four subgroups were assessed preoperatively 1 month after reoperation and at the final follow-up using the Japanese Orthopedic Association (JOA) score, Oswestry Disability Index (ODI), and Visual Analog Scale (VAS) for back and leg pain. Medical records were searched for operative data and complications.

2.5. Ethics Approval and Consent to Participate

This study was conducted in accordance with the principles of the Declaration of Helsinki for Clinical Research [12]. The trial protocol was approved by Nippon Koukan Hospital Ethics Committee (No. 202115). Informed consent was obtained in the form of opt-out on the website.

2.6. Data Analysis

For numerical variables, means and standard deviations were calculated, and comparisons were made using a two-tailed Student t-test. Categorical variables were compared using a χ^2 test. A p value of <0.05 was defined as statistically significant, and two-sided 90% confidence intervals were calculated.

3. Results

3.1. Demographics and Clinical Characteristics

Among the 909 patients who had undergone FED-IL for lumbar disc herniation, 65 patients (7.2%) experienced recurrent lumbar disc herniation and required reoperation. Mean age, BMI, and sex did not differ significantly between recurrent and non-recurrent groups, whereas smoking and DM showed higher rates in the recurrent group (Table 1).

Sixty-five patients with reoperation were allocated: 7 to the VE group, 14 to the E group, 17 to the M group, and 27 to the L group (Table 2). One patient in the L group had re-recurrent herniation. No significant differences in sex or BMI were evident among subgroups, but mean age was significantly lower in the VE group (42.9 years) in comparison to the L group (54.1 years, $p = 0.045$) (Table 2). FED-IL was performed for all 7 cases in the VE group, 9 of 14 cases in the E group, 12 of 17 cases in the M group, and 15 of 27 cases in the L group, whereas fusion surgeries were performed on 0, 3, 3, and 10 cases, respectively (Table 2). Operation time for primary FED-IL did not differ significantly between subgroups, but operation time for re-FED-IL was significantly shorter in the VE group (average 26.4 min) than in the other groups (E, 66.7 min; M, 74.9 min; L, 73.0 min; $p < 0.01$ each) (Table 2). Duration of postoperative hospitalization was similar among subgroups at primary FED-IL but was significantly shorter in the VE group (4 days) in comparison to the L group (10.7 days; $p = 0.011$) at re-FED-IL (Table 2). JOA score showed similar trends in improvement among the four subgroups after secondary FED-IL (Figure 4a). VAS scores for limb and lumbar pain were decreased at one month and final follow-up after the secondary FED-IL (Figure 4b,c). ODI was improved at the 1-month and final follow-up (Figure 4d).

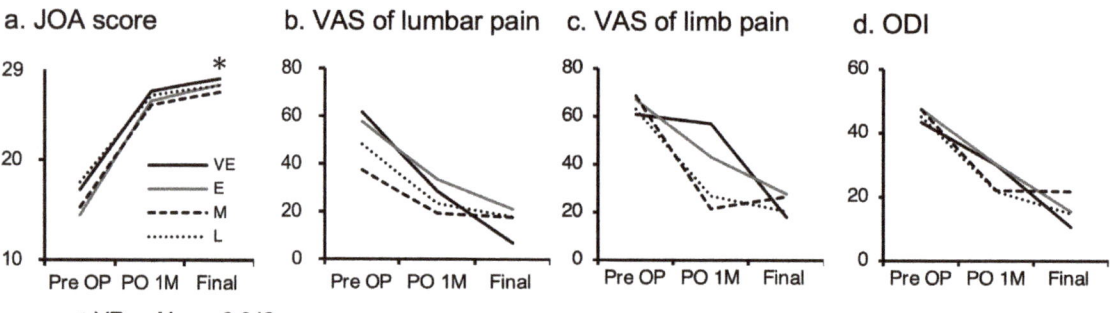

Figure 4. (**a**) JOA score improved similarly among the four groups after secondary FED-IL. Conversely, the VE group had significantly higher JOA scores compared to M groups at the final follow-up (* $p = 0.042$). (**b**) VAS of lumbar pain decreased similarly among the groups. (**c**) The VAS of limb pain also decreased similarly. (**d**) ODI improved equally among the groups. JOA = Japanese Orthopedic Association; ODI = Oswestry Disability Index; VAS = visual analog scale.

3.2. Radiological Characteristics

Recurrent group patients had lower disc height, a greater number of subligamentous extrusion (SE) type herniation, and increased Modic change compared to the non-recurrent population. However, LL, Cobb angle, and disc migration did not reach statistical significance (Table 1).

3.3. Case of Very Early Group

A 51-year-old woman underwent FED-IL using a standard procedure (Figure 2) for left-sided L4/5 SE type lumbar disc herniation. Pain relief was obtained immediately after surgery, and discharge was therefore scheduled for 2 days after. However, limb pain reappeared while showering on postoperative day 2. Recurrent disc herniation was confirmed by computed tomography after myelography. Re-FED-IL was performed 7 days after the primary FED-IL (Figure 3). Operation time for this case was 12 min. Pain again improved, and she was discharged 4 days after the reoperation.

4. Discussion

Lumbar disc herniation is one of the common pathologies encountered in routine practice. Surgical intervention is usually indicated for unsuccessful conservative treatment. Surgery for lumbar disc herniation offers several advantages over conservative treatment, such as greater improvement of ADL [13,14] and rapid pain relief [15]. Moreover, advances in surgical techniques and equipment over recent years have enabled endoscopic lumbar discectomy, thereby reducing the burden of surgical invasiveness on the patient and facilitating a rapid return to daily life and work [16].

FED has become even more popular since FED-IL was described by Ruetten [6] and Choi [17] in 2006. Before the interlaminar approach was introduced, the transforaminal approach (FED-TF) was the only option; but this method is technically demanding for spinal surgeons who are unfamiliar with endoscopic spine surgery. Enlarged endoscopes and high-speed drills enabled an interlaminar approach that is similar to conventional open procedures. As the FED-IL is still relatively new, few long-term observational studies of large populations have been reported [4,6,18]. Ruetten et al. [6] provided the first description of full endoscopic resection of the herniated lumbar disc using an interlaminar approach on 331 patients with 2 years of follow-up. In that study, 82% of patients no longer reported leg pain after surgery, and recurrent herniation was observed in 2.7% [6]. Wasinpongwanich et al. retrospectively reviewed clinical outcomes from 545 patients for over 4 years, finding 66 recurrences (12.11%) throughout follow-up, with 7.3% of patients requiring a second operation, although the type of reoperations was not disclosed [18]. Xie reported on 479 patients with a mean follow-up of 44.3 months, with 9 cases (1.9%) showing recurrent herniation. Four cases improved with conservative treatment and five cases underwent reoperation (open surgery in three, FED-IL in two) [19]. In the present study, we followed up on 909 cases for a mean of 46.3 months, with 65 patients (7.2%) developing recurrent herniation. This was similar to previous reports with recurrence rates of 1.9–10.3% [4,19–24]. As the follow-up for patients approaches 5 years after FED-IL, the recurrence rate after FED-IL is likely to approximate the true recurrence rate.

Risk factors for recurrence after FED include old age and obesity [22,25]. Yao et al. identified age > 50 years and BMI > 25 kg/m^2 as risk factors for recurrent herniation [25], and Kim et al. reported a mean age of 47.4 years in the recurrent group, while a mean age of 34.4 years was reported in the non-recurrent group [22]. Similarly, BMI was 24.9 kg/m^2 in the recurrent group and 22.9 kg/m^2 in the non-recurrent group [22]. In the present study, no difference was evident between recurrent and non-recurrent groups (Table 1). Many previous reports have described similar findings [26,27], and the apparently discrepant findings reported by Yao et al. may be explained by their use of FED-TF [22,25].

A significant correlation of smoking with the incidence of recurrent herniation has been found by several authors [28]. Nicotine plays a role in the degeneration of the intervertebral disc through narrowing the reduction in local blood flow followed by tissue hypoxia [29]. Moreover, nicotine, a small substance, can enter the intervertebral disc by diffusion and exert toxic effects directly on the intervertebral disc that causes disc degeneration [29]. In the present study, the smoking rate in the recurrent group was significantly higher in comparison to the non-recurrent group. Advanced disc degeneration by smoking may have played a role in recurrent herniation and contributed to recurrent herniation. Whether smoking cessation may reduce the recurrence of herniation remains an interesting topic for the future study.

The rate of DM patients in the recurrent group was higher in the present study than in the non-recurrent group (Table 1). Mobbs et al. also reported the rate of reoperation in the diabetic population was 28%, whereas the control group was 3.5% [30]. Interestingly, Robinson et al. reported fewer proteoglycans in the intervertebral discs of diabetic patients compared to nondiabetics, suggesting a potential mechanism underlying the higher rates in DM patients [31]. This pathological change might contribute to a decrease in the strength of the disc collagen matrix and cause susceptibility for the recurrent herniation in DM patients. Strict control of blood sugar after FED-IL is expected to reduce the recurrence of herniation.

Radiological measurements in the present study have elucidated several risk factors for recurrent herniation. Among these, disc height was lower in the recurrent group (Table 1). Kim et al. also found decreased disc height as a risk factor and hypothesized that an impaired healing process of the annulus contributes to the pathogenesis of recurrence [32]. Moreover, LL and Cobb angles were recorded, but no difference was found between groups. Large LL was suggested as the risk factor for recurrence in L5/S1 level herniation [33], whereas other levels were included in the present study. Chaojie et al. speculated wide lumbar lordosis increased shear force on the L5-S1 segment [33].

In an MRI study, subligamentous extrusion type herniation was found as the risk factor for recurrence (Table 1). Carragee et al. reported extrusion and sequestration were the end-stage in the process of fragmentation of disc material [34]. Protrusion or subligamentous extrusion-type herniation may have residual disc material that could serve as a candidate for the next herniation. Migration of disc material had no influence on recurrence, whereas Modic change was found as the risk factor for the recurrence (Table 1). Lu et al. showed recurrent herniation preferentially occurred when Modic change exists [35]. Thus, the weak connection between the cartilage and the vertebral body was the possible cause for the relapse.

Among the 65 cases, 19 patients (29.2%; VE+E groups) received reoperation within 3 months, and 46 cases (70.8%; M+L group) underwent reoperation after 3 months (Table 2). This result conflicts with the report by Kim et al. that 1001 of 2578 reoperations (38.8%) were performed within 3 months [36]. Cheng et al. followed FED-TF cases and found that 76.5% of reoperations were performed within 0.5 years after primary surgery [37]. We encountered more reoperations performed later than those reports [36,37]. This may represent differences in the approaches applied, as FED-IL or FED-TF, or in the indications for reoperation for recurrent lumbar disc herniation. Further research is needed to explain this discrepancy.

Among the four subgroups of recurrence (VE, E, M, and L groups), age, sex, and BMI were similar, except the VE group was significantly younger than the L group (Table 2). High levels of activity might cause early prolapse of disc material after the surgery. All patients in the VE group underwent FED-IL for reoperation, whereas more fusion surgeries were performed for cases with later recurrence. Surgical options for recurrent lumbar disc herniation include re-discectomy using conventional or minimally invasive techniques, with or without fusion. To determine the technique to be applied for reoperation, factors such as degeneration (including instability or deformity) and presenting symptoms (including limb or lumbar pain) are considered. Re-discectomy via a conventional [38] or minimally invasive technique [39,40] alone is the first choice for reoperation in terms of minimizing operation time, intraoperative blood loss, and total cost of the procedure [41].

Patients with back pain show significantly better improvement with fusion compared to discectomy alone, so patients with significant back pain should consider spinal fusion [41–43]. In addition, fusion surgeries, such as transforaminal lumbar interbody fusion, offer the advantage that discectomy can be performed through unscarred virgin tissues with no adhesions and through the lateral aspect of the dura mater with minimal retraction of the dura. While reoperation for recurrent lumbar disc herniation in previous studies [38–43] has demonstrated favorable clinical outcomes, high-quality evidence supporting indications for operative techniques remains limited, and the methods selected to treat recurrent lumbar disc herniation, for the most part, remain dependent on the preference of the surgeon.

The reoperation time for FED-IL was significantly shorter in the VE group than in the other groups. The process of scar formation and repair has been classified into three phases [44]. The first phase is the local inflammatory reaction in the first 3–5 days after surgery, involving hemostasis and coagulation. The second phase lasts 2–3 weeks for the formation of granulation tissue. The third phase involves the subsequent tissue reconstruction, transforming to scar tissue in the region of the defect [44]. The operation time for FED-IL was thus significantly shorter for the VE group than for even the E group. Reoperation performed later than 2 weeks after primary FED-IL is technically demanding for deal with adhesive soft tissues, whereas re-herniation before 2 weeks is easily removed by FED-IL without any adhesions present. In addition, the duration of hospitalization after reoperation was shorter in the VE group than in the other groups (Table 2), and clinical outcomes after reoperation were favorable (Figure 4c). These results indicate that reoperation can be positively recommended for patients with re-herniation before 2 weeks, especially since the symptoms of re-herniation are often more severe than the initial symptoms.

5. Study Limitations

This was a retrospective study, so key limitations in this study were selection bias and incomplete data. In the future, a prospective investigation would provide sufficient data to better clarify issues identified in this study.

6. Conclusions

Disc height, smoking, diabetes mellitus (DM), subligamentous extrusion (SE) type, and Modic change were identified as risk factors for recurrent lumbar disc herniation after FED-IL. The procedure selected to treat recurrent lumbar disc herniation mostly depends on the surgeon's preference. Revision FED-IL is the first choice for the recurrent herniation in terms of minimizing surgical burden, whereas fusion surgery offers the advantage that discectomy can be performed through unscarred tissues. FED-IL is recommended for recurrent herniation within 2 weeks before adhesion progress.

Author Contributions: Conceptualization, K.O. (Koichiro Ono); methodology, K.O. (Koichiro Ono); Supervision, K.O. (Kazuo Ohmori) and T.M.; Visualization, R.Y. and O.M.; writing—original draft preparation, K.O. (Koichiro Ono); writing—review and editing, K.O. (Koichiro Ono); supervision, K.O. (Kazuo Ohmori) and T.M. All authors have read and agreed to the published version of the manuscript.

Funding: No funding was received for this study. No benefits in any form have been or will be received from a commercial party related directly or indirectly to the subject of this paper.

Institutional Review Board Statement: The study was conducted according to the guidelines of the Declaration of Helsinki, approved by the Nippon Koukan Hospital Ethics Committee (202115, 4 January 2022).

Informed Consent Statement: Informed consent was obtained in the form of opt-out on the website.

Data Availability Statement: The data used to support the funding of this study are available from the corresponding author upon request.

Conflicts of Interest: The authors declare that there is no conflict of interest regarding the publication of this paper.

References

1. Lurie, J.D.; Tosteson, T.D.; Tosteson, A.N.; Zhao, W.; Morgan, T.S.; Abdu, W.A.; Herkowitz, H.; Weinstein, J.N. Surgical versus nonoperative treatment for lumbar disc herniation: Eight-year results for the spine patient outcomes research trial. *Spine* **2014**, *39*, 3–16. [CrossRef] [PubMed]
2. Ruan, W.; Feng, F.; Liu, Z.; Xie, J.; Cai, L.; Ping, A. Comparison of percutaneous endoscopic lumbar discectomy versus open lumbar microdiscectomy for lumbar disc herniation: A meta-analysis. *Int. J. Surg.* **2016**, *31*, 86–92. [CrossRef] [PubMed]
3. Minamide, A.; Yoshida, M.; Yamada, H.; Nakagawa, Y.; Hashizume, H.; Iwasaki, H.; Tsutsui, S. Clinical outcomes after microendoscopic laminotomy for lumbar spinal stenosis: A 5-year follow-up study. *Eur. Spine J.* **2015**, *24*, 396–403. [CrossRef] [PubMed]
4. Ruetten, S.; Komp, M.; Merk, H.; Godolias, G. Full-endoscopic interlaminar and transforaminal lumbar discectomy versus conventional microsurgical technique: A prospective, randomized, controlled study. *Spine* **2008**, *208*, 931–939. [CrossRef]
5. Ruetten, S.; Komp, M.; Merk, H.; Godolias, G. Use of newly developed instruments and endoscopes: Full-endoscopic resection of lumbar disc herniations via the interlaminar and lateral transforaminal approach. *J. Neurosurg. Spine* **2007**, *6*, 521–530. [CrossRef]
6. Ruetten, S.; Komp, M.; Godolias, G. A New full-endoscopic technique for the interlaminar operation of lumbar disc herniations using 6-mm endoscopes: Prospective 2-year results of 331 patients. *Minim. Invasive Neurosurg.* **2006**, *49*, 80–87. [CrossRef]
7. Ruetten, S.; Komp, M.; Godolias, G. An extreme lateral access for the surgery of lumbar disc herniations inside the spinal canal using the full-endoscopic uniportal transforaminal approach-technique and prospective results of 463 patients. *Spine* **2005**, *30*, 2570–2578. [CrossRef]
8. Phan, K.; Xu, J.; Schultz, K.; Alvi, M.A.; Lu, V.M.; Kerezoudis, P.; Maloney, P.R.; Murphy, M.E.; Mobbs, R.J.; Bydon, M. Full-endoscopic versus micro-endoscopic and open discectomy: A systematic review and meta-analysis of outcomes and complications. *Clin. Neurol. Neurosurg.* **2017**, *154*, 1–12. [CrossRef]
9. Mobbs, R.J.; Sivabalan, P.; Li, J. Minimally invasive surgery compared to open spinal fusion for the treatment of degenerative lumbar spine pathologies. *J. Clin. Neurosci.* **2012**, *19*, 829–835. [CrossRef]
10. Dabbs, V.M.; Dabbs, L.G. Correlation between disc height narrowing and low back pain. *Spine* **1990**, *15*, 1366–1369. [CrossRef]
11. Pesenti, S.; Lafage, R.; Stein, D.; Elysee, J.C.; Lenke, L.G.; Schwab, F.J.; Kim, H.J.; Lafage, V. The amount of proximal lumbar Lordosis is related to pelvic incidence. *Clin. Orthop. Relat. Res.* **2018**, *476*, 1603–1611. [CrossRef] [PubMed]
12. Fuson, R.L.; Sherman, M.; Vleet, J.V. The conduct of orthopaedic clinical trials. *J. Bone Jt. Surg. Am.* **1997**, *79*, 1089–1098. [CrossRef] [PubMed]
13. Weinstein, J.N.; Lurie, J.D.; Tosteson, T.D.; Skinner, J.S.; Hanscom, B.; Tosteson, A.N.; Herkowitz, H.; Fischgrund, J.; Cammisa, F.P.; Albert, T.; et al. Surgical vs. nonoperative treatment for lumbar disk herniation: The Spine Patient Outcomes Research Trial (SPORT) observational cohort. *JAMA* **2006**, *296*, 2451–2459. [CrossRef] [PubMed]
14. Atlas, S.J.; Keller, R.B.; Chang, Y.; Deyo, R.A.; Singer, D.E. Surgical and nonsurgical management of sciatica secondary to a lumbar disc herniation: Five-year outcomes from the Maine Lumbar Spine Study. *Spine* **2001**, *26*, 1179–1187. [CrossRef] [PubMed]
15. Peul, W.C.; van Houwelingen, H.C.; van den Hout, W.B.; Brand, R.; Eekhof, J.A.; Tans, J.T.; Thomeer, R.T.; Koes, B.W. Leiden-The Hague Spine Intervention Prognostic Study Group. Surgery versus prolonged conservative treatment for sciatica. *N. Engl. J. Med.* **2007**, *356*, 2245–2256. [CrossRef] [PubMed]
16. Choi, K.C.; Kim, J.S.; Park, C.K. Percutaneous Endoscopic Lumbar Discectomy as an Alternative to Open Lumbar Microdiscectomy for Large Lumbar Disc Herniation. *Pain Physician.* **2016**, *19*, E291–E300. [PubMed]
17. Choi, G.; Lee, S.H.; Raiturker, P.P.; Lee, S.; Chae, Y.S. Percutaneous endoscopic interlaminar discectomy for intracanalicular disc herniations at L5-S1 using a rigid working channel endoscope. *Neurosurgery* **2006**, *58*, ONS59–ONS68. [CrossRef]
18. Wasinpongwanich, K.; Pongpirul, K.; Lwin, K.M.M.; Kesornsak, W.; Kuansongtham, V.; Ruetten, S. Full-Endoscopic Interlaminar Lumbar Discectomy: Retrospective Review of Clinical Results and Complications in 545 International Patients. *World Neurosurg.* **2019**, *132*, e922–e928. [CrossRef]
19. Xie, T.H.; Zeng, J.C.; Li, Z.H.; Wang, L.; Nie, H.F.; Jiang, H.S.; Song, Y.M.; Kong, Q.Q. Complications of Lumbar Disc Herniation Following Full-endoscopic Interlaminar Lumbar Discectomy: A Large, Single-Center, Retrospective Study. *Pain Physician* **2017**, *20*, E379–E387.
20. Choi, K.C.; Kim, J.S.; Ryu, K.S.; Kang, B.U.; Ahn, Y.; Lee, S.H. Percutaneous endoscopic lumbar discectomy for L5-S1 disc herniation: Transforaminal versus interlaminar approach. *Pain Physician* **2013**, *16*, 547–556.
21. Yin, S.; Du, H.; Yang, W.; Duan, C.; Feng, C.; Tao, H. Prevalence of Recurrent Herniation Following Percutaneous Endoscopic Lumbar Discectomy: A Meta-Analysis. *Pain Physician* **2018**, *21*, 337–350. [PubMed]
22. Kim, J.M.; Lee, S.H.; Ahn, Y.; Yoon, D.H.; Lee, C.D.; Lim, S.T. Recurrence after successful percutaneous endoscopic lumbar discectomy. *Minim. Invasive Neurosurg.* **2007**, *50*, 82–85. [CrossRef] [PubMed]
23. Marković, M.; Živković, N.; Milan, S.; Gavrilović, A.; Stojanović, D.; Aleksić, V.; Ruetten, S. Full-endoscopic interlaminar operations in lumbar compressive lesions surgery: Prospective study of 350 patients—"ENDOS" Study. *J. Neurosurg. Sci.* **2020**, *64*, 16–24. [CrossRef] [PubMed]
24. Passacantilli, E.; Lenzi, J.; Caporlingua, F.; Pescatori, L.; Lapadula, G.; Nardone, A.; Santoro, A. Endoscopic interlaminar approach for intracanal L5-S1 disc herniation: Classification of disc prolapse in relation to learning curve and surgical outcome. *Asian J. Endosc. Surg.* **2015**, *8*, 445–453. [CrossRef] [PubMed]

25. Yao, Y.; Liu, H.; Zhang, H.; Wang, H.; Zhang, C.; Zhang, Z.; Wu, J.; Tang, Y.; Zhou, Y. Risk Factors for Recurrent Herniation After Percutaneous Endoscopic Lumbar Discectomy. *World Neurosurg.* **2017**, *100*, 1–6. [CrossRef]
26. Shimia, M.; Babaei-Ghazani, A.; Sadat, B.E.; Habibi, B.; Habibzadeh, A. Risk factors of recurrent lumbar disk herniation. *Asian J. Neurosurg.* **2013**, *8*, 93–96.
27. Kim, K.T.; Lee, D.H.; Cho, D.C.; Sung, J.K.; Kim, Y.B. Preoperative Risk Factors for Recurrent Lumbar Disk Herniation in L5-S1. *J. Spinal Disord. Tech.* **2015**, *28*, E571–E577. [CrossRef]
28. Miwa, S.; Yokogawa, A.; Kobayashi, T.; Nishimura, T.; Igarashi, K.; Inatani, H.; Tsuchiya, H. Risk factors of recurrent lumbar disc herniation: A single center study and review of the literature. *J. Spinal Disord Tech.* **2015**, *28*, E265–E269. [CrossRef]
29. Akmal, M.; Kesani, A.; Anand, B.; Singh, A.; Wiseman, M.; Goodship, A. Effect of nicotine on spinal disc cells: A cellular mechanism for disc degeneration. *Spine* **2004**, *29*, 568–575. [CrossRef]
30. Mobbs, R.J.; Newcombe, R.L.; Chandran, K.N. Lumbar discectomy and the diabetic patient: Incidence and outcome. *J. Clin. Neurosci.* **2001**, *8*, 10–13. [CrossRef]
31. Robinson, D.; Mirovsky, Y.; Halperin, N.; Evron, Z.; Nevo, Z. Changes in proteoglycans of intervertebral disc in diabetic patients. A possible cause of increased back pain. *Spine* **1998**, *23*, 849–856. [CrossRef] [PubMed]
32. Kim, K.T.; Park, S.W.; Kim, Y.B. Disc height and segmental motion as risk factors for recurrent lumbar disc herniation. *Spine* **2009**, *34*, 2674–2678. [CrossRef] [PubMed]
33. Chaojie, Y.; Xinli, Z.; Chong, L.; Shian, L.; Jinming, X.; Tuo, L.; Zide, Z.; Jiarui, C. Risk Factors for Recurrent L5–S1 Disc Herniation After Percutaneous Endoscopic Transforaminal Discectomy: A Retrospective Study. *Med. Sci. Monit.* **2020**, *26*, e919888-1–e919888-12.
34. Carragee, E.J.; Han, M.Y.; Suen, P.W.; Kim, D. Clinical outcomes after lumbar discectomy for sciatica: The effects of fragment type and annular competence. *J. Bone Jt. Surg Am.* **2003**, *85*, 102–108. [CrossRef]
35. Lu, H.; Shengwen, L.; Junhui, L.; Zhi, S.; Shunwu, F.; Fengdong, Z. Recurrent disc herniation following percutaneous endoscopic lumbar discectomy preferentially occurs when Modic changes are present. *J. Orthop. Surg. Res.* **2020**, *15*, 176.
36. Kim, C.H.; Chung, C.K.; Park, C.S.; Choi, B.; Kim, M.J.; Park, B.J. Reoperation rate after surgery for lumbar herniated intervertebral disc disease: Nationwide cohort study. *Spine* **2013**, *38*, 581–590. [CrossRef] [PubMed]
37. Cheng, J.; Wang, H.; Zheng, W.; Li, C.; Wang, J.; Zhang, Z.; Huang, B.; Zhou, Y. Reoperation after lumbar disc surgery in two hundred and seven patients. *Int. Orthop.* **2013**, *37*, 1511–1517. [CrossRef]
38. Patel, M.S.; Braybrooke, J.; Newey, M.; Sell, P. A comparative study of the outcomes of primary and revision lumbar discectomy surgery. *Bone Jt. J.* **2013**, *95-B*, 90–94. [CrossRef]
39. Hoogland, T.; van den Brekel-Dijkstra, K.; Schubert, M.; Miklitz, B. Endoscopic transforaminal discectomy for recurrent lumbar disc herniation: A prospective, cohort evaluation of 262 consecutive cases. *Spine* **2008**, *33*, 973–978. [CrossRef]
40. Smith, J.S.; Ogden, A.T.; Shafizadeh, S.; Fessler, R.G. Clinical outcomes after microendoscopic discectomy for recurrent lumbar disc herniation. *Clin. Spine Surg.* **2010**, *23*, 30–34. [CrossRef]
41. El Shazly, A.A.; El Wardany, M.A.; Morsi, A.M. Recurrent lumbar disc herniation: A prospective comparative study of three surgical management procedures. *Asian J. Neurosurg.* **2013**, *8*, 139–146. [CrossRef] [PubMed]
42. Dower, A.; Chatterji, R.; Swart, A.; Winder, M.J. Surgical management of recurrent lumbar disc herniation and the role of fusion. *J. Clin. Neurosci.* **2016**, *23*, 44–50. [CrossRef]
43. Shepard, N.; Cho, W. Recurrent Lumbar Disc Herniation: A Review. *Glob. Spine J.* **2019**, *9*, 202–209. [CrossRef] [PubMed]
44. Wang, H.; Sun, W.; Fu, D.; Shen, Y.; Chen, Y.Y.; Wang, L.L. Update on biomaterials for prevention of epidural adhesion after lumbar laminectomy. *J. Orthop. Translat.* **2018**, *13*, 41–49. [CrossRef] [PubMed]

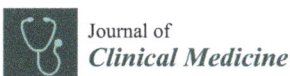

Editorial

Current Advances in Spinal Diseases of the Elderly: Introduction to the Special Issue

Takashi Hirai [1,*,†], Masashi Uehara [2,†], Masayuki Miyagi [3,†], Shinji Takahashi [4,†] and Hiroaki Nakashima [5,†]

1. Department of Orthopaedic Surgery, Tokyo Medical and Dental University, Tokyo 113-8519, Japan
2. Department of Orthopaedic Surgery, Shinshu University School of Medicine, Nagano 390-8621, Japan; masashi_u560613@yahoo.co.jp
3. Department of Orthopaedic Surgery, Kitasato University School of Medicine, Kanagawa 252-0375, Japan; masayuki008@aol.com
4. Department of Orthopedic Surgery, Osaka City University Graduate School of Medicine, Osaka 545-8585, Japan; shinji@med.osaka-cu.ac.jp
5. Department of Orthopedic Surgery, Nagoya University Graduate School of Medicine, Aichi 466-8550, Japan; hirospine@med.nagoya-u.ac.jp
* Correspondence: hirai.orth@tmd.ac.jp
† All members contributed equally to this editorial.

Citation: Hirai, T.; Uehara, M.; Miyagi, M.; Takahashi, S.; Nakashima, H. Current Advances in Spinal Diseases of the Elderly: Introduction to the Special Issue. *J. Clin. Med.* **2021**, *10*, 3298. https://doi.org/10.3390/jcm10153298

Received: 22 July 2021
Accepted: 23 July 2021
Published: 26 July 2021

Publisher's Note: MDPI stays neutral with regard to jurisdictional claims in published maps and institutional affiliations.

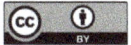

Copyright: © 2021 by the authors. Licensee MDPI, Basel, Switzerland. This article is an open access article distributed under the terms and conditions of the Creative Commons Attribution (CC BY) license (https://creativecommons.org/licenses/by/4.0/).

Spine-related disorders often impair quality of life (QOL) and the ability to perform activities of daily living and are a problem in rapidly aging societies. Motor deficits, poor balance, and neuropathic pain are known to be major causes of frailty in the elderly population. Spine surgeons and neurosurgeons must interpret these pathologies accurately to make a correct diagnosis and aim for an optimal solution when treating such patients. Therefore, they must be able to recognize the spinal diseases that lead to severe disorders in the elderly. This Special Issue of the *Journal of Clinical Medicine* is dedicated to current topics in spine-related disorders of the elderly (Figure 1). This narrative review focuses on present perspectives and future directions concerning refractory spinal disorders, including spinal tumors, osteoporosis, spinal metastasis, spinal deformity, and ossification of the spinal ligaments.

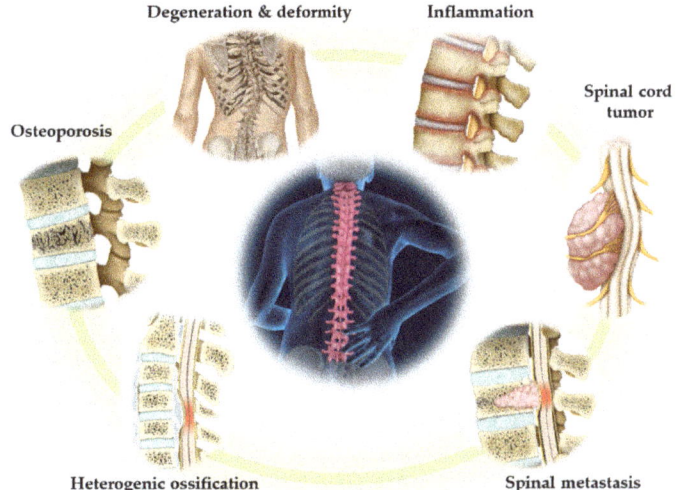

Figure 1. Typical spine-related disorders in the elderly.

1. Spinal Deformity

In 1994, Dubousset et al. [1] introduced the "cone of economy" concept, which has since been applied when evaluating balance in elderly patients with spinal deformity. According to this concept, when the gravity line is within the cone of economy, minimal muscle activation is needed to maintain balance, but in patients with severe spinal deformity, the gravity line is outside the cone of economy, such that greater muscle energy is required and maintaining a standing posture becomes difficult [2]. Patients with spinal malalignment often complain of a variety of symptoms, including intermittent claudication due to severe low back pain, gastroesophageal reflux disease caused by excessive pressure on the abdomen due to spinal kyphosis, and depression and the resulting deterioration of QOL [3]. Schwab et al. reported that global spinal sagittal malalignment, high pelvic tilt, and spinopelvic alignment mismatch lead to the deterioration of health-related QOL in elderly patients with spinal deformity [4] and devised the well-known SRS-Schwab classification of adult spinal deformity. Recent improvements in spinal instrumentation and surgical strategies have meant that surgeons are better able to correct spinal alignment and perform long spinal fusion surgery to improve low back pain, gait, and health-related QOL [5]. However, surgery for spinal deformity has a high complication rate [6], and there are some concerns about performing highly invasive surgery in elderly patients. Therefore, we should also focus on intervention in the early stages of spinal deformity.

One of the most important factors in spinal deformity is vertebral fractures, which are prevalent in the elderly because of osteoporosis. Vertebral fractures contribute to spinal malalignment [7], and sagittal spinal malalignment is a potential risk factor for new vertebral fractures in patients with osteoporosis [8]. Therefore, treatment of osteoporosis to avoid vertebral fractures is important in terms of preserving spinal alignment.

Another frequently encountered cause of spinal deformity is the age-related decrease in muscle mass, known as sarcopenia. In a study by Eguchi et al., the incidence of sarcopenia was significantly higher in patients with spinal deformity than in those with lumbar spinal stenosis [9]. Moreover, strong correlations were found between decreased trunk muscle mass, global spinal sagittal malalignment, and poor low back pain, and health-related QOL scores [10]. These findings indicate that the measurement of skeletal muscle mass is required for a diagnosis of sarcopenia. However, the measurement of trunk muscle mass may also be needed in patients with spinal deformity. Furthermore, the management of spinal deformity should include early intervention to improve both skeletal and trunk muscle mass.

2. Osteoporotic Vertebral Fractures

Osteoporotic fractures are particularly common in vertebrae, and their diagnosis and treatment are very important in our aging society. An osteoporotic vertebral fracture (OVF) not only reduces QOL by causing chronic low back pain and a decrease physical activity but also increases the mortality risk by about 15% [11]. Although an OVF is not difficult to diagnose, there are some points that need to be taken into account so that these fractures are not missed or misdiagnosed. Considering that the risk of a future OVF is markedly increased in patients with a prior OVF, the correct diagnosis and treatment of osteoporosis are important to reduce the risk of a future fracture. The first 1–2 years after OVF is a time of increased risk for further fractures and is known as the imminent fracture risk period [12]. Therefore, therapeutic intervention for osteoporosis should be initiated promptly at the time of an OVF. The goals of treatment are pain relief and the achievement of the pre-injury QOL and activities of daily living (ADL) performance level. Although conservative measures are the mainstay of treatment for OVF, there is still no gold standard approach in terms of bracing and physical therapy. The choice of treatment must be tailored to the patient's general condition and previous level of physical activity.

At present, there is no OVF classification that can be used to guide treatment. Although the Genant classification [13] is the most widely used in epidemiological and clinical studies because of its simplicity, it does not categorize OVF according to morphology, making it difficult to use for treatment decisions. More recently, the German Society for Orthopaedics and Trauma has proposed a classification that can be used to decide feasible treatment [14,15]. However, in elderly patients, the treatment goals will vary greatly depending on overall health status and the pre-fracture ability to perform ADL, so the extent to which this scoring system is actually useful needs further validation.

It is well known that elderly patients are at high risk of surgical complications. Vertebral augmentation, posterior fixation, osteotomy, and anterior fixation are the surgical options for OVF. It is necessary to understand the advantages and disadvantages of these techniques before selecting a surgical method. Vertebral augmentation or local fixation is indicated when the aim is to reduce back pain caused by a local fracture or pseudoarthrosis, whereas decompression fixation is indicated for neurological symptoms. However, there are some potential problems with implant surgery, such as loss of correction, adjacent vertebral fracture, leakage and migration of cement, and a need for revision surgery [16,17]. Preoperative imaging evaluation is important to minimize the risk of these complications.

The risk of complications with implant surgery increases in patients over 80 years of age [18]. Posterior fusion is indicated when the vertebral body shows mobility but is judged to be poorly improved by vertebral augmentation alone based on imaging findings or when neurological symptoms are present. If the mobility of the vertebral body is observed, vertebral body augmentation can be used to support the anterior column. However, the correction effect is poor [19]. Loss of correction after posterior fusion is caused by loosening of the screw on either the cephalad or caudal side. For posterior fixation, the pedicle screw alone may pull out, and a combination of various hook systems and wire ring taping should be considered. Augmentation of fenestrated pedicle screws is also an option but has been reported to have a high cement leak rate [18].

Anterior column reconstruction is necessary when the fractured vertebral body is unstable but not amenable to vertebral augmentation, when there is instability at the disc level, and when there is prominent vertebral body deformation that requires resection. The anterior column can be reconstructed by a posterior osteotomy or anterior discectomy, but posterior anchoring is essential for the correction of kyphosis. According to one report [20], an operating time of 3 h and blood loss of less than 500 mL is acceptable in patients over 80 years of age. Therefore, the anterior reconstruction can be performed if short fusion is possible but is not otherwise indicated in this age group.

OVF is basically treated conservatively in elderly patients, but surgery should be considered for those who are resistant to conservative measures and those with neurological symptoms. Given that OVF is often difficult to treat, it is important to start screening for osteoporosis at a relatively young age and initiate treatment as early as possible.

3. Tumors of the Spinal Cord

Spinal cord tumors are rare and account for 4–16% of all tumors in the central nervous system [21–24]. A previous study in our orthopedic department identified 678 patients with spinal cord tumors over a 10-year period. Most of the patients who required surgery were in their 50 s or 60 s, with a mean age at the time of surgery of 52.4 years.

Intramedullary spinal cord tumors (ImSCTs) comprise approximately 5–20% of all spinal cord tumors [21–24]. Although glioma and astrocytoma are common ImSCTs in pediatric patients, ependymomas are the most common ImSCT in adults. Ependymomas tend to be located in the cervical or cervicothoracic region in adults, whereas most are myxopapillary ependymomas in the conus medullaris in pediatric patients. Other ImSCTs commonly found in adults are hemangioma and hemangioblastoma [23]. Most hemangiomas are found at the cervical and thoracic levels and are typically observed in patients aged older than 50 years. Three-quarters of hemangiomas are intramedullary, and the remainder are at intradural or epidural sites. Adult hemangioblastoma is most likely to occur in those in their 30s [23]. Approximately 90% of hemangioblastomas are ImSCTs, and the remainder are intradural-extramedullary tumors. Moreover, 40% of hemangioblastomas are associated with von Hippel–Lindau disease and whole-body computed tomography is needed to confirm the diagnosis.

Intradural-extramedullary tumors are the most common spinal cord tumors. In Asian populations, most intradural-extramedullary tumors are schwannomas followed by meningiomas [23]. However, in non-Asian countries, the incidence of meningioma is at least as high as that of schwannoma. Schwannoma is typically diagnosed after the age of 30, with the highest incidence in those aged 50–59 years [23]. In contrast, meningioma typically occurs after the age of 50, and its highest incidence is among those aged 60–69 years [23].

Recent progress in research on spinal cord tumors includes advances in the genetic analysis and identification of causative genes for various tumors [21]. Meningioma is one of the most common spinal cord tumors, and the most consistent genetic abnormality found in patients with these tumors is a complete or partial loss of chromosome 22, followed by the loss of 1p, 9p, and 10q and gain of 5p and 17q [21]. Further advances are expected in the field of genetic analysis, and in addition to arranging the pathological classification of tumors, developments in gene therapy for malignant tumors are anticipated.

4. Spinal Metastasis

In recent years, there has been an increase in the number of patients with metastatic spine tumors due to advances in the treatment of their primary cancers and population aging. Metastatic spinal cord compression occurs in 5–14% of all patients with cancer [25]. Therefore, it is important to detect and treat compression because it may lead to pathological fractures and paralysis, both of which can greatly impair ADLs [26]. Nonetheless, many patients develop severe paralysis due to spinal cord compression and require emergency hospitalization. In such cases, improvement after surgery is poor, and the risk of complications is high. Therefore, it is necessary to establish a comprehensive treatment plan that takes into account the likely prognosis and the patient's overall state of health.

In 2005, Patchell et al. reported a randomized trial in which they found that surgery was more effective than radiotherapy for metastatic spinal cord compression in terms of maintaining the ability to walk [25]. However, a subsequent study [27] found that the therapeutic outcome of radiation was inferior to that previously reported. Rades et al. investigated 11 prognostic factors in a cohort of 2296 patients with metastatic spinal cord compression. Using matched-pair analysis, they were able to compare the outcomes between 108 patients who underwent surgery plus radiotherapy and 216 patients who received radiation alone [28]. They found no significant difference in terms of improvement in motor function or the ambulation rate between the two groups and reported a surgery-related complication rate of 11%. They concluded that patients over 65 years of age with metastatic spinal cord compression did not benefit remarkably from the addition of surgery to radiotherapy in terms of functional outcome, local control of metastatic spinal cord compression, or survival [29]. In a systematic review of metastatic spine tumors, the incidence of complications from radiotherapy alone was unknown, and few studies had documented the progression of the systemic disease during treatment [27]. The overall surgical complication rate was 29% (range, 5–65%), and the 30-day postoperative mortality rate was 5% (range, 0–22%) [27]. The guidelines for diagnosis and treatment of bone metastasis published by the relevant Japanese societies weakly recommend surgery for functional improvement [30].

Further prospective randomized trials are needed to establish the value of surgery for metastatic spinal cord compression. In recent years, minimally invasive techniques, such as percutaneous pedicle screw fixation, have become popular and are reportedly useful in patients with high-risk metastatic spinal tumors [31,32]. Advances in surgical techniques and minimally invasive surgery are expected to improve surgical outcomes in the future.

5. Ossification of Spinal Ligaments

The spinal ligaments stabilize the structure of the entire spine and are known to work together to allow spinal mobility. Ossification of the spinal ligaments (OSL) is a result of heterotopic bone formation in the spine. This pathologic state is well known to be more prevalent in Asian countries than in the West. Basic studies have identified several genetic factors that are associated with the onset and extension of ossification of the posterior longitudinal ligament (OPLL). Karasugi et al. [33] performed a genome-wide linkage study based on 214 sibling pairs with OPLL and identified loci with suggestive linkage on 1p21, 2p22–2p24, 7q22, 16p24, and 20p12. Furthermore, Nakajima et al. identified six putative genes in a genome-wide association study (GWAS) that included 1130 patients with OPLL and 7125 controls [34]. Given that the GWAS could explain less than 2% of the total genetic variance of OPLL, further information is necessary to understand the mechanisms.

Current advances in diagnostic imaging technology have improved our understanding of the distribution and extension of OSL. Hirai et al. investigated the distribution of ossified lesions throughout the whole spine using low-dose radiation computed tomography (CT) and demonstrated that the prevalence of OPLL in the whole spine is correlated with female sex, body mass index, and the degree of OPLL in the cervical spine [35]. They also found a strong association between OSL and other concomitant ossified lesions in the cervical and thoracic spine [36–40]. Katsumi et al. evaluated the chronologic progression of ossified lesions on three-dimensional CT images for patients with OPLL. They reported a mean annual increase in the lesion rate of 4.1% in non-surgically treated patients and identified younger age and obesity to be risk factors for progression. Interestingly, they also showed that the mean annual increase in the lesion rate was significantly lower in patients who underwent posterior decompression with fusion surgery than in those who underwent laminoplasty without fusion (2.0% vs. 7.5%). Considering that OPLL often results in the onset and deterioration of spinal disorders with increasing size, it is important for physicians and spine surgeons to conduct future investigations to identify significant predictors of extension and thickening of ossification.

Clinically, surgery is indicated in patients with cervical OPLL who have progressive myelopathic symptoms, such as clumsy hands, a spastic gait, and bowel or bladder impairment that lead to severe restriction of everyday activities. Two major surgical strategies, namely, laminoplasty and anterior decompression with fusion, have been used in patients with OPLL and myelopathy. Laminoplasty was developed in Japan as a minimally invasive and effective posterior strategy that is relatively easy and safe to perform [41] and is now used throughout the world. However, despite these advantages, laminoplasty is not suitable for patients with extensive ossified lesions (with a canal occupying ratio > 60%), beak-type OPLL, or cervical kyphotic alignment because of decompression at the ventral portion of the spinal cord [42,43]. The anterior technique essentially decompresses the ossification and stabilizes the structures of the cervical spine. Compared with laminoplasty, anterior corpectomy with fusion achieves better clinical outcomes in patients with extensive OPLL and/or kyphotic alignment [44]. Posterior decompression with fusion is a further strategy that can be used to achieve decompression and stability in these patients with outcomes similar to those achieved using the anterior method [45]. However, to obtain a good clinical outcome, it is best to operate on a patient with OPLL before the spinal cord is damaged irreversibly. We, therefore, should weigh the benefits of these three types of surgery in patients with a spinal disorder caused by ossified lesions.

Funding: This research received no external funding.

Conflicts of Interest: The authors declare no conflict of interest.

References

1. Dubousset, J.; Weinstein, S. The pediatric spine: Principles and practice. In *Three-Dimensional Analysis of the Scoliotic Deformity*; Raven Press: New York, NY, USA, 1994; Volume 479, p. 496.
2. Haddas, R.; Satin, A.; Lieberman, I. What is actually happening inside the "cone of economy": Compensatory mechanisms during a dynamic balance test. *Eur. Spine J.* **2020**, *29*, 2319–2328. [CrossRef]
3. Matsuyama, Y. Surgical treatment for adult spinal deformity: Conceptual approach and surgical strategy. *Spine Surg. Relat. Res.* **2017**, *1*, 56–60. [CrossRef]

4. Schwab, F.; Ungar, B.; Blondel, B.; Buchowski, J.; Coe, J.; Deinlein, D.; DeWald, C.; Mehdian, H.; Shaffrey, C.; Tribus, C.; et al. Scoliosis Research Society-Schwab adult spinal deformity classification: A validation study. *Spine* **2012**, *37*, 1077–1082. [CrossRef]
5. Kondo, R.; Yamato, Y.; Nagafusa, T.; Mizushima, T.; Hasegawa, T.; Kobayashi, S.; Togawa, D.; Oe, S.; Kurosu, K.; Matsuyama, Y. Effect of corrective long spinal fusion to the ilium on physical function in patients with adult spinal deformity. *Eur. Spine J.* **2017**, *26*, 2138–2145. [CrossRef]
6. Yamato, Y.; Matsuyama, Y.; Hasegawa, K.; Aota, Y.; Akazawa, T.; Iida, T.; Ueyama, K.; Uno, K.; Kanemura, T.; Kawakami, N.; et al. A Japanese nationwide multicenter survey on perioperative complications of corrective fusion for elderly patients with adult spinal deformity. *J. Orthop. Sci.* **2017**, *22*, 237–242. [CrossRef]
7. Zhang, Y.-L.; Shi, L.-T.; Tang, P.-F.; Sun, Z.-J.; Wang, Y.-H. Correlation analysis of osteoporotic vertebral compression fractures and spinal sagittal imbalance. *Orthopade* **2017**, *46*, 249–255. [CrossRef]
8. Kobayashi, T.; Takeda, N.; Atsuta, Y.; Matsuno, T. Flattening of sagittal spinal curvature as a predictor of vertebral fracture. *Osteoporos. Int.* **2007**, *19*, 65–69. [CrossRef]
9. Eguchi, Y.; Suzuki, M.; Yamanaka, H.; Tamai, H.; Kobayashi, T.; Orita, S.; Yamauchi, K.; Suzuki, M.; Inage, K.; Fujimoto, K.; et al. Associations between sarcopenia and degenerative lumbar scoliosis in older women. *Scoliosis Spinal Disord.* **2017**, *12*, 1–7. [CrossRef]
10. Hori, Y.; Hoshino, M.; Inage, K.; Miyagi, M.; Takahashi, S.; Ohyama, S.; Suzuki, A.; Tsujio, T.; Terai, H.; Dohzono, S.; et al. Issls prize in clinical science 2019: Clinical importance of trunk muscle mass for low back pain, spinal balance, and quality of life—A multicenter cross-sectional study. *Eur. Spine J.* **2019**, *28*, 914–921. [CrossRef]
11. Tosteson, A.N.A.; Gabriel, S.E.; Grove, M.R.; Moncur, M.M.; Kneeland, T.S.; Iii, L.J.M. Impact of Hip and Vertebral Fractures on Quality-Adjusted Life Years. *Osteoporos. Int.* **2001**, *12*, 1042–1049. [CrossRef]
12. Roux, C.; Briot, K. Imminent fracture risk. *Osteoporos. Int.* **2017**, *28*, 1765–1769. [CrossRef]
13. Genant, H.K.; Wu, C.Y.; Van Kuijk, C.; Nevitt, M.C. Vertebral fracture assessment using a semiquantitative technique. *J. Bone Miner. Res.* **2009**, *8*, 1137–1148. [CrossRef]
14. Kerttula, L.I.; Serlo, W.S.; Tervonen, O.A.; Pääkkö, E.L.; Vanharanta, H.V. Post-traumatic findings of the spine after earlier vertebral fracture in young patients: Clinical and MRI study. *Spine* **2000**, *25*, 1104–1108. [CrossRef]
15. Blattert, T.R.; Schnake, K.J.; Gonschorek, O.; Gercek, E.; Hartmann, F.; Katscher, S.; Mörk, S.; Morrison, R.; Müller, M.; Partenheimer, A.; et al. Nonsurgical and Surgical Management of Osteoporotic Vertebral Body Fractures: Recommendations of the Spine Section of the German Society for Orthopaedics and Trauma (DGOU). *Glob. Spine J.* **2018**, *8*, 50S–55S. [CrossRef]
16. Takahashi, S.; Hoshino, M.; Yasuda, H.; Hori, Y.; Ohyama, S.; Terai, H.; Hayashi, K.; Tsujio, T.; Kono, H.; Suzuki, A.; et al. Characteristic radiological findings for revision surgery after balloon kyphoplasty. *Sci. Rep.* **2019**, *9*, 1–7. [CrossRef]
17. Takahashi, S.; Hoshino, M.; Yasuda, H.; Hori, Y.; Ohyama, S.; Terai, H.; Hayashi, K.; Tsujio, T.; Kono, H.; Suzuki, A.; et al. Development of a scoring system for predicting adjacent vertebral fracture after balloon kyphoplasty. *Spine J.* **2019**, *19*, 1194–1201. [CrossRef]
18. Saleh, A.; Thirukumaran, C.; Mesfin, A.; Molinari, R.W. Complications and readmission after lumbar spine surgery in elderly patients: An analysis of 2320 patients. *Spine J.* **2017**, *17*, 1106–1112. [CrossRef]
19. Katsumi, K.; Hirano, T.; Watanabe, K.; Ohashi, M.; Yamazaki, A.; Ito, T.; Sawakami, K.; Sano, A.; Kikuchi, R.; Endo, N. Surgical treatment for osteoporotic thoracolumbar vertebral collapse using vertebroplasty with posterior spinal fusion: A prospective multicenter study. *Int. Orthop.* **2016**, *40*, 2309–2315. [CrossRef]
20. Yoshida, G.; Hasegawa, T.; Yamato, Y.; Kobayashi, S.; Oe, S.; Banno, T.; Mihara, Y.; Arima, H.; Ushirozako, H.; Yasuda, T.; et al. Predicting Perioperative Complications in Adult Spinal Deformity Surgery Using a Simple Sliding Scale. *Spine* **2018**, *43*, 562–570. [CrossRef]
21. Abd-El-Barr, M.M.; Huang, K.; Moses, Z.B.; Iorgulescu, J.B.; Chi, J.H. Recent advances in intradural spinal tumors. *Neuro-Oncology* **2017**, *20*, 729–742. [CrossRef]
22. Azad, T.D.; Pendharkar, A.V.; Nguyen, V.; Pan, J.; Connolly, I.D.; Veeravagu, A.; Popat, R.; Ratliff, J.K.; Grant, G.A. Diagnostic Utility of Intraoperative Neurophysiological Monitoring for Intramedullary Spinal Cord Tumors: Systematic Review and Meta-Analysis. *Clin. Spine Surg.* **2018**, *31*, 112–119. [CrossRef] [PubMed]
23. Hirano, K.; Imagama, S.; Sato, K.; Kato, F.; Yukawa, Y.; Yoshihara, H.; Kamiya, M.; Deguchi, M.; Kanemura, T.; Matsubara, Y.; et al. Primary spinal cord tumors: Review of 678 surgically treated patients in Japan. A multicenter study. *Eur. Spine J.* **2012**, *21*, 2019–2026. [CrossRef] [PubMed]
24. Shrivastava, R.K.; Epstein, F.J.; Perin, N.I.; Post, K.D.; Jallo, G.I. Intramedullary spinal cord tumors in patients older than 50 years of age: Management and outcome analysis. *J. Neurosurg. Spine* **2005**, *2*, 249–255. [CrossRef]
25. Patchell, R.A.; Tibbs, P.A.; Regine, W.F.; Payne, R.; Saris, S.; Kryscio, R.J.; Mohiuddin, M.; Young, B. Direct decompressive surgical resection in the treatment of spinal cord compression caused by metastatic cancer: A randomised trial. *Lancet* **2005**, *366*, 643–648. [CrossRef]
26. Crnalic, S.; Hildingsson, C.; Bergh, A.; Widmark, A.; Svensson, O.; Löfvenberg, R. Early diagnosis and treatment is crucial for neurological recovery after surgery for metastatic spinal cord compression in prostate cancer. *Acta Oncol.* **2012**, *52*, 809–815. [CrossRef]
27. Kim, J.M.; Losina, E.; Bono, C.M.; Schoenfeld, A.J.; Collins, J.E.; Katz, J.N.; Harris, M.B. Clinical outcome of metastatic spinal cord compression treated with surgical excision ± radiation versus radiation therapy alone: A systematic review of literature. *Spine* **2012**, *37*, 78–84. [CrossRef]

28. Rades, D.; Huttenlocher, S.; Dunst, J.; Bajrovic, A.; Karstens, J.H.; Rudat, V.; Schild, S. Matched Pair Analysis Comparing Surgery Followed By Radiotherapy and Radiotherapy Alone for Metastatic Spinal Cord Compression. *J. Clin. Oncol.* **2010**, *28*, 3597–3604. [CrossRef]
29. Rades, D.; Huttenlocher, S.; Evers, J.N.; Bajrovic, A.; Karstens, J.H.; Rudat, V.; Schild, S.E. Do elderly patients benefit from surgery in addition to radiotherapy for treatment of metastatic spinal cord compression? *Strahlenther. Onkol.* **2012**, *188*, 424–430. [CrossRef]
30. Shibata, H.; Kato, S.; Sekine, I.; Abe, K.; Araki, N.; Iguchi, H.; Izumi, T.; Inaba, Y.; Osaka, I.; Kawai, A.; et al. Diagnosis and treatment of bone metastasis: Comprehensive guideline of the Japanese Society of Medical Oncology, Japanese Orthopedic Association, Japanese Urological Association, and Japanese Society for Radiation Oncology. *ESMO Open* **2016**, *1*, e000037. [CrossRef] [PubMed]
31. Hamad, A.; Vachtsevanos, L.; Cattell, A.; Ockendon, M.; Balain, B. Minimally invasive spinal surgery for the management of symptomatic spinal metastasis. *Br. J. Neurosurg.* **2017**, *31*, 526–530. [CrossRef]
32. Gu, Y.; Dong, J.; Jiang, X.; Wang, Y. Minimally Invasive Pedicle Screws Fixation and Percutaneous Vertebroplasty for the Surgical Treatment of Thoracic Metastatic Tumors with Neurologic Compression. *Spine* **2016**, *41*, B14–B22. [CrossRef] [PubMed]
33. Karasugi, T.; Genetic Study Group of Investigation Committee on Ossification of the Spinal Ligaments; Nakajima, M.; Ikari, K.; Tsuji, T.; Matsumoto, M.; Chiba, K.; Uchida, K.; Kawaguchi, Y.; Mizuta, H.; et al. A genome-wide sib-pair linkage analysis of ossification of the posterior longitudinal ligament of the spine. *J. Bone Miner. Metab.* **2012**, *31*, 136–143. [CrossRef] [PubMed]
34. Nakajima, M.; Genetic Study Group of Investigation Committee on Ossification of the Spinal Ligaments; Takahashi, A.; Tsuji, T.; Karasugi, T.; Baba, H.; Uchida, K.; Kawabata, S.; Okawa, A.; Shindo, S.; et al. A genome-wide association study identifies susceptibility loci for ossification of the posterior longitudinal ligament of the spine. *Nat. Genet.* **2014**, *46*, 1012–1016. [CrossRef] [PubMed]
35. Hirai, T.; Yoshii, T.; Iwanami, A.; Takeuchi, K.; Mori, K.; Yamada, T.; Wada, K.; Koda, M.; Matsuyama, Y.; Takeshita, K.; et al. Prevalence and Distribution of Ossified Lesions in the Whole Spine of Patients with Cervical Ossification of the Posterior Longitudinal Ligament A Multicenter Study (JOSL CT study). *PLoS ONE* **2016**, *11*, e0160117. [CrossRef]
36. Hirai, T.; Yoshii, T.; Nagoshi, N.; Takeuchi, K.; Mori, K.; Ushio, S.; Iwanami, A.; Yamada, T.; Seki, S.; Tsuji, T.; et al. Distribution of ossified spinal lesions in patients with severe ossification of the posterior longitudinal ligament and prediction of ossification at each segment based on the cervical OP index classification: A multicenter study (JOSL CT study). *BMC Musculoskelet. Disord.* **2018**, *19*, 107. [CrossRef]
37. Mori, K.; Yoshii, T.; Hirai, T.; Iwanami, A.; Takeuchi, K.; Yamada, T.; Seki, S.; Tsuji, T.; Fujiyoshi, K.; Furukawa, M.; et al. Prevalence and distribution of ossification of the supra/interspinous ligaments in symptomatic patients with cervical ossification of the posterior longitudinal ligament of the spine: A CT-based multicenter cross-sectional study. *BMC Musculoskelet. Disord.* **2016**, *17*, 492. [CrossRef]
38. Mori, K.; Yoshii, T.; Hirai, T.; Nagoshi, N.; Takeuchi, K.; Ushio, S.; Iwanami, A.; Yamada, T.; Seki, S.; Tsuji, T.; et al. The characteristics of the patients with radiologically severe cervical ossification of the posterior longitudinal ligament of the spine: A CT-based multicenter cross-sectional study. *J. Orthop. Sci.* **2020**, *25*, 746–750. [CrossRef]
39. Nishimura, S.; Nagoshi, N.; Iwanami, A.; Takeuchi, A.; Hirai, T.; Yoshii, T.; Takeuchi, K.; Mori, K.; Yamada, T.; Seki, S.; et al. Prevalence and Distribution of Diffuse Idiopathic Skeletal Hyperostosis on Whole-spine Computed Tomography in Patients with Cervical Ossification of the Posterior Longitudinal Ligament: A Multicenter Study. *Clin. Spine Surg.* **2018**, *31*, E460–E465. [CrossRef]
40. Yoshii, T.; Hirai, T.; Iwanami, A.; Nagoshi, N.; Takeuchi, K.; Mori, K.; Yamada, T.; Seki, S.; Tsuji, T.; Fujiyoshi, K.; et al. Co-existence of ossification of the nuchal ligament is associated with severity of ossification in the whole spine in patients with cervical ossification of the posterior longitudinal ligament -A multi-center CT study. *J. Orthop. Sci.* **2019**, *24*, 35–41. [CrossRef]
41. Chiba, K.; Ogawa, Y.; Ishii, K.; Takaishi, H.; Nakamura, M.; Maruiwa, H.; Matsumoto, M.; Toyama, Y. Long-term Results of Expansive Open-Door Laminoplasty for Cervical Myelopathy—Average 14-Year Follow-up Study. *Spine* **2006**, *31*, 2998–3005. [CrossRef]
42. Iwasaki, M.; Okuda, S.; Miyauchi, A.; Sakaura, H.; Mukai, Y.; Yonenobu, K.; Yoshikawa, H. Surgical Strategy for Cervical Myelopathy due to Ossification of the Posterior Longitudinal Ligament: Part 1: Clinical results and limitations of laminoplasty. *Spine* **2007**, *32*, 647–653. [CrossRef] [PubMed]
43. Seichi, A.; Hoshino, Y.; Kimura, A.; Nakahara, S.; Watanabe, M.; Kato, T.; Ono, A.; Kotani, Y.; Mitsukawa, M.; Ijiri, K.; et al. Neurological Complications of Cervical Laminoplasty for Patients with Ossification of the Posterior Longitudinal Ligament—A multi-Institutional Retrospective Study. *Spine* **2011**, *36*, E998–E1003. [CrossRef] [PubMed]
44. Sakai, K.; Okawa, A.; Takahashi, M.; Arai, Y.; Kawabata, S.; Enomoto, M.; Kato, T.; Hirai, T.; Shinomiya, K. Five-year Follow-up Evaluation of Surgical Treatment for Cervical Myelopathy Caused by Ossification of the Posterior Longitudinal Ligament: A prospective comparative study of anterior decompression and fusion with floating method versus laminoplasty. *Spine* **2012**, *37*, 367–376. [CrossRef] [PubMed]
45. Yoshii, T.; Sakai, K.; Hirai, T.; Yamada, T.; Inose, H.; Kato, T.; Enomoto, M.; Tomizawa, S.; Kawabata, S.; Arai, Y.; et al. Anterior decompression with fusion versus posterior decompression with fusion for massive cervical ossification of the posterior longitudinal ligament with a ≥50% canal occupying ratio: A multicenter retrospective study. *Spine J.* **2016**, *16*, 1351–1357. [CrossRef] [PubMed]

MDPI
St. Alban-Anlage 66
4052 Basel
Switzerland
Tel. +41 61 683 77 34
Fax +41 61 302 89 18
www.mdpi.com

Journal of Clinical Medicine Editorial Office
E-mail: jcm@mdpi.com
www.mdpi.com/journal/jcm

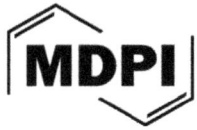

www.ingramcontent.com/pod-product-compliance
Lightning Source LLC
LaVergne TN
LVHW070445100526
838202LV00014B/1671